Anabolic Therapy in Modern Medicine

Anabolic Therapy in Modern Medicine

by William N. Taylor, M.D.

McFarland & Company, Inc., Publishers

Jefferson, North Carolina, and London

Library of Congress Cataloguing-in-Publication Data

Taylor, William N.
   Anabolic therapy in modern medicine / by William N.
Taylor.
      p.   cm.
   Includes bibliographical references and index.
   ISBN 0-7864-1241-0 (softcover : 50# alkaline paper) ∞
   1. Anabolic steroids—Therapeutic use. I.   Title.
   [DNLM: 1. Anabolic Steroids—therapeutic use.
   WK150T247a2002]
   RM297.S74T39   2002
   615'.36—dc21   2001007859

British Library cataloguing data are available

Manufactured in the United States of America

Cover: anatomical drawing ©2002 Art Today

McFarland & Company, Inc., Publishers
  Box 611, Jefferson, North Carolina 28640
   www.mcfarlandpub.com

This book is dedicated to my wife,
Judith Jones Taylor, my eternal love,
who inspires me with her creativity, understanding,
wisdom, tenderness, and passion.

Contents

PART 4: Anabolic Therapy for Other Catabolic Diseases and Conditions

Preface

The major purpose of this book is to compile evidence-based information on anabolic therapy from various disciplines in medicine and science and illustrate areas in which use of anabolic agents can contribute to better patient care, especially in the area of physical medicine and rehabilitation. Many modalities in rehabilitation apply graduated and progressive physical and mental stressors to patients in order to improve their overall health and physical activities. Patients' ability to respond to these applied stressors is influenced by many factors, including their biochemical status as they enter the rehabilitative processes. To make improvements, patients must be able to respond with anabolic and biochemical responses. The ability to respond in a constructive fashion to the applied stressors of rehabilitation is regulated by anabolic hormones, growth factors, and anabolic peptides that influence the genetic machinery to make adaptive changes.

Traditionally, the prescription of anabolic agents for patients has been one of the most underused modalities in medicine. Likewise, in the field of rehabilitative medicine, the practice of physiatry has been focused mostly on blending the supervision of allied physical and mental health professionals with the sciences of exercise physiology, polymer engineering, metallurgy, and medical management. Little effort has been paid to the growing body of evidence-based information that illustrates the positive outcomes that can be achieved when patients are given pharmacologic anabolic stimuli to maximize the outcomes and hasten the processes of rehabilitation. Too often poor rehabilitative outcomes are accepted as a matter of course when physicians' and allied health professionals' expectations are based on results obtained without the application of anabolic agents. In other words, the standard of care has been set without realization of the positive outcomes that can be achieved with the use of anabolic agents.

1

It is hoped that this book will provide the stimulus for physicians to offer a higher standard of care for their patients. Providing anabolic agents can improve the positive outcomes when they are added to preventive and therapeutic medicine, as well as to the process of rehabilitative from disease and injury.

Part 1

Androgens: Synthesis and Scope of Chemical Potentials

1

Introduction: Anabolic Therapy and the Body's Catabolic Responses to Ill-Health Conditions

The majority of diseases and ill-health conditions tend to induce catabolic biochemical reactions within the human body. For many diseases, such as autoimmune diseases, coronary artery disease, stroke, and Type II diabetes in men, there are pre-existing catabolic changes that make individuals more prone to certain illnesses. For other diseases, such as cancer, acquired immunodeficiency syndrome (AIDS), and chronic renal failure (CRF), the disease process itself induces antianabolic and catabolic reactions in the body. In other diseases and conditions, such as major trauma, spinal cord injuries, and major thermal injuries, the body's response to these insults is to shut down anabolic mechanisms and encourage catabolism. Finally, some diseases are treated with medications and other therapeutic modalities, such as corticosteroids, cytotoxic chemotherapy, and radiotherapy, that reduce the body's anabolic functions.

Historically, it was hoped or speculated that the human body would accelerate the biochemical mechanisms that promote anabolic activities, and, furthermore, by promoting these anabolic mechanisms, it would then be in an improved position to combat the catabolic changes brought on by disease and injury. Unfortunately, these hopes and speculations have been shown to be wishful thinking.

There are several major questions that must be asked regarding the body's catabolic reactions to disease, traumatic conditions, immobilization and microgravity conditions, and advancing age. Some of these questions are:

(1) Why would the human body respond to the insults of disease or trauma with catabolic responses when it needs anabolic responses?

(2) How do disease and injurious conditions induce catabolic responses within the body?

(3) Wouldn't the body increase its chances of surviving or limiting these insults by responding in an anabolic manner?

(4) Why doesn't the body respond to disease and injury insults by upregulating its anabolic biochemical mechanisms?

(5) If the body responds to disease and injurious insults with endogenous catabolic mechanisms, then why doesn't the medical care of these conditions involve methods to reverse catabolism and encourage anabolism?

(6) Why doesn't the medical profession provide anabolic therapies for diseases and injuries that can reverse the catabolic responses caused by these conditions and the body's response to these conditions?

(7) Why isn't more research conducted on anabolic therapies for catabolic diseases and traumatic injuries?

(8) Why is aging associated with an accelerated increase risk for common diseases such as cancer, heart disease, stroke, osteoporosis, dementia, and disabling conditions?

One of the major purposes of this book is to answer some of these questions and apply the answers to patient care.

The human body is programmed to equate optimal health and anabolic potentials with the ability to procreate. Many conditions, such as advanced age, disease conditions, and major traumatic insults are associated with a reduction in the ability to procreate. Perhaps this programmed response is a remnant of the "survival of the fittest" phenomenon. Disease conditions and major injuries are associated with major losses in both anabolic potentials and procreation abilities. In other words, during illness or advancing age the body responds with chemical messages that translate to signals that discourage procreation but also reduce anabolic potentials.

In the human body, anabolic potentials and procreation abilities are inexorably linked by common biochemical messengers. These common biochemical messengers make up the class of sex steroids referred to as androgens, which are among the most powerful anabolic chemicals in the human body. Androgens are also among the most powerful endogenous chemicals involved with libido and procreation. Therefore, androgens regulate both anabolic mechanisms and procreative mechanisms in the human body.

It should not be surprising that, when the human body is faced with disease or traumatic injury, it responds by reducing serum androgen levels both acutely and chronically. This decreased androgen production tends to emphasize reducing procreation ability over the beneficial anabolic potentials that could be helpful in combating these conditions.

The concept of prescribing anabolic agents to counteract the catabolic state of disease processes reverses the natural catabolic processes that are triggered by the body. In effect, anabolic therapy, particularly with androgens, overrides the body's catabolic responses to disease, trauma, and aging, that often result in reduced androgen production. Many major diseases are associated with reduced serum androgen levels (hypoandrogenemia). Therefore, androgen therapy, as anabolic replacement therapy, seems to be appropriate treatment for combating many disease conditions.

Some diseases and conditions, such as congestive heart failure, major thermal injury, some neuromuscular diseases, and frailty, are associated with decreased serum levels of insulin-like growth factor-1 (formerly called somatomedin-C) that is referred to as hyposomatomedinemia. Insulin-like growth factor-1 (IGF-1) is an anabolic agent that regulates growth and trophic mechanisms throughout the body. Hyposomatomedinemia, that is associated with ill-health conditions and advancing age, usually stems from a depressed growth hormone-releasing hormone (GHRH)-growth hormone (GH)-insulin-like growth factor (IGF)-insulin-like growth factor binding protein (IGFBP) axis, or GHRH-GH-IGF-IGFBP axis. The blunted response of this axis results in significant losses of anabolic potential. Therefore, correcting hyposomatomedinemia, with anabolic agents that stimulate this axis or by replacing the components of this axis, seems to be a logical measure for enhancing anabolic potentials in patients with a variety of diseases and age-related conditions. In recent years, the recombinantly produced synthetic components of the GHRH-GH-IGF-IGFBP axis have become available and have been used in investigational studies.

Agents that stimulate the GHRH-GH-IGF-IGFBP axis include androgens, synthetic GHRH hormone analogs, synthetic GH secretagogues, and other drugs. These agents are available and the clinical investigation of some of them is just beginning. Other approaches to anabolic therapy for some diseases involve gene therapy techniques. These investigational modalities utilize the insertion (into tissues like skeletal muscles) of genes that code for and produce one or more anabolic hormones or agents.

Regardless of the mode and sophistication of anabolic therapies, it is safe to say that modern medicine has powerful anabolic agents to apply to disease conditions. The investigational studies regarding the clinical uses of anabolic therapies are rapidly growing, expanding, and evolving. Much of the information that has been obtained from these studies is currently being considered for therapies that may delay or reverse aging processes.

In the following chapters in this book, the evidence-based rationale for the use of anabolic therapies will be presented for a number of disease conditions. In most cases, androgen therapy is proposed to correct the underlying androgen deficiency, correct hyposomatomedinemia, and increase anabolic potentials.

Correcting hypoandrogenemia, with androgen therapy, for many diseases and ill-health conditions, is the first and most important anabolic measure that affects outcomes. The well-referenced chapters on a variety of diseases should help convince modern physicians of the advantages of the therapeutic use of anabolic therapy in their patients. Maximizing anabolic potentials via pharmacologic anabolic therapies should be considered for most patients who are undergoing traditional rehabilitation modalities.

Another goal of this book is to provide a collective body of international references regarding the evidence-based information on anabolic therapy for allied health care providers and the patients and family members of patients who are afflicted with specific diseases. Much of the general public is becoming more aware of anabolic therapies via the Internet and other sources that have become available. An increasing number of patients, and patients' family members, use the Internet to gain access to the most current information on specific diseases. More Americans are becoming critical consumers of health care and have become familiar with technical medical terminology and concepts involved with medical therapies. Some of this information is derived from scientific investigations in countries where there are fewer restrictions on scientists. Also, several anabolic agents are available for purchase over the Internet and an increasing number of Americans are buying them in this manner. A significant number of Americans purchase anabolic agents from other countries, such as Mexico or the Netherlands, for use in the United States.

This book also contains sections that address some of the historical highlights of anabolic therapies in medicine. In past decades, critical mistakes and political dogma influenced the progression of anabolic therapies in the United States. The advent of several newly discovered scientific techniques and machines has paved the way for re-evaluating some of the older studies that were conducted. These newer methods for evaluating anabolic therapies have led to an improved understanding of the mechanisms of action of these agents. Some knowledge of the early history of anabolic therapies and the recent knowledge of their mechanisms of action may have future implications for policy decisions that are likely to be made in this area.

2

Historical Use of Anabolic Agents in Medicine

Introduction: Defining the Breadth of Anabolic Agents

Anabolic agents in medicine date back over 100 years and involved then the use of glandular extracts (primarily testicular extracts and pituitary extracts). In 1935, testosterone became the first anabolic agent that was synthesized from chemical reactions. During the 1950s and 1960s nearly two dozen analogs of testosterone (anabolic steroids) were synthesized by a rapidly expanding pharmaceutical industry. Synthetic testosterone and anabolic steroids have been referred to collectively as synthetic anabolic-androgenic steroids or androgens. A comprehensive history of the abuse of testosterone and anabolic steroids has been compiled by this author in other books and will not be presented here.[1, 2, 3, 4]

Other anabolic agents, including extracted versions of human chronic gonadotrophin (hCG) and human growth hormone (hGH), have been used in clinical medicine for over 50 years. However, the advent of genetic engineering techniques has expanded the menu of therapeutic anabolic agents to include:

(1) recombinant human growth hormones (rhGHs).

(2) recombinant human insulin-like growth factor-1 (rhIGF-1).

(3) recombinant human growth hormone-releasing hormone (rhGHRH).

(4) recombinant human luteinizing hormone (rhLH).

(5) recombinant human luteinizing hormone-releasing hormone (rhLHRH).

(6) recombinant human insulin-like growth factor binding proteins (rhIGFBPs).

(7) recombinant polypeptide molecules that function as growth hormone-releasing hormone (GHRH) analogs or growth hormone (GH) secretagogues.

In very recent times, with the invention of gene therapy, genetically altered genes can be introduced into the body, code for, and produce a wide variety of the aforementioned anabolic agents in diseases where catabolism dominates the clinical picture.

Other biochemical molecules have been recently considered anabolic agents within the human body; they include anabolic globulins, anabolic cytokines, certain chemokines, specific tissue growth factors, various neuropeptides, and a number of trophic or growth factors. Some of these anabolic molecules have been recombinantly synthesized and the clinical trials with these products have recently begun.

Defining the Scope of Patients Who Require Anabolic Therapies

Providing the optimal anabolic stimulus for patients with catabolic conditions should have been an obvious goal in the overall treatment of patients for decades. However, physicians (especially American physicians) have been exceedingly slow to accept the fact that many of their patients require anabolic therapies to survive and fully recover from catabolic disease states or conditions. There are several general categories of patients for whom the use of anabolic therapy may be considered. These include:

(1) patients who have defined anabolic stimuli inadequacies.

(2) patients who have disease conditions where anabolic stimuli inadequacies are known to be prevalent.

(3) patients where mildly supraphysiologic doses of anabolic agents should be utilized to maximize recovery and outcome from catabolic or chronic diseases.

(4) most patients who are undergoing traditional physical medicine and rehabilitation modalities, to shorten recovery periods and improve outcomes.

(5) patients with chronic wasting syndromes due to chronic catabolic diseases and conditions.

(6) patients with various conditions where anabolic therapy has been

shown to improve libido, mood, overall mental health, physical functioning, and quality of life issues.

(7) patients with poor body composition profiles where anabolic therapies have been shown to improve body composition and reduce the risks for diseases and conditions that arise from frailty, sarcopenia, osteoporosis, and obesity.

(8) patients with age-related reductions in anabolic hormones or agents which enhance longevity, improve quality of life, and reduce catabolic disease risks.

(9) patients with immune system alterations whose immune system functioning improves with anabolic agents.

Summary: Anabolic Therapy Is the Future of Medicine

The use of anabolic therapy will likely revolutionize the practice of medicine over the next decade and beyond. As with antibiotic therapy and antiviral therapies in the past, the optimal use of anabolic therapies will become commonplace and a permanent fixture in the way medicine is practiced in the 21st century. Anabolic therapies are probably the most important ingredients in the next phase of the extension of human life and the raising of its quality. These therapies have not been fully exploited to date.

In the chapters that follow, the progress in the use of anabolic therapies will be detailed for a large number of diseases. The rationale and science-based information regarding anabolic therapy has been expanding rapidly (especially over the past five years). It is hoped that this book will form a substantive capitulation of the published international work in these areas.

Notes

1. Taylor, W.N. *Anabolic Steroids and the Athlete.* Jefferson, N.C.: McFarland & Company, Inc., Publishers (1982).
2. Taylor, W.N. *Hormonal Manipulation: A New Era of Monstrous Athletes.* Jefferson, N.C.: McFarland & Company, Inc., Publishers (1985).
3. Taylor, W.N. *Macho Medicine: A History of the Anabolic Steroid Epidemic.* Jefferson, N.C.: McFarland & Company, Inc., Publishers (1991).
4. Taylor, W.N. *Anabolic Steroids and the Athlete, 2nd Edition.* Jefferson, N.C.: McFarland & Company, Inc., Publishers (2001).

Part 2

Anabolic Therapy for Sarcopenia, Osteoporosis, and Hormone Replacement Therapy

3

Rationale for Anabolic Therapy in Sarcopenia and Frailty Conditions

Introduction: Sarcopenia: The Condition of the 21st Century

Advancing adult age is associated with profound changes in body composition, the principal component of which is a decrease in skeletal muscle mass. This age-related loss in skeletal muscle mass has been referred to as sarcopenia.[1] It is a consequence of normal aging, and does not require a disease to occur, although muscle mass loss can be accelerated by many chronic illnesses. At the present time, there is only a limited understanding of the public health significance of sarcopenia. However, the well-recognized functional consequences of sarcopenia include gait and balance problems, increased risk for fall, and loss of physical functional independence.[2]

Most aging individuals die from atherosclerosis, cancer, or dementia; but in the oldest of the old, loss of muscle strength resulting in frailty is the factor which limits an individual's chances of living an independent life until death.[3] Since the theoretical potential human lifespan has be estimated to be over 125 years,[4] efforts to prevent or reverse sarcopenia will likely become more paramount in the years ahead.

The development of sarcopenia is a complex, multifaceted process that begins in midlife and accelerates after the age of 75 years.[5] It has been shown that the prevalence of sarcopenia increases dramatically with age, from 13–24 percent in persons less than 70 years of age to greater than 50 percent in persons over 80 years of age. Sarcopenia has been significantly associated with self-reported physical disability in both men and women, independent of ethnicity, age, morbidity, obesity, income, and health behaviors.[6]

Attempts have been made to standardize the definition of sarcopenia by using a variety of measurements.[7] The most specific and accurate definition of estimated muscle mass has been shown to be measured by dual-energy x-ray absorptiometry (DEXA). Using DEXA, sarcopenia has been arbitrarily defined as muscle mass of more than 2 standard deviations below the gender-specific young-normal mean.[8]

There are many candidate mechanisms leading to sarcopenia, including age-related declines in alpha-motor neurons, growth hormone (GH) production, androgen production, and physical activity. In addition, body fat gain, production of catabolic and inflammatory cytokines, and inadequate intake of dietary protein are also potentially important contributing factors of wasting and sarcopenia.[9]

The Need to Reeducate Health Care Providers

A major challenge in preventing an epidemic of sarcopenia-induced frailty is to deliver an anabolic stimulus to the muscles of elderly adults on a mass scale.[10] This challenge (addressed by the National Institute on Aging) behooves physicians to create an improved dialogue between several areas of science and medicine, including endocrinology, neuroendocrinology, immunology, exercise physiology, clinical nutrition, and clinicians in order to use multidisciplinary approaches to make solutions available to patients.[11]

Adequate training and retraining of physicians and changes in the present approaches and attitudes in caring for patients with sarcopenic states may be the greatest obstacles to overcome if application of anabolic agents, including biosynthetic hormones, to patient care is to be realized.[12] Participants in competitive sports have demonstrated that the use of androgens, growth factors, and other anabolic agents enhance human performance, yet physicians continue to be slow to adopt this approach in patients who have age-related or disease-related decrease in strength and activity.[13] It has been shown that the use of anabolic agents can, at the same time, both decrease the loss of body proteins and muscle mass, and promote and accelerate the recovery from debilitating conditions, thereby shortening hospital stay and reducing rehabilitation and convalescence time.[14]

Hypoandrogenemia and Hyposomatomedinemia in Sarcopenia

It is now recognized that sarcopenia in men and women is caused primarily by hypoandrogenemia (low serum level of androgens) and hyposomatomedinemia (low serum levels of insulin-like growth factor-1, IGF-1). It has been shown that androgen and IGF-1 levels correlate positively with, and are predictive of, muscle mass and strength in elderly people.[15] It is also recognized that, from cross-sectional studies, that elderly men and women, who have adequate circulating androgen and IFG-1 levels, have more skeletal muscle mass, better physical fitness levels, and greater activity levels compared to those with hypoandrogenemia and hyposomatomedinemia.[16, 17, 18, 19]

Age-related changes in muscle mass and strength begin in midlife and have been shown to be related to a decline in synthetic rates of mixed muscle proteins, myosin heavy chains, and mitochondrial proteins consequent to a decline in androgen and IGF-1 levels.[20] These age-related skeletal muscle changes have been shown to be greatest in type II muscle fibers.[21] These observations indicate that sarcopenia is a progressive process that even occurs in healthy independently living older adults who may not manifest weight loss.[22]

Three integrated hormonal systems, which decline with aging, are involved in the major pathogenesis of age-related sarcopenia. These are:[23, 24, 25, 26, 27]

(1) reduced hypothalamic-pituitary-gonadal axis function. Depression of this axis function results in reduced sex steroid levels of estrogens and androgens (in perimenopause, menopause and andropause) in women, and androgens (andropause) in men and contributes to hypoandrogenemia.

(2) altered hypothalamic-pituitary-adrenal axis functions. Depression of this axis results in reduced androgen production: dehydroepiandrosterone (DHEA) and its sulfate (adrenopause) in both genders. However, adrenopause may be clinically more important in women, especially after menopause. Age-related changes in adrenal function have been well-documented and result in a decreased androgen-cortisol ratio. Changes in this ratio contribute to hypoandrogenemia that is associated with aging and acute and chronic illnesses.

(3) altered hypothalamic-pituitary functions that are known as somatopause. The age-related reduction function of the growth hormone-releasing hormone (GHRH)-growth hormone (GH)-insulin-like, IGF-growth

factor insulin-like growth factor binding protein (IGFBP) axis, GHRH-GH-IGF-IGFBP axis, has been referred to as somatopause in both men and women. Somatopause results in a reduction in circulating levels of IGF-1 (hyposomatomedinemia) and bioavailability of IGF-1. Reduced anabolic potential from somatopause can occur with aging and chronic illnesses.

Androgen and Other Anabolic Therapies for Sarcopenia

The systems involved with preventing and reversing sarcopenia are integrated and modulated by androgens, thus making androgen therapy the most cost-effective, safe, cornerstone for preventing or reversing sarcopenia. Therefore, androgen therapy should be an obvious choice for treating hypoandrogenemia and sarcopenia related to age and chronic illness.[28] Although physical training in persons with hypoandrogenemia and sarcopenia can have moderate effects at reversing losses in muscle mass,[29, 30, 31, 32] it has been shown that maintaining regular physical activity and adequate protein intake, in general, will not offset the age-related loss of skeletal muscle mass.[33] Androgens play an important role in determining the muscular response to aging, acute and chronic illness, and strength training.[34]

In recent years, advances in scientific modalities have provided insight into the multifaceted mechanisms of action that androgens have on muscle mass and strength as summarized in Table 3-1. Androgens act directly and indirectly on androgen and other receptors in skeletal muscle cells and other tissues located throughout the body. Androgen administration has been shown to enhance muscle mass and strength by the following mechanisms:

(1) by a direct stimulation of skeletal muscle cell ribosomes via androgen receptors (AR) resulting in an increased activity of RNA-polymerase within skeletal muscle cell nuclei without utilizing IGF-1 receptors. This results in an increased content of skeletal muscle protein, including myosin, myofibrillar, and sarcoplasmic fractions.[35, 36, 37]

(2) by enhancing skeletal muscle cell amino acid uptake and protein synthesis, and fractional synthetic rates of muscle cell protein (statistically significant) over and above hyperaminoacidemia therapy alone and *without a training stimulus*.[38]

(3) by reducing the outward transport of amino acids (statistically

significant) from skeletal muscle cells and improving intracellular reutilization of amino acids *without a training stimulus*.[39]

(4) by exerting their anabolic effects on skeletal muscles specifically which does not depend on the physical training.[40]

(5) by exerting a combined effect with progressive resistance exercise resulting in an increased number of AR and AR density over and above resistance training alone (statistically significant).[41]

(6) by possessing a key anabolic function that can activate satellite cells in skeletal muscle to cause an increased muscle fiber number, or hyperplasia, along with the hypertrophy of existing muscle fibers.[42, 43]

(7) by enhancing the incorporation of carbohydrate and protein during the physical training recovery phase, further enhancing their anabolic mechanisms.[44]

Androgen therapy can also have major anabolic effects that are independent of AR in skeletal muscles. It has been shown that androgen therapy directly stimulates the GHRH-GH-IGF-IGFBP axis by increasing GH secretion and elevating circulating IGF-1, free IGF-1 levels, and IGFBP-3 levels in normal, hypogonadal, and aging individuals[45, 46, 47, 48, 49, 50, 51, 52] by a direct stimulatory effect on the hypothalamus that increases GHRH pulse amplitudes.[53]

Insulin-like growth factors have major anabolic influences on cell growth and tissue repair.[54] These growth factors promote anabolic and growth actions via binding to IGF-1 receptors. [55] The presence of IGF-1 receptors (IGFR) in skeletal muscle cells indicates that IGF-1 acts independently of the androgen receptors to stimulate protein and glycogen synthesis.[56] IGF-1 receptor stimulation results in elevated levels of IGF-1 messenger RNAs that translates into increased protein synthesis in skeletal muscle[57] and inhibition of catabolism.[58]

Androgen therapy increases circulating IGF-1 levels and IGF-1 bioavailability. Therefore, androgen therapy has both direct (via androgen receptors) and indirect (via IGF-1 receptors) anabolic effects in skeletal muscle acting on two distinct types of genetic machinery. This double receptor effect acts in an additive or synergistic manner to enhance protein synthesis, skeletal muscle mass, and neuromuscular strength. Because the correction of androgen and IGF-1 deficiencies improves muscle mass, work capacity, and quality of life, treatment with androgens, with or without GH or IGF-1 administration, can be a useful adjunct to the conventional rehabilitation protocols for preventing or reversing sarcopenia.[59]

Table 3-1: Direct and Indirect Androgen
Effects on Skeletal Muscle Function

Target Receptors	Mechanisms of Action
Muscle cell androgen receptors	(1) Upregulation of genetic machinery in muscle cells: (a) enhanced amino acid uptake (b) enhanced amino acid utilization (c) enhanced protein synthesis without a training stimulus (d) additional protein synthesis when combined with a training stimulus (2) Upregulation of androgen receptor activity and androgen receptor concentration in muscle cells: (a) normalizes age-related reduction in androgen receptor concentrations (b) normalizes age-related reduction in protein synthesis
Muscle satellite cell receptors	Stimulates satellite cells to produce an increased muscle fiber number (hyperplasia)
Muscle cell IGF-1 receptors	Indirectly and independently stimulates IGF-1 receptor activity and IGF-1 genetic machinery in muscle cells: (a) improves insulin sensitivity (b) stimulates glycogen synthesis (c) stimulates protein synthesis (d) provides protective and trophic effects
Hypothalamic GHRH receptors	Stimulates the GHRH-GH-IGF-IGFBP axis to increase circulating IGF-1 levels and activities
Leukocyte receptors	Modulates inflammatory and catabolic cytokine production
Nervous tissue receptors	Androgens act as direct and indirect neurotransmitters and enhance nerve cell communications

Besides its stimulation of GHRH release that elevates systemic IGF-1 levels, androgen therapy has also been shown to stimulate local tissue IGF-1 levels, and provide subsequent anabolic and trophic activities in various tissues and cells.[60, 61, 62, 63] These local IGF-1 molecules have been shown to be essential for the differentiation of many cell types, and to have anabolic and protective roles in a number of tissues, including those in the integumentary, musculoskeletal, nervous, immune, cardiovascular, and pulmonary systems.[64, 65, 66, 67, 68, 69, 70, 71]

Androgen therapy in older individuals has been associated with anabolic effects that reverse catabolic and sarcopenic states by increasing lean body mass, muscle mass, neuromuscular strength, improving body composition, and improving sense of well-being.[72, 73, 74, 75, 76, 77, 78, 79, 80, 81] These findings have provided the physiological evidence that androgens should be considered as pharmacological intervention against losses in lean body mass associated with aging, disease, trauma, and burn injury.[82]

Androgen therapy has been shown to be safe and effective treatment for elderly patients (60- to 80-year-old men and women).[83, 84] In a large double-blind, placebo-controlled study, androgen therapy (DHEA 50mg/day for one year in aging men and women) has been confirmed to lack harmful consequences. The study also showed that low-dose androgen therapy does not create "supermen or superwomen" as seen with androgen abuse by bodybuilders.[85]

Androgen therapy can provide a pharmacologic, anabolic assist in the rehabilitation of older men and women with a variety of illnesses.[86, 87, 88, 89, 90] It has also been shown, in randomized, placebo-controlled, double-blind studies, that androgen therapy improves the outcomes in ill or disabled older men and women who are undergoing conventional rehabilitative modalities; it does so by reversing sarcopenia.[91, 92]

Other authors have suggested that therapy with a variety of other anabolic agents should be considered to prevent or reverse sarcopenia in elderly patients, including, recombinant GHRH, GHRH secretagogues, GH, GH secretagogues and analogues, IGF-1, IGFBP-3, combinations of androgens with GH and/or IGF-1, and skeletal muscle gene therapy with genes that secrete one or more of these agents.[93, 94, 95, 96, 97, 98, 99, 100, 101 102, 103, 104, 105, 106] It has been shown that GH therapy increases muscle mass and strength in healthy elderly people, but it does not restore a youthful rate of myofibrillar protein synthesis.[107] However, when GH therapy is combined with progressive strength training exercise in elderly subjects, substantial (statistically significant) increases in muscle mass and strength (24–62 percent depending on muscle groups) have been measured in 14 weeks of training during a double-blind, placebo-controlled study.[108] These studies have indicated promising results and further indicate that stimulating the GHRH-GH-IGF-IGFBP axis can prevent or reverse sarcopenic states alone[109] or in combination with strength training exercises, such as with physical therapy. Ongoing trials should further delineate which anabolic agents will be the most cost-effective and safest.

Androgen Therapy for Sarcopenic States Associated with Chronic Illnesses

Besides sarcopenia in the elderly, a variety of diseases, injuries, and illnesses are associated with musculoskeletal wasting syndromes and sarcopenic states. Reversing the hypoandrogenemia and hyposomato-medinemia in these patients, with androgen (including testosterone, stanozolol, oxandrolone, nandrolone, oxymetholone, and DHEA) or GH therapy or both, has been shown to increase muscle protein synthesis, lean body mass, muscle mass, and neuromuscular strength, decrease body fat, reduce fatigue, and elevate mood.[110, 111, 112, 113, 114, 115, 116, 117, 118, 119, 120, 121, 122, 123, 124, 125, 126, 127, 128, 129, 130, 131, 132, 133, 134, 135, 136, 137, 138, 139, 140, 141] This range of diseases and conditions (specifically covered in other chapters) includes, adrenal insufficiency, Type II diabetes, multiple sclerosis, rheumatoid arthritis, Sjogren's syndrome, scleroderma, muscular dystrophy, spinal cord injury, major burns, renal dialysis, stroke, angina, cardiac and pulmonary rehabilitation, valvular cardiac disorders, Addison's disease, Graves disease, Klinefelter's syndrome, Raynaud's syndrome, corticosteroid-induced sarcopenia, osteoporosis, chronic fatigue syndrome, fibromyalgia, AIDS, decubitus ulcers, short bowel syndrome, TPN therapy, prolonged immobilization, and others.

Additional Health Benefits of Androgen Therapy in Sarcopenic States

Several beneficial health-related effects of androgen therapy have been shown when hypoandrogenemia has been identified. These benefits are presented in detail in other chapters of this book. A summary of the additional health-related benefits is contained in Table 3-2.

Table 3-2: Summary of Health-Related Benefits of Androgen Therapy in Sarcopenic States

Increases libido and sexual function

Increases energy level, elevates mood, and improves self-esteem

Improves lipid and lipoprotein profiles that reduces risks for cardiovascular diseases including heart attack

Enhances fibrinolysis that reduces risks for thromboembolic events and diseases including stroke

Improves modulation of the neuroimmune system

Improves anemic conditions by elevating hemoglobin and hematocrit concentrations

Stimulates osteoblasts to improve bone mineral density and osteoporosis treatment

Improves angina and improves exercise tolerance

Improves insulin sensitivity and reduces insulin requirements in acquired diabetic states

Decreases risks for and has beneficial effects in autoimmune diseases by modulating pathogenic cytokine profiles

Provides neuroprotective and neuroregenerative potentials

Improves cognition and reflex responses

Improves vasomotor symptoms in menopausal and postmenopausal women

Improves rehabilitation outcomes and hastens recovery from a variety of conditions

Counteracts the catabolic effects of corticosteroid therapy and reduces corticosteroid requirements for patients undergoing corticosteroid therapy

Provides other anabolic and anti-aging effects

Summary

In this chapter, the rationale for anabolic therapy in sarcopenic states has been presented. It is safe to say that providing an anabolic agent during the rehabilitation of many diseases and injuries, and for preventing or reversing catabolic and sarcopenic conditions, has come of age and will progress in the near future. Even the most conservative physiatrists will soon be converted to administering anabolic agents for their rehabilitation patients.

Androgen therapy continues to be the cornerstone of preventing and reversing sarcopenia, wasting conditions, and sarcopenic states. Mildly supraphysiologic doses of androgens have been shown to be safe, effective, cost-effective, and readily available for prescription use for treating these conditions in both men and women. Androgen therapy prevents and corrects sarcopenia via direct androgen receptor binding in skeletal muscle, upregulating the genetic machinery, and correcting hypoandrogenemia. Exogenous androgen therapy also corrects hyposomatomedinemia by stimulating the GHRH-GH-IGF-IGFBP axis via upregulating GHRH pulse amplitudes, thereby increasing GH secretion, elevating circulating IGF-1, IGFBP-3, and free IGF-1 levels, which provides a substantial anabolic effect.

Furthermore, androgen therapy stimulates tissue and cell secretions of IGF-1 and various neurotrophins that provide local and systemic anabolic, regenerative, and protective functions.

Prudent androgen therapy for sarcopenia or wasting syndromes in men includes:

(1) testosterone preparations, such as long-acting esters (testosterone cypionate [200–300mg IM biweekly], oral esters such as methyltestosterone [5–15mg/day], or sublingual or transdermal applications.

(2) nandrolone decanoate (200–300mg IM biweekly).
(3) oral stanozolol (6–20mg/day).
(4) oral oxandrolone (7.5–20mg/day).

For women, androgen therapy for sarcopenia or wasting syndromes includes:

(1) nandrolone decanoate (50–100mg IM biweekly).
(2) oral tibolone (2.5–5mg/day; unavailable in the US).
(3) oral stanozolol (2–8mg/day).
(4) oral oxandrolone (2.5–7.5 mg/day).
(5) oral DHEA (50–100mg/day; available over the counter).

Short-term adverse conditions associated with judicious androgen therapy are generally mild, reversible, dose-related, and duration-related. They include mildly decreased HDL-C levels, mild acne, mild hoarseness, minimal facial hair increase, mild fluid retention, and oily skin. It should be apparent that the benefits of androgen therapy for the treatment of sarcopenia, wasting syndromes, and sarcopenic states significantly outweigh the mild associated potential risks to patients.

Notes

1. Evans, W.J. What is sarcopenia? *J. Gerontol. A. Biol. Sci. Med. Sci.* 1995; 50 (Spec. No.): 5–8.

2. Dutta, C. Significance of sarcopenia in the elderly. *J. Nutr.* 1997; 127 (5 Suppl.): 992S–993S.

3. Lamberts, S.W., A.W. van den Beld, and A.J. van der Lely. The endocrinology of aging. *Science* 1997; 278 (5337): 419–424.

4. Guyot, R.S. A new theory about the ages of man. *Int. J. Aging Hum. Dev.* 1992; 36 (2): 91–98.

5. Waters, D.L., R.N. Baumgartner, and P.J. Garry. Sarcopenia: current prospectives. *J. Nutr. Health Aging* 2000; 4 (3): 133–139.

6. Baumgartner, R.N., K.M. Koehler, D. Gallagher, et al. Epidemiology of sarcopenia among the elderly in New Mexico. *Am. J. Epidemiol.* 1998; 147 (8): 755–763.

7. Melton, L.J., K. Khosla, and B.L. Riggs. Epidemiology of sarcopenia. *Mayo Clin. Proc.* 2000; 75 (Suppl.): S10–12.

8. Melton, L.J., S. Khosla, C.S. Crowson, et al. Epidemiology of sarcopenia. *J. Am. Geriatr. Soc.* 2000; 48 (6): 625–630.

9. Roubenoff, R. The pathophysiology of wasting in the elderly. *J. Nutr.* 1999; 129 (1 Suppl.): 256S–259S.

10. Roubenoff, R. Sarcopenia: a major modifiable cause of frailty in the elderly. *J. Nutr. Health Aging* 2000; 4 (3): 140–142.

11. Dutta, C., and E.C. Hadley. The significance of sarcopenia in old age. *J. Gerontol. A. Biol. Sci. Med. Sci.* 1995; 50 (Spec. No.): 1–4.

12. Wilmore, D.W. Impediments to the successful use of anabolic agents in clinical care. *J. Parenter. Enteral Nutr.* 1999; 23 (6 Suppl.): S210–213.

13. Wilmore, D.W. Deterrents to the successful clinical use of growth factors that enhance protein anabolism. *Curr. Opin. Clin. Nutr. Metab. Care* 1999; 2 (1): 15–21.

14. Garcia de Lorenzo, A., and J.M. Culebras. [Hormones, growth factors, and drugs in metabolism and nutrition.] *Nutr. Hosp.* 1995; 10 (5): 297–305.

15. Baumgartner, R.N., D.L. Walters, D. Gallagher, et al. Predictors of skeletal muscle mass in elderly men and women. *Mech. Ageing Dev.* 1999; 107 (2): 123–136.

16. Ravaglia, G., P. Forti, M. Maioli, et al. The relationship of dehydroepiandrosterone sulfate (DHEAS) to endocrine-metabolic parameters and functional status in the oldest-old. Results from an Italian study on healthy free-living over ninety-year-olds. *J. Clin. Endocrinol. Metab.* 1996; 81 (3): 1173–1178.

17. Bonnefoy, M., T. Kostka, M.C. Patricot, et al. Physical activity and dehydroepiandrosterone sulfate, insulin-like growth factor-1 and testosterone in healthy active elderly people. *Age Ageing* 1998; 27 (6): 745–751.

18. Abbasi, A., E.H. Duthie, L. Sheldahl, et al. Association of dehydroepiandrosterone sulfate, body composition, and physical fitness in independent community-dwelling older men and women. *J. Am. Geriatr. Soc.* 1998; 46 (3): 263–273.

19. Lostka, T., L.M. Arsac, M.C. Patricott, et al. Leg extensor power and dehydroepiandrosterone sulfate, insulin-like growth factor-1 and testosterone in healthy active elderly people. *Eur. J. Appl. Physiol.* 2000; 82 (1–2): 83–90.

20. Proctor, D.N., P. Balagopal, and K.S. Nair. Age-related sarcopenia in humans is associated with reduced synthetic rates of specific muscle proteins. *J. Nutr.* 1998; 128 (2 Suppl.): 351S–355S.

21. Singh, M.A., W. Ding, T.J. Manfredi, et al. Insulin-like growth factor-1 in skeletal muscle after weight-lifting exercise in frail elders. *Am. J. Physiol.* 1999; 277 (1 Pt 1): E135–143.

22. Gallagher, D., E. Ruts, M. Visser, et al. Weight stability masks sarcopenia in elderly men and women. *Am. J. Physiol. Endocrinol. Metab.* 2000; 279 (2): E366–E375.

23. Cohen, P., I. Ocrant, P.J. Fielder, et al. Insulin-like growth factors (IGFs): implications for aging. *Psychoneuroendocrinology* 1992; 17 (4): 335–342.

24. Lamberts, S.W., A.W. van den Beld, and A.J. van der Lely. The endocrinology of aging. *Science* 1997; 278 (5337): 419–424.

25. Rosen, C.J., J. Glowacki, and W. Craig. Sex steroids, the insulin-like growth factor regulatory system, and aging: implications for the management of older post-menopausal women. *J. Nutr. Health Aging* 1998; 2 (1): 39–44.

26. Harper, A.J., J.E. Buster, and P.R. Casson. Changes in adrenocortical function with aging and therapeutic implications. *Semin. Reprod. Endocrinol.* 1999; 17 (4): 327–338.

27. Short, K.R., and K.S. Nair. Mechanisms of sarcopenia in aging. *J. Endocrinol. Invest.* 1999; 22 (5 Suppl.): 95–105.

28. Wolfe, R., A. Ferrando, M. Sheffield-Moore, et al. Testosterone and muscle protein metabolism. *Mayo Clin. Proc.* 2000; 75 (Suppl.): S55–59.

29. Graves, J.E., M.L. Pollock, and J.F. Carroll. Exercise, age, and skeletal muscle function. *South. Med. J.* 1994; 87 (5): S17–22.

30. Fielding, R.A. The role of progressive resistance training and nutrition in the preservation of lean body mass in the elderly. *J. Am. Coll. Nutr.* 1995; 14 (6): 587–594.

31. Evans, W.J. Reversing sarcopenia: how weight training can build strength and vitality. *Geriatrics* 1996; 51 (5): 46–47.

32. Frischknecht, R. Effect of training on muscle strength and motor function in the elderly. *Reprod. Nutr. Dev.* 1998; 38 (2): 167–174.

33. Starling, R.D, P.A. Ades, and E.T. Poehlman. Physical activity, protein intake, and appendicular skeletal muscle mass in older men. *Am. J. Clin. Nutr.* 1999; 70 (1): 91–96.

34. Roth, S.M., R.F. Ferrell, and B.F. Hurley. Strength training for the prevention and treatment of sarcopenia. *J. Nutr. Health Aging* 2000; 4 (3): 143–155.

35. Bullock, G., A.M. White, and J. Worthington. The effects of catabolic and anabolic steroids on amino acid incorporation by skeletal-muscle ribosomes. *Biochem. J.* 1968; 108 (3): 417–425.

36. Rogozkin, V. Metabolic effects of anabolic steroid on skeletal muscle. *Med. Sci. Sports* 1979; 11 (2): 160–163.

37. Wu, F.C. Endocrine aspects of anabolic steroids. *Clin. Chem.* 1997; 43 (7): 1289–1292.

38. Sheffield-Moore, M., R.R. Wolfe, D.C Gore, et al. Combined effects of hyperaminoacidemia and oxandrolone on skeletal muscle protein synthesis. *Am.J. Physiol. Endocrinol. Metab.* 2000; 278 (2): E273–279.

39. Sheffield-Moore, M., R.J. Urban, S.E. Wolf, et al. Short-term oxandrolone administration stimulates net muscle protein synthesis in young men. *J. Clin. Endocrinol. Metab.* 1999; 84 (8): 2705–2711.

40. Dzamukov, R.A., and V.V. Valiullin. [Response of skeletal muscles to anabolic steroid is specific and does not depend on the motor activity regime.] *Bull. Eksp. Biol. Med.* 1999; 127 (4): 406–408.

41. Kadi, F., P. Bonnerud, A. Eriksson, et al. The expression of androgen receptors in human neck and limb muscles: effects of training and self-administration of androgenic-anabolic steroids. *Histochem. Cell. Biol.* 2000; 113 (1): 25–29.

42. Kadi, F., A. Eriksson, S. Holmner, et al. Effects of anabolic steroids on the muscle cells of strength-trained athletes. *Med. Sci. Sports Exerc.* 1999; 31 (11): 1528–1534.

43. Kadi, F. Adaptation of human skeletal muscle to training and anabolic steroids. *Acta Physiol. Scand. Suppl.* 2000; 646: 1–52.

44. Houston, M.E. Gaining weight: the scientific basis of increasing skeletal muscle mass. *Can. J. Appl. Physiol.* 1999; 24 (4): 305–316.

45. Hobbs, C.J., S.R. Plymate, C.J. Rosen, et al. Testosterone administration increases insulin-like growth factor-1 levels in normal men. *J. Clin. Endocrinol. Metab.* 1994; 78 (6): 1360–1367.

46. Morales, A.J., J.J. Nolan, J.C. Nelson, et al. Effects of replacement dose of dehydroepiandrosterone in men and women of advancing age. *J. Clin. Endocrinol. Metab.* 1994; 78 (6): 1360–1367.

47. Gelato, M.C., and R.A. Frost. IGFBP-3. Functional and structural implications in aging and wasting syndromes. *Endocrine* 1997; 7 (1): 81–85.

48. Casson, P.R., N. Santoro, K. Elkind-Hirsch, et al. Postmenopausal dehydroepiandrosterone administration increases free insulin-like growth factor-1 and decreases high-density lipoprotein: a six month trial. *Fertil. Steril.* 1998; 70 (1): 107–110.

49. Jorgensen, J.O., N. Vahl, T.B. Hansen, et al. Determinants of serum insulin-like growth factor 1 in growth hormone deficient adults as compared to healthy subjects. *Clin. Endocrinol. (Oxf.)* 1998; 48 (4): 479–486.

50. Morales, A.J., R.H. Haubrich, J.Y. Hwang, et al. The effects of six months treatment with 100mg daily dose of dehydroepiandrosterone (DHEA) on circulating sex steroids, body composition, and muscle strength, in age-advanced men and women. *Clin. Endocrinol. (Oxf.)* 1998; 49 (4): 421–434.

51. Span, J.P., G.F. Pieters, C.G. Sweep, et al. Gender difference in insulin-like growth factor 1 response to growth hormone (GH) treatment and GH-deficient adults: role of sex hormone replacement. *J. Clin. Endocrinol. Metab.* 2000; 85 (3): 1121–1125.

52. Savine, R., and P. Sonksen. Growth hormone replacement for somatopause? *Horm. Res.* 2000; 53 (Suppl. S3): 37–41.

53. Eakman, G.D., J.S. Dallas, S.W. Ponder, et al. The effects of testosterone and dihydrotestosterone on hypothalamic regulation of growth hormone secretion. *J. Clin. Endocrinol. Metab.* 1996; 81 (3): 1217–1223.

54. Zapf, J., M.Y. Donath, C. Schmid. [Spectrum of effectiveness of insulin-like growth factors.] *Schweiz. Med. Wochenschr.* 2000; 130 (6): 190–195.

55. Hall, K., P. Bang, and K. Brismar. [Insulin-like growth factors. Future treatment in catabolism?] *Lakartidningen* 1995; 92 (26–27): 2668–2671.

56. Baxter, R.C. The insulin-like growth factors and their binding proteins. *Comp. Biochem. Physiol. B.* 1998; 91 (2): 229–235.

57. Binoux, M. The IGF system in metabolism regulation. *Diebete. Metab.* 1995; 21 (5): 330–337.

58. Froesch, E.R., and M. Hussain. Recombinant human insulin-like growth factor-1: a therapeutic challenge for diabetes mellitus. *Diabetologia* 1994; 37 (Suppl. 2): S179–185.

59. Abbasi, A., D.E. Mattson, M. Cilusinier, et al. Hyposomatomedinemia and hypogonadism in hemiplegic men who live in nursing homes. *Arch. Phys. Med. Rehabil.* 1994; 75 (5): 594–599.

60. Bitar, M.S., C.W. Pilcher, I. Kahn, et al. Diabetes-induced suppression of IGF-1 and its receptor mRNA levels in rat superior cervical ganglia. *Diabetes Res. Clin. Pract.* 1997; 38 (2): 73–80.

61. Gori, F., L.C. Hofbauer, C.A. Conover, et al. Effects of androgens on the insulin-like growth factor system in an androgen-responsive human osteoblastic cell line. *Endocrinology* 1999; 149 (12): 5579–5586.

62. Solerte, S.B., M. Fioravanti, G. Vignati, et al. Dehydroepiandrosterone sulfate enhances natural killer cell cytotoxicity in humans via locally generated immunoreactive insulin-like growth factor-1. *J. Clin. Endocrinol. Metab.* 1999; 84 (9): 3260–3267.

63. Solerte, S.B., R. Gornati, L. Cravello, et al. Dehydroepiandrosterone-sulfate (DHEA-S) restores the release of IGF-1 from natural killer cells (NK) in old patients with dementia of Alzheimer's type (DAT). *J. Endocrinol. Invest.* 1999; 22 (10 Suppl.): 32–34.

64. Ren, J., W.K. Samson, and J.R. Sowers. Insulin-like growth factor 1 as a cardiac hormone: physiological and pathophysiological implications in heart disease. *J. Mol. Cell. Cardiol.* 1999; 31 (11): 2049–2061.

65. Smith, L.E., W. Shen, C. Perruzzi, et al. Regulation of vascular endothelial growth factor-dependent retinal neovascularization by insulin-like growth factor-1 receptor. *Nat. Med.* 1999; 5 (12): 1390–1395.

66. Russell, J.W., and E.L. Feldman. Insulin-like growth factor-1 prevents apoptosis in sympathetic neurons exposed to high glucose. *Horm. Metab. Res.* 1999; 31 (2–3): 90–96.

67. Winkler, R., F. Paseau, N. Boussif, et al. [The IGF system: summary and recent data.] *Rev. Med. Liège.* 2000; 55 (7): 725–739.

68. Blakytny, R., E.B. Jude, J. Martin Gibson, et al. Lack of insulin-like growth factor 1 (IGF1) in the basal keratinocyte layer of diabetic skin and diabetic foot ulcers. *J. Pathol.* 2000; 190 (5): 589–594.

69. Ferreira, I.M., I.T. Vereschi, L.E. Nery, et al. The influence of 6 months of oral anabolic steroids on body mass and respiratory muscles in undernourished COPD patients. *Chest* 1998; 114 (1): 19–28.

70. Casaburi, R. Skeletal muscle function in COPD. *Chest* 2000; 117 (5 Suppl. 1): 267S–271S.

71. Schols, A.M. Nutrition in chronic obstructive pulmonary disease. *Curr. Opin. Pulm. Med.* 2000; 6 (2): 110–115.

72. Tenover, J.S. Effects of testosterone supplementation in the aging male. *J. Clin. Endocrinol. Metab.* 1992; 75 (4): 1092–1098.

73. Lovejoy, J.C., G.A. Bray, C.S. Greeson, et al. Oral anabolic steroid treatment, but not parenteral androgen treatment, decreases abdominal fat in obese, older men. *Int. J. Obes. Relat. Metab. Disord.* 1995; 19 (9): 614–624.

74. Wolf, O.T., O. Neumann, D.H. Hellhammer, et al. Effects of a two-week physiological dehydroepiandrosterone substitution on cognitive performance and well-being in healthy elderly women and men. *J. Clin. Endocrinol. Metab.* 1997; 82 (7): 2363–2367.

75. Bross, R., C. Casaburi, T.W. Storer, et al. Androgen effects on body composition and muscle function: implications for the use of androgens as anabolic agents in sarcopenic states. *Baillieres Clin. Endocrinol. Metab.* 1998; 12 (3): 365–378.

76. Bross, R., T. Storer, and S. Bhasin. Aging and muscle loss. *Trends Endocrinol. Metab.* 1999; 10 (5): 194–195.

77. Tenover, J.S. Androgen replacement therapy to reverse and/or prevent age-related sarcopenia in men. *Baillieres Clin. Endocrinol. Metab.* 1998; 12 (3): 419–425.

78. Creutzberg, E.C., and A.M. Schols. Anabolic steroids. *Curr. Opin. Clin. Nutr. Metab. Care* 1999; 2 (3): 243–253.

79. Lund, B.C., K.A. Bever-Stille, and P.J. Perry. Testosterone and andropause: the feasibility of testosterone replacement in elderly men. *Pharmacotherapy* 1999; 19 (8): 951–956.

80. Snyder, P.J., H. Peachey, P. Hannoush, et al. Effect of testosterone treatment on body composition and muscle strength in men over 65 years of age. *J. Clin. Endocrinol. Metab.* 1999; 84 (4): 2647–2653.

81. Pineiro, V., X. Casabiell, R. Peino, et al. Dihydrotestosterone, stanozolol, androstenedione and dehydroepiandrosterone sulfate inhibit leptin secretion in female but not in male samples of omental adipose tissue in vitro: lack of effect of testosterone. *J. Endocrinol.* 1999; 160 (3): 425–432.

82. Sheffield-Moore, M. Androgens in the control of skeletal muscle protein synthesis. *Ann. Med.* 2000; 32 (3): 181–186.

83. Casson, P.R., N. Santoro, K. Eldind-Hirsh, et al. Postmenopausal dehydroepiandrosterone administration increases free insulin-like growth factor-1 and decreases high-density lipoprotein: a six month trial. *Fertil. Steril.* 1998; 70 (1): 107–110.

84. Legrain, S., C. Massien, N. Lahlou, et al. Dehydroepiandrosterone replacement administration: pharmacokinetic and pharmacodynamic studies in healthy elderly subjects. *J. Clin. Endocrinol. Metab.* 2000; 85 (9): 3208–3217.

85. Baulieu, E.E., G. Thomas, S. Legrain, et al. Dehydroepiandrosterone (DHEA), DHEA sulfate, and aging: contribution of the DHEAge Study to a sociobiomedical issue. *Proc. Natl. Acad. Sci. USA* 2000; 97 (8): 4279–4284.

86. Lye, M.D., and A.E. Ritch. A double-blind trial of an anabolic steroid (stanozolol) in the disabled elderly. *Rheumatol. Rehabil.* 1977; 16 (1): 62–69.

87. Ferreira, I.M., I.T. Vereschi, L.E. Nery, et al. The influence of 6 months of oral anabolic steroids on body mass and respiratory muscles in undernourished COPD patients. *Chest* 1998; 114 (1): 19–28.

88. Shapiro, J., J. Christiana, and W.H. Frishman. Testosterone and other anabolic steroids as cardiovascular drugs. *Am. J. Ther.* 1999; 6 (3): 167–174.

89. Tomoda, H. Effect of oxymetholone on left ventricular dimensions in heart failure secondary to idiopathic dilated cardiomyopathy or to mitral or aortic regurgitation. *Am J. Cardiol.* 1999; 83 (1): 123–125.

90. English, K.M. Low-dose transdermal testosterone therapy improves angina threshold in men with chronic stable angina: a randomized, double-blind, placebo-controlled study. *Circulation* 2000; 102: 1096–1911.

91. Lye, M.D., and A.E. Ritch. A double-blind trial of an anabolic steroid (stanozolol) in the disabled elderly. *Rheumatol. Rehabil.* 1977; 16 (1): 62–69.

92. Bashski, V., M. Elliot, A. Gentili, et al. Testosterone improves rehabilitation outcomes of ill older men. *J. Am. Geriatr. Soc.* 2000; 48 (5): 550–553.

93. Corpas, E., S.M. Harman, M.A. Pineyro, et al. Growth hormone (GH)-releasing hormone-(1–29) twice daily reverses the decreased GH and insulin-like growth factor-1 levels in old men. *J. Clin. Endocrinol. Metab.* 1992; 75 (2): 530–535.

94. Kupfer, S.R., L.E. Underwood, R.C. Baxter, et al. Enhancement of the anabolic effects of growth hormone and insulin-like growth factor 1 by use of both agents simultaneously. *J. Clin. Invest.* 1993; 91 (2): 391–396.

95. Goth, M., I. Szabolcs, and F. Peter. [Growth hormone therapy in adults.] *Orv. Hetil.* 1995; 136 (23): 1243–1247.

96. Berneis, K., and U. Keller. Metabolic actions of growth hormone: direct and indirect. *Baillieres Clin. Endocrinol. Metab.* 1996; 10 (3): 337–352.

97. Chapman, I.M., M.A. Bach, E. van Cauter, et al. Simulation of growth hormone (GH)-insulin-like growth factor 1 by daily oral administration of a GH secretagogue (MK-677) in healthy elderly subjects. *J. Clin. Endocrinol. Metab.* 1996; 81 (12): 4249–4257.

98. Ghigo, E., E. Arvat, L. Gianotti, et al. Short-term administration of intranasal or oral Hexarelin, a synthetic hexapeptide, does not desensitize the growth hormone responsiveness in human aging. *Eur. J. Endocrinol.* 1996; 135 (4): 407–412.

99. Korbonits, M., and A.B. Grossman. [Growth hormone-releasing peptides (GHRP) and their analogues.] *Orv. Hetil.* 1996; 137 (45): 2503–2509.

100. Vittone, J., M.R. Blackman, J. Busby-Whitehead, et al. Effects of single nightly injections of growth hormone-releasing hormone (GHRH 1-29) in healthy elderly men. *Metabolism* 1998; 46 (1): 89–96.

101. Camanni, F., E. Ghigo, and E. Arvat. Growth hormone-releasing peptides and their analogues. *Front. Neuroendocrinol.* 1998; 19 (1): 47–72.

102. Anwer, K., M. Shi, M.F. French, et al. Systemic effect of human growth hormone after intramuscular injection of a single dose of a muscle-specific gene medicine. *Hum. Gene Ther.* 1998; 9 (5): 659–670.

103. Ghigo, E., E. Arvat, and F. Camanni. Orally active growth hormone secretagogues: state of the art and clinical perspectives. *Ann. Med.* 1998; 30 (2): 159–168.

104. Hoffman, D.M, R. Pallasser, M. Duncan, et al. How is whole body protein turnover perturbed in growth hormone-deficient adults? *J. Clin. Endocrinol. Metab.* 1998; 83 (12): 4344–4349.

105. Cummings, D.E., and G.R. Merriam. Age-related changes in growth hormone secretion: should the somatopause be treated? *Semin. Reprod. Endocrinol.* 1999; 17 (4): 311–325.

106. Bross, R., M. Javanbakht, and S. Bhasin. Anabolic interventions for aging-associated sarcopenia. *J. Clin. Endocrinol. Metab.* 1999; 84 (10): 3420–3430.

107. Welle, S., C. Thornton, M. Statt, et al. Growth hormone increases muscle mass and strength but does not rejuvenate myofibrillar protein synthesis in healthy subjects over 60 years old. *J. Clin. Endocrinol. Metab.* 1996; 81 (9): 3239–3243.

108. Taffe, D.R., L. Pruitt, J. Reim, et al. Effect of recombinant human growth hormone on the muscle strength response to resistance exercise in elderly men. *J. Clin. Endocrinol. Metab.* 1994; 79 (5): 1361–1366.

109. Soloman, F., R. Cuneo, and P.H. Sonksen. Growth hormone and protein

metabolism. *Horm. Res.* 1991; 36 (Suppl 1): 41–43.

110. Szabo, S., R.C. Wagner, E.G. Malatinszky, et al. [The effect of anabolic steroids on blood proteins and autoantibodies in multiple sclerosis.] *Stud. Cercet. Neurol.* 1967; 12 (6): 457–461.

111. Mall, G., A. Heibrunn, H.F. Paarmann, et al. [The treatment of multiple sclerosis with anabolic steroids.] *Med. Klin.* 1968; 63 (51): 2075–2077.

112. Cendrowski, W., W. Kuran. [Results of combined administration of anabolic steroids in patients with multiple sclerosis. *Neurol. Neurochir.* 1972; 6 (4): 573–576.

113. Belch, J.J., R. Madhok, B. McArdle, et al. The effect of increasing fibrinolysis in patients with rheumatoid arthritis: a double blind study of stanozolol. *Q.J. Med.* 1986; 58 (225): 19–27.

114. Drosos, A.A., P. van Vliet-Dascolpoulou, A.P. Andonopoulos, et al. *Clin. Exp. Rheumatol.* Nandrolone decanoate (deca-durabolin) in primary Sjogren's syndrome: a double-blind study. 1988; 6 (1): 53–57.

115. Jayson, M.I., C.D. Holland, A. Keegan, et al. A controlled study of stanozolol in primary Raynaud's phenomenon and systemic sclerosis. *Ann. Rheum. Dis.* 1991; 50 (1): 41–47.

116. Shizgal, H.M. Anabolic steroids and total parenteral nutrition. *Wien. Med. Wochenschr.* 1993; 143 (14–15): 375–380.

117. Sartorio, A., and M.V. Narici. Growth hormone (GH) treatment in GH-deficient adults: effects on muscle size, strength and neural activation. *Clin. Physiol.* 1994; 14 (5): 527–537.

118. Schols, A.M., P.B. Soeters, R. Mostert, et al. Physiological effects of nutritional support and anabolic steroids in patients with chronic obstructive pulmonary disease. A placebo-controlled randomized trial. *Am. J. Respir. Crit. Care Med.* 1995; 152 (4 Pt. 1): 1268–1274.

119. Schambelan, M., K. Mulligan, C. Grunfeld, et al. Recombinant human growth hormone in patients with HIV-associated wasting. A randomized, placebo-controlled trial. Serostim Study Group. *Ann. Intern. Med.* 1996; 125 (11): 873–882.

120. Baum, H.B., B.M. Biller, J.S. Finkelstein, et al. Effects of physiologic growth hormone therapy on bone density and body composition in patients with adult-onset growth hormone deficiency. A randomized, placebo-controlled trial. *Ann. Intern. Med.* 1996; 125 (11): 883–890.

121. Reid, I.R., D.J. Wattie, M.C. Evans, et al. Testosterone therapy in glucocorticoid-treated men. *Arch. Intern. Med.* 1996; 156 (11): 1173–1173.

122. Fenichel, G., A. Pestronk, J. Florence, et al. A beneficial effect of oxandrolone in the treatment of Duchenne muscular dystrophy: a pilot study. *Neurology* 1997; 48 (5): 1225–1226.

123. Demling, R.H., and L. DeSanti. Oxandrolone, an anabolic steroid, significantly increases the rate of weight gain in the recovery phase after major burns. *J. Trauma* 1997; 43 (1): 47–51.

124. Bhasin, S., T.W. Storer, N. Asbel-Sethi, et al. Effects of testosterone replacement with a nongenital, transdermal system, Androderm, in human immunodeficiency virus-infected men with low testosterone levels. *J. Clin. Endocrinol. Metab.* 1998; 83 (9): 3155–3162.

125. Grinspoon, S., C. Corcoran, H. Askari, et al. Effects of androgen administration in men with the AIDS wasting syndrome. A randomized, double-blind, placebo-controlled trial. *Ann. Intern. Med.* 1998; 129 (1): 18–26.

126. Ferreira, I.M., I.T. Verreschi, L.E. Nery, et al. The influence of 6 months of oral anabolic steroids on body mass and respiratory muscles in undernourished COPD patients. *Chest* 1998; 114 (1): 19–28.

127. Russell-Jones, D.L., S.B. Bowes, S.E. Rees, et al. Effect of growth hormone treatment on postprandial protein metabolism in growth hormone-deficient adults. *Am. J. Physiol.* 1998; 274 (6): E1050–1056.

128. Mulligan, K., V.W. Tai, and M. Schambelan. Use of growth hormone and other anabolic agents in AIDS wasting. *J. Parenter. Enteral Nutr.* 1999; 23 (6 Suppl.): S202–209.

129. Shapiro, J., J. Christiana, and W.H. Frishman. Testosterone and other anabolic steroids as cardiovascular drugs. *Am. J. Ther.* 1999; 6 (3): 167–174.

130. Demling, R.H. Comparison of the anabolic effects and complications of human growth hormone and the testosterone analogue, oxandrolone, after severe burn injury. *Burns* 1999; 25 (3): 215–221.

131. van Vollenhhoven, R.F., J.L. Park, M.C. Genovese, et al. A double-blind, placebo-controlled, clinical trial of dehydroepiandrosterone in severe systemtic lupus erythematosus. *Lupus* 1999; 8 (3): 181–187.

132. Spungen, A. M., D.R. Grimm, M. Strakhan, et al. Treatment with an anabolic agent is associated with improvement in respiratory function in persons with tetraplegia: a pilot study. *Mt. Sinai, J. Med.* 1999; 66 (3): 201–205.

133. Johansen, K.L., K. Mulligan, and M. Schambelan. Anabolic effects of nandrolone decanoate in patients receiving dialysis: a randomized controlled trial. *JAMA* 1999; 281 (14): 1275–1281.

134. Strawford, A., T. Barbieri, M. van Loan, et al. Resistance exercise and supraphysiologic androgen therapy in eugonadal men with HIV-related weight loss: a randomized controlled trial. *JAMA* 1999; 281 (14): 1282–1290.

135. Scolapio, J.S. Effect of growth hormone, glutamine, and diet on body composition in short bowel syndrome: a randomized, controlled study. *J. Parenter. Enteral. Nutr.* 1999; 23 (6): 309–312.

136. Berger, J.R. Resistance exercise and oxandrolone for men with HIV-related weight loss. *JAMA* 2000; 284 (2): 176.

137. Romeyn, M., and N. Gunn. Resistance exercise and oxandrolone for men with HIV-related weight loss. *JAMA* 2000; 284 (2): 176.

138. Wang, C., R.S. Swedloff, A. Iranmanesh, et al. Transdermal testosterone gel improves sexual function, mood, muscle strength, and body composition parameters in hypogonadal men. Testosterone Gel Study Group. *J. Clin. Endocrinol. Metab.* 2000; 85 (8): 2839–2853.

139. Demling, R.H., and D.P. Orgill. The anticatabolic and wound healing effects of the testosterone analogue oxandrolone after severe burn injury. *J. Crit. Care* 2000; 15 (1): 12–17.

140. Cutolo, M. Sex hormone adjuvant therapy in rheumatoid arthritis. *Rheum. Dis. Clin. North Am.* 2000; 26 (4): 881–895.

141. English, K.M. Low-dose transdermal testosterone therapy improves angina threshold in men with chronic stable angina: a randomized, double-blind, placebo-controlled study. *Circulation* 2000; 102: 1906–1911.

4

Rationale for Anabolic Therapy in Corticosteroid-Induced Osteoporosis

Introduction: Iatrogenic Bone Disease

Osteoporosis is a very common and serious condition that has often been mistakenly thought to be confined to postmenopausal osteoporosis in women or senile osteoporosis in elderly men. However, osteoporosis can occur in a variety of conditions, including drug therapies that accelerate bone mineral density (BMD) loss by interfering with bone metabolism homeostasis. Pharmacological interventions that are used in the treatment of a variety of illnesses have been shown to cause, contribute to, or accelerate the osteoporosis process, especially with concurrent age-related and gonadal involution-related reduction of BMD.

The most common drug-induced cause of osteoporosis results from or is associated with prolonged corticosteroid therapy in patients for the treatment of a variety of disease conditions.[1, 2] Corticosteroid-induced (CST-induced) osteoporosis has been recognized for nearly 60 years. For patients with it, CST-induced osteoporosis often results in bone fractures and chronic pain with little or no associated trauma. It is the most common form of iatrogenic osteoporosis.

In younger people, prolonged or repetitive corticosteroid therapy is the most common form of osteoporosis.[3] CST-induced osteoporosis can occur with oral, inhaled, intramuscular, or intravenous corticosteroid therapies. Although the true incidence of CST-induced osteoporosis varies, *it has been reported that as many as 90 percent of patients treated with prolonged corticosteroid therapy develop osteoporosis.*[4] Patients with rheumatoid arthritis, systemic lupus erythematosus, scleroderma, and other neuroendocrine, autoimmune inflammatory arthritis, together with patients with chronic asthmatic conditions,[5] account for nearly half of all patients treated with prolonged or repetitive corticosteroid therapy.[6] CST-induced osteoporosis continues to be a major problem faced by rheumatologists, with up to 50 percent of patients at risk for vertebral fractures.[7]

Although most physicians are aware of this condition, recent studies have indicated that fewer than 50 percent of patients on prolonged or repetitive corticosteroid therapy receive the appropriate anabolic therapies they require to prevent or reverse the catabolic consequences, including significant BMD losses.[8, 9, 10, 11] Care of patients on prolonged or repeated doses of corticosteroids makes up a significant percentage of the practice in physical medicine and rehabilitation.

Hypoandrogenemia and Hyposomatomedinemia in CST-Induced Osteoporosis

It is now well recognized that hypoandrogenemia in both men and women can be a major predictor of BMD and osteoporosis that is associated with aging, chronic disease, and significant corticosteroid therapy.[12, 13, 14, 15, 16, 17] Therefore, androgen therapy represents a rational, convenient, effective, and safe strategy for preventing and treating CST-induced osteoporosis.[18, 19] It has been suggested that androgen therapy is advisable for all patients with CST-induced osteoporosis,[20] especially for those patients who have already had fractures or who have ongoing BMD losses.[21] Androgen therapy has been shown (statistically significant) to reverse the deleterious BMD losses and other catabolic effects, such as loss of lean body mass and increased body fat gains caused by prolonged corticosteroid treatment.[22]

Prolonged use of or repetitive corticosteroid therapy alters bone metabolism homeostasis and accelerates BMD loss by several specific mechanisms as listed in Table 4-1. Many of these mechanisms are intertwined with androgen metabolism or androgen deficiency states. The greatest rate of BMD loss has been shown to occur within the first six to 12 months of corticosteroid therapy.[23] It has also been shown that it is not unusual for these patients to lose as much as 20 percent or more of their BMD within the first 12 months of corticosteroid therapy.[24]

Prolonged corticosteroid therapy causes accelerated BMD losses via several interacting mechanisms that affect hormonal, systemic, and local tissue networks. These interactive mechanisms have been shown to

Table 4-1. Overview of Specific Mechanisms for CST-Induced Osteoporosis

Pathogenic Abnormality	Pathologic Mechanism.
Reduced bone formation	Reduced osteoblast stimulation due to: (1) hypoandrogenemia due to adrenal suppression (2) hypoandrogenemia from blunted LH secretion (3) hyposomatomedinemia from reduced androgen stimulation of GHRH and reduced IGF-1 levels (4) competitive inhibition of androgen receptors by corticosteroids (5) inhibition of osteoblast stimulating cytokines
Increased bone resorption	Increased osteoclast activities: (1) hypoestrogenemia (in women) from blunted LH secretion (2) competitive inhibition of estrogen receptors by corticosteroids (3) secondary hyperparathyroidism (4) hypoandrogenemia that results in reduced inhibition of proresorptive cytokines
Altered calcium metabolism	(1) reduced calcium absorption from the intestines (2) hypercalcuria due to reduction of renal tubular reabsorption of calcium causing secondary hyperparathyroidism.
Altered bone architecture	(1) disproportionate BMD loss from trabecular bone (2) disproportionate increased risk for bone fracture

result in pathological changes exhibited in: reduced bone formation, increased bone resorption, detrimental alterations in calcium metabolism, and detrimental changes to bone architecture on a histomorphometric basis.[25]

Reduced Bone Formation

It is now well recognized that osteoblasts are bone-forming cells that are stimulated by androgens, GH, IGF-1, and other anabolic agents and cytokines. Androgens bind to osteoblast receptors, and this finding has stimulated renewed interest in androgen effects on bone, an interest that has been overshadowed by conventional wisdom's interest in estrogen-related effects.[26] Other androgen-related osteoblast stimulating effects produced are mediated, in part, by androgen-dependent IGF-1 production and differential regulation of circulating IGFBPs.[27]

The anabolic effects of androgens on osteoblast bioactivities have been indicated by a number of specific molecules in the serum of patients.[28] These biochemical markers of bone formation and osteoblast activities include serum osteocalcin (Oc), bone-specific alkaline phosphatase (bAP), N- and C-terminal propeptide of type 1 procollagen (PINP and PICP respectively), and others.[29,30,31,32,33,34] These bone markers have been shown to indicate osteoblast activity that reflects formation of organic matrix in bone.[35] The discovery of these biochemical markers, along with improved imaging techniques, including dual-energy x-ray absorptiometry (DEXA), have provided updated methods to assess the pharmacological therapies that stimulate osteoblast activities and result in increases in BMD.[36,37,38] These developments have also allowed an improved understanding of the mechanisms that endogenous hormone interactions have on bone formulation and homeostasis.

Recent studies have shown that the androgen-induced effect on osteoblasts is both prolonged and restorative, and that the osteoblast stimulation continues for a period of time after androgen therapy is discontinued.[39] Androgen therapy has also been shown to restore serum osteocalcin levels to the normal range in patients with CST-induced osteoporosis.[40] These measures of direct osteoblast stimulation have been shown by in vitro studies with human osteoblastlike cells[41] and with serial bone biopsy (before and after androgen treatment) conformation with osteoporotic men and women patients treated with androgen (stanozolol) therapy.[42] In this latter study, histological examination of bone tissue showed:

(1) active-appearing osteoblasts within the trabecular bone tissue.

(2) increased trabecular bone turnover and increased trabecular bone mass (statistically significant).

(3) increased endocortical turnover and increased cortical and endocortical bone masses (statistically significant).

These site-specific and differential effects of androgen therapy result in normal bone morphology and have important implications for its long-term use in the management of osteoporosis. The increase in trabecular bone mass has been shown to be of particular importance for CST-induced osteoporosis where patients tend to have a specific acceleration of trabecular bone mass losses.[43]

Corticosteroids tend to interact competitively and in an antagonistic manner with androgens for receptor sites in osteoblasts.[44] When androgens bind to osteoblast receptors, the osteoblast is stimulated to increase anabolic bone metabolism. However, when corticosteroids bind to these same receptors, the osteoblastic anabolic functions are suppressed.[45] Corticosteroids act directly, via osteoblast receptors, to suppress the anabolic genetic machinery.[46] Corticosteroid therapy also alters cytokine balance to favor the stimulation of osteoclasts that increase resorption of bone.[47]

Besides competing for osteoblast receptor sites with androgens, *corticosteroid therapy can cause hypoandrogenemia* by the following three mechanisms:

(1) by blunting the luteinizing hormone (LH) response to luteinizing hormone-releasing hormone (LHRH).[48] In this manner, corticosteroid therapy alters the LHRH-LH-gonadal axis that reduces androgen synthesis in and release from the gonadal tissues in both genders.[49, 50] However, this mechanism of CST-induced hypoandrogenemia has been shown to be more clinically significant in men.[51] In a recent, controlled, prospective study of normal men, corticosteroid therapy was correlated (statistically significant) with reduced bone formation markers, losses in BMD, increased SHBG, and reduced free testosterone levels.[52] Low free androgen levels in men have been shown (statistically significant) to be associated with osteoporotic vertebral fractures.[53]

(2) by suppressing the synthesis and secretion of testosterone, dehydroepiandrosterone (DHEA), and androstenedione from the adrenal glands. It has been shown that corticosteroid administration suppresses the hypothalamic-pituitary-adrenal axis, alters the cortisol-androgen synthesis and secretion ratios, and can aggravate the age-related shift in steroid biosynthesis within the adrenal glands, all of which further increase cortisol in the cortisol-androgen ratios.[54, 55] This effect has been shown to be more clinically relevant in women.

In normal women, it has been shown that there is a parallel adrenal activity in response to trophic stimuli without invoking an adrenal-gonadal interaction. Thus, *decreased adrenal androgen production is not paralleled by an increased ovarian androgen production.*[56] In postmenopausal women, adrenal steroid production has been shown to selectively increase cortisol levels during acute illness, while selectively decreasing androgen levels that are not counterbalanced by ovarian androgen production.[57] Furthermore, it has been shown that estrogen monotherapy for hormone replacement therapy (HRT) results in a profound reduction in free, bioavailable androgen levels, causing a significant hypoandrogenic state[58] by increasing sex hormone binding globulin (SHBG) levels by 160 percent.[59] Estrogen plus androgen therapy decreases SHBG and allows for lower estrogen replacement doses while increasing the bioavailability of androgens.[60] Therefore, corticosteroid therapy for acute or chronic illness in women, especially in postmenopausal women, treated with or without estrogen monotherapy for HRT, can result in significant hypoandrogenemia that results in reduced osteoblast activity and loss of BMD.

In contrast, it has been shown that, in men, there is an independent secretion of androgens by the adrenals and testes. Deficits in adrenal androgen production are generally paralleled by increased testicular androgen secretion.[61]

(3) by elevating the circulating levels of sex hormone binding globulin (SHBG) that provides additional binding sites for androgens and reduces levels of free, bioavailable circulating androgens.[62]

Corticosteroid-induced hypoandrogenemia can result in loss of the anabolic stimuli which affect bone formation and which are independent of competition with androgens for bone receptors. Hypoandrogenemia can result in a depressed GHRH-GH-IGF-IGFBP axis. Androgens have been shown to directly stimulate the GHRH-GH-IGF-IGFBP axis at the hypothalamic level by a direct stimulatory effect that increases GHRH pulse amplitudes.[63, 64] Such androgen stimulation has been shown to elevate circulating IGF-1, free IGF-1, and IGFBP-3 levels in normal, hypogonadal, hyposomatotrophic, and aging individuals.[65, 66, 67, 68, 69, 70, 71, 72] Normalizing GH secretory patterns or administering GHRH or GH has been shown to elevate IGF-1, free IGF-1, and IGFBP-3 levels.[73, 74] Besides having a direct stimulatory effect on IGF-1 synthesis,[75] it has been shown that GH may have a direct stimulatory function on IGFBP-3 by enhancing its synthesis.[76]

Growth hormone stimulates osteoblasts in vitro[77] and increases osteoblast activity in vivo as determined by serum markers of osteoblast activities.[78, 79, 80] GH increases bone formation both via a direct interaction with GH receptors located on osteoblasts and via locally produced IGF-1 (autocrine/paracrine action).[81, 82] As a result, individuals with GH-deficient states have been shown to have a reduction in osteoblast activities that often results in low BMD and osteoporosis.[83]

Corticosteroid administration and hypercortisolemia have been shown to significantly inhibit the GHRH-GH-IGF-IGFBP axis by blunting the GH response to GHRH and GHRH analogues.[84] A blunted GH response to GHRH has also been shown to decrease circulating levels of insulin-like growth factor-1 (IGF-1), insulin-like-growth-factor binding protein-3 (IGFBP-3) levels, and free bioavailable IGF-1.[85,86] In vitro studies have shown that corticosteroids decrease IGF-1 synthesis[87] and expression[88] which is reflected in decreased IGF-1 mRNA activities.[89]

It has been suggested that various cytokines, such as IL-6, may play a role in osteoblast stimulation.[90] In vitro examination of corticosteroid effects on osteoblast cytokine synthesis has shown that osteoblast-stimulating cytokines are reduced and their resultant activities, reflected by reduced mRNA levels, are blunted.[91]

Increased Bone Resorption

Corticosteroid therapy increases bone resorption by five or more mechanisms. First, it can cause hypoestrogenemia by blunting the LH release from LHRH stimulation. Estrogens have been shown to be inhibitors of osteoclast activity. Low estrogen levels can reduce the inhibition of the bone dissolving osteoclasts. Second, corticosteroids and estrogenic steroids compete for osteoclast receptor sites, and corticosteroid binding to osteoclasts stimulates bone resorption. Third, corticosteroid therapy induces an increase of SHBG that subsequently reduces free estrogenic and androgenic steroid levels thereby reducing the levels of sex steroid bioavailability. Fourth, it can induce a secondary hyperparathyroidism that further stimulates osteoclasts resulting in increased bone resorption.[92, 93] Finally, corticosteroid therapy can cause hypoandrogenemia that results in reduced inhibition of proresorptive cytokines which results in accelerated bone resorption.[94]

Altered Calcium Metabolism

Corticosteroid therapy has been shown to alter calcium homeostasis by two mechanisms.[95, 96] First, corticosteroids decrease the calcium and phosphate absorption from the small intestine thereby reducing the efficiency of calcium absorption from the diet or from calcium supplementation.[97, 98] Second, corticosteroid therapy affects renal function by increasing the urinary excretion of calcium by decreasing renal tubular resorption of calcium.[99] These two effects cause a negative calcium balance that causes the secretion of parathyroid hormone (PTH) and induces secondary hyperparathyroidism that results in osteoclast activation.[100] It has been shown that approximately 30 percent of patients treated with prolonged corticosteroid therapy develop secondary hyperparathyroidism resulting in hypercalcuria.[101]

Altered Bone Architecture

Studies of bone biopsies taken from patients treated with prolonged corticosteroid therapy and examined by histological methods have shown that that BMD losses are greater in the trabecular bone regions when compared to other types of osteoporosis.[102] This means that for any clinically measured decrease in bone mineral density, there is a greater risk for fracture with CST-induced osteoporosis than with osteoporosis from other causes.

In summary, with all of the aforementioned mechanisms presented, it is readily apparent that CST-induced osteoporosis can be the most dangerous and "brittle" type of osteoporosis. The first symptom that a patient may have with CST-induced osteoporosis is a nontraumatic vertebral or rib fracture that may result in chronic pain. Unlike with postmenopausal osteoporosis, where lumbar spine fractures are more common, the usual fractures with CST-induced osteoporosis are more common in the thoracic spine, ribs, distal forearm, and femur.[103, 104]

Studies with Anabolic Therapy for CST-Induced Osteoporosis

Perhaps the best mode of pharmacologic prevention and treatment of CST-induced osteoporosis has been known for many years. Androgen therapy for patients of both genders with CST-induced osteoporosis has been used empirically for several decades, as well as for all other types of osteoporosis. However, some of the early studies that reported the beneficial use of androgen therapy for osteoporosis did not distinguish between CST-induced osteoporosis and other types, including postmenopausal osteoporosis. As anabolic steroids were added to the list of available androgens for clinical use in the late 1950s, a study was published that indicated that androgen therapy was an effective treatment for preventing and reversing the catabolic bone effects induced by prolonged and concurrent corticosteroid therapy in men and women patients with rheumatoid arthritis.[105] By 1963, over a dozen androgens and/or anabolic steroids had been approved by the FDA for clinical use.[106]

During the 1960s and early 1970s, several major medical textbooks recommended androgen therapy for HRT in women and for osteoporosis treatment in both men and women, including CST-induced osteoporosis. The following quotations illustrate these recommendations.

"In menopausal women estrogen-androgen combination improves physical, mental, and emotional status."— Parsons and Sommers, *Gynecology* (1962).[107]

"Endocrine therapy consists of administration of estrogen or estrogen plus androgen."— Williams, *Textbook of Endocrinology* (1962).[108]

For CST-induced osteoporosis "androgens or estrogen-androgen combination is the therapy of choice."— Cecil-Loeb, *Textbook of Medicine* (1963).[109]

"The current consensus seems to be that androgens and their various anabolic steroids are useful in the treatment of osteoporosis. In women, estrogen given concurrently with small doses of androgen minimizes virilization."— Goodman and Gilman, *The Pharmacological Basis of Therapeutics* (1970).[110]

"Although several medical approaches to treatment are recommended for osteoporosis, the most unanimously endorsed, as well as the most definitive, is the use of anabolic steroids."— Krusen, *Physical Medicine and Rehabilitation* (1971).[111]

These recommendations from several major medical textbooks were echoed by the information contained in the *Physician's Desk Reference (PDR)* and the package inserts for these steroids, approved by the U.S. Food and Drug Administration (FDA), regarding androgen therapy for osteoporosis, such as: "anabolic steroids are indicated for osteoporosis from corticosteroid therapy"[112] and "anabolic steroids are probably effective for postmenopausal and senile osteoporosis."[113, 114] However, in 1984, the FDA removed the osteoporosis indication from the *PDR* and package insert materials during a federal mandate to "clean up" the approved indications for a number of prescription drugs. Accompanying the FDA action was the enactment of generic drug laws that discouraged pharmaceutical companies from reapplying for previously FDA-approved indications. These two federal actions influenced the responses of the pharmaceutical industry and *resulted in no reapplications for the osteoporosis indication for androgens being submitted to the FDA.*

The result of the FDA's decision to withdraw the osteoporosis indication for androgens was that physicians who were prescribing androgens for CST-induced osteoporosis were essentially left with no other effective medication to prevent and reverse the BMD losses associated with corticosteroid therapy. In a letter to the editor, published in the *New England Journal of Medicine*, a prominent physician stated:

"The recent decision of the FDA to withdraw approval for the use of anabolic steroids in treating osteoporosis appears counterproductive and unjustified by the available research."[115] Questions remain as to why the

FDA removed the osteoporosis indication for androgens from the package inserts and *PDR*.

The FDA's decision was made several years prior to the development of DEXA, serum bone markers for bone activities, updated bone histomorphometric, bioassay, immunochemical, and cell receptor techniques that have now been utilized to prove many of the mechanisms that androgen therapy has on bone formation and homeostasis. These technical advancements have provided for a renewed interest in androgen therapy for CST-induced osteoporosis, and "anabolic steroids have recently made a comeback."[116] This "comeback" has primarily occurred in the international medical science community minus the United States.

Physicians in the United States have been slow to utilize anabolic therapies for CST-induced osteoporosis and other catabolic, disabling diseases.[117] A number of barriers have recently been identified, including inadequate training of physicians, poor coordination between medical specialties, improper and prevailing physician attitudes, third-party reimbursement practices, concerns regarding "off-label" use of prescription medications, and others.[118, 119] In the face of this poor record of utilization in the U.S., use of anabolic agents may decrease catabolic states, promote and accelerate the recovery, shorten hospital stay, and reduce the convalescence time of disabling diseases and conditions.[120]

Recently, several authors have recommended the use of androgen therapy for the prevention and reversal of CST-induced osteoporosis,[121, 122, 123, 124, 125, 126] especially for patients who have hypoandrogenemia,[127, 128, 129] who have had osteoporotic fractures or have ongoing BMD losses,[130, 131] or who have not responded to other pharmacologic or therapeutic modalities.[132] Androgen therapy has been shown to reverse BMD deficits and other catabolic influences associated with corticosteroid therapy.[133, 134, 135, 136, 137]

It has been concluded that, to prevent CST-induced osteoporosis and its dramatic complications, the therapeutic challenge is to preserve functional capacity while using the lowest possible dosage of corticosteroids.[138] Androgen therapy has been shown to reduce corticosteroid requirements and assist in corticosteroid tapering for patients undergoing prolonged or recurrent corticosteroid therapy for chronic illnesses.[139, 140, 141, 142, 143, 144, 145]

Other anabolic hormones and growth factors, which stimulate the GHRH-GH-IGF-IGFBP axis, may prove to be beneficial in preventing and reversing CST-induced osteoporosis.[146, 147] Growth hormone, GH secretagogues, and IGF-1 therapies have been shown to increase serum bone formation markers and BMD in elderly patients.[148, 149, 150, 151] Thus far, the results from these studies have not been extrapolated to indicate the specific use for the prevention and reversal of CST-induced osteoporosis.

Summary

This extensive discussion of CST-induced osteoporosis clearly indicates that androgen therapy should continue to play a predominant therapeutic role in the treatment of this condition. In the past, androgen therapy has been considered to be the *treatment of choice for CST-induced osteoporosis* and should continue to be recognized in this manner. However, recent surveys have indicated that androgen therapy has been significantly underutilized in the prevention and treatment of CST-induced osteoporosis. Recent surveys have also indicated that more than 50 percent of the patients undergoing prolonged or recurrent cyclical therapy with corticosteroids are not receiving diagnostic, preventive, or appropriate therapy for CST-induced osteoporosis.[152, 153]

Androgen therapy has been shown to prevent and reverse BMD losses and other catabolic losses by several mechanisms, including:

(1) the correction of hypoandrogenemia (gonadal or adrenal) that can be induced by or be associated with corticosteroid therapy.

(2) the correction of hyposomatomedinemia that can be induced by or be associated with corticosteroid therapy. Androgen therapy has been shown to stimulate an increase in GH secretion by directly enhancing GHRH pulse amplitudes. Androgen therapy also increases serum levels of IGF-1, free IGF-1, and IGFBP-3, and stimulates bone tissue IGF-1 levels and activities.

(3) the restoration of BMD, normal bone mass, and normal bone morphology with increased osteoblast stimulation that continues for a period of time after androgen therapy cessation.

(4) the direct stimulation of osteoblast activity and by the direct competitive and antagonistic (with corticosteroids) binding to osteoblast receptor sites.

(5) the inhibition of osteoclast activity by modulating proresorptive cytokines.

(6) the correction of CST-induced elevations in SHBG which results in increased free serum androgen levels.

(7) the reduction of the corticosteroid requirements for patients who are undergoing corticosteroid therapy.

(8) the assistance in corticosteroid tapering regimens which reduces the signs and symptoms of corticosteroid withdrawal.

(9) the prevention and reversal of other CST-induced catabolic effects, such as sarcopenia and losses of neuromuscular strength.

Androgen therapy should be considered as a routine therapeutic choice for all patients with CST-induced osteoporosis. This includes patients with autoimmune diseases, spinal cord injury, neuromuscular diseases, chronic asthmatic conditions, and others who are treated with high-dose, prolonged, or repetitive cyclical regimens of corticosteroids. With adrogen therapy, rehabilitation outcomes with androgen therapy are likely to be improved for patients with these conditions.

Notes

1. Johnson, B.E., B. Lucasey, R.G. Robinson, et al. Contributing diagnosis in osteoporosis. The value of a complete medical evaluation. *Arch. Intern. Med.* 1989; 149: 1069–1072.

2. Laan, R.F., W.C. Bujis, L.J. Erning, et al. Differential effects of glucocorticoids on the cortical and appendicular and cortical vertebral bone mineral content. *Calcif. Tissue Int.* 1993; 52: 5–9.

3. Khosla, S., E.G., S.F. Lufkin, S.F. Hodgston, et al. Epidemiology and clinical features of osteoporosis in young individuals. *Bone* 1994; 15: 551–555.

4. Lukert, B.P. Glucocorticoid-induced osteoporosis. *Southern Med. J.* 1992; 85: 2548–2551.

5. Bonala, S.B., B.M. Reddy, and B.A. Silverman. Bone mineral density in women with asthma on long-term inhaled corticosteroid therapy. *Ann. Allergy Asthma Immunol.* 2000; 85 (6): 494–500.

6. Walsh, L.J., C.A. Wong, M. Pringle, et al. Use of oral corticosteroids in the community and the prevention of secondary osteoporosis; a cross sectional study. *Brit. Med. J.* 1996; 313: 344–346.

7. Adachi, J.D., Bensen, W.G., and A.B. Hodsman. Corticosteroid-induced osteoporosis. *Semin. Arthritis Rheum.* 1993; 22 (6): 375–384.

8. Peat, I.D., S. Healy, D.M. Reid, et al. Steroid induced osteoporosis: an opportunity for prevention? *Ann. Rheum. Dis.* 1995; 54: 66–68.

9. Bell, R., A. Carr, and P. Thompson. Managing corticosteroid induced osteoporosis in medical outpatients. *J. Royal Coll. Physicians Lond.* 1997; 31: 158–161.

10. Buckley, L.M., M. Marquez, R. Feezor, et al. Prevention of corticosteroid-induced osteoporosis: results of a patient survey. *Arthritis Rheum.* 1999; 42 (8): 1736–1739.

11. Hougardy, D.M., G.M, M.D. Bleasel, et al. Is enough attention being given to the adverse effects of corticosteroid therapy? *J. Clin. Pharm. Ther.* 2000; 25 (3): 227–234.

12. Swerdloff, R.S., and C. Wang. Androgen deficiency and aging in men. *West. J. Med.* 1993; 159 (5): 579–585.

13. Miklos, S. Dehydroepiandrosterone sulfate in the diagnosis of osteoporosis. *Acta Biomed. Ateneo Parmense.* 1995; 66 (3–4): 139–146.

14. Longcope, C. Androgen metabolism and the menopause. *Semin. Reprod. Endocrinol.* 1998; 16 (2): 111–115.

15. De Lorenzo, A., S. Lello, A. Andreoli, et al. Body composition and androgen pattern in early period of postmenopause. *Gyencol. Endocrinol.* 1998; 12 (3): 171–177.

16. Lund, B.C., K.A. Bever-Stille, and P.J. Perry. Testosterone and andropause: the feasibility of testosterone replacement therapy in elderly men. *Pharmacotherapy* 1999; 19 (8): 951–956.

17. Ravaglia, G., P. Forti, F. Maioli, et al. Body composition, sex steroids, IGF-1,

and bone mineral status in aging men. *J. Gerontol. A. Biol. Sci. Med. Sci.* 2000; 55 (9): M516–521.

18. Adami, S., and M. Rossini. Anabolic steroids in corticosteroid-induced osteoporosis. *Wien. Med. Wochenschr.* 1993; 143 (15–15): 395–397.

19. Olbricht, T., and G. Benker. Glucocorticoid-induced osteoporosis: pathogenesis, prevention and treatment, with special regard to the rheumatic diseases. *J. Intern. Med.* 1993; 234 (3): 237–244.

20. Geusens, P. Nandrolone decanoate: pharmacological properties and therapeutic use in osteoporosis. *Clin. Rheumatol.* 1995; 14 (Suppl. 3): 32–39.

21. Adachi, J.D., W.G. Bensen, and A.B. Hodsman. Corticosteroid-induced osteoporosis. *Semin. Arthritis Rheum.* 1993; 22 (6): 375–384.

22. Reid, I., D.J. Wattie, M.C. Evans, et al. Testosterone therapy in glucocorticoid-treated men. *Arch. Intern. Med.* 1996; 156 (11): 1173–1177.

23. LoCascio, V., E. Bonucci, B. Imhimbo, et al. Bone loss in response to long-term glucocorticoid therapy. *Bone. Miner.* 1990; 8: 39–51.

24. Reid, I.R., and A.B. Grey. Corticosteroid osteoporosis. *Baillieres Clin. Rheumatol.* 1993; 7: 573–587.

25. Zaqqa, D., and R.D. Jackson. Diagnosis and treatment of glucocorticoid-induced osteoporosis. *Cleveland Clin. J. Med.* 1999; 66 (4): 221–230.

26. Khosla, S. The effects of androgens on osteoblast function in vitro. *Mayo Clin. Proc.* 2000; 75 (Suppl): S51–54.

27. Gori, F., L.C. Hofbauer, C.A. Conover, et al. Effects of androgens on the insulin-like growth factor system in an androgen-responsive human osteoblastic cell line. *Endocrinology* 1999; 140 (12): 5579–5586.

28. Labrie, F., A. Belanger, V. Luu-The, et al. DHEA and the incracrine formation of androgens and estrogens in peripheral target tissues: its role during aging. *Steroids* 1998; 63 (5–6): 322–328.

29. Cosman, F., J. Nieves, C. Wilkinson, et al. Bone density change and biochemical indicies of skeletal turnover. *Calcif. Tissue Int.* 1996; 58 (4): 236–243.

30. Dresner-Pollak, R., R.A. Parker, M. Poku, et al. Biochemical markers of bone turnover reflect femoral bone loss in elderly women. *Calcif. Tissue Int.* 1996; 59 (5): 328–333.

31. Garnero, P., and P.D. Delmas. New developments in biochemical markers for osteoporosis. *Calc. Tissue Int.* 1996; 59 (7): 2–9.

32. Russell, R.G. The assessment of bone metabolism in vivo using biochemical approaches. *Horm. Metab. Res.* 1997; 29 (3): 138–144.

33. Ganero, P., and P.D. Delmas. Biochemical markers of bone turnover. Applications for osteoporosis. *Endocrinol. Metab. Clin. North Am.* 1998; 27 (2): 303–323.

34. Fink, E., C. Cormier, P. Steinmetz, et al. Differences in the capacity of several biochemical bone markers to assess high bone turnover in early menopause and response to alendronate therapy. *Osteoporos. Int.* 2000; 11 (4): 295–303.

35. Christenson, R.H. Biochemical markers of bone metabolism: an overview. *Clin. Biochem.* 2000; 30 (8): 573–593.

36. Adachi, J.D. The correlation of bone mineral density and biochemical markers to fracture risk. *Calcif. Tissue. Int.* 1996; 59 (7): 16–19.

37. Seibel, M.J., and H.W. Woitge. Basic principles and clinical applications of biochemical markers of bone metabolism: biochemical and technical aspects. *J. Clin. Densitom.* 1999; 2 (3): 299–321.

38. Hunter, D.J., and P.N. Sambrook. Bone loss: Epidemiology of bone loss. *Arthritis Res.* 2000; 2 (6): 441–445.

39. Couch, M., F.E. Preston, R.G. Malia, et al. Changes in plasma osteocalcin

concentrations following treatment with stanozolol. *Clin. Chim. Acta* 1986; 158: 43–47.

40. Adami, S., V. Fossaluzza, R. Suppi, et al. The low osteocalcin levels of glucocorticoid-treated patients can be brought to normal by nandrolone decanoate administration. In C. Christiansen, J.S. Johansen, and B.J. Riss, eds. *Osteoporosis 1987.* Copenhagen: Osteopress ApS., pp. 1039–1049,1987.

41. Vaishnav, R., J.N. Beresford, J.A. Gallagher, et al. Effects of the anabolic steroid stanozolol on cells derived from human bone. *Clin. Sci.* 1988; 74: 455–460.

42. Beneton, M.N.C., A.J.P. Yates, S. Rogers, et al. Stanozolol stimulates remodeling of trabecular bone and net formation of bone at the endocortical surface. *Clin. Sci.* 1991; 81: 543–549.

43. Chappard, D., E. Legrand, M.F. Basle, et al. Altered trabecular architecture induced by corticosteroids: a bone histomorphometric study. *J. Bone Miner. Res.* 1996; 11: 676–685.

44. Bland, R. Steroid hormone receptor expression and action in bone. *Clin. Sci. (Colch.)* 2000; 98 (2): 217–240.

45. Ziegler, R., and C. Kasperk. Glucocorticoid-induced osteoporosis: prevention and treatment. *Steroids* 1998; 63 (5–6)344–348.

46. Delany, A.M., Y. Dong, and E. Canalis. Mechanisms of glucocorticoid action in bone cells. *J. Cell. Bichem.* 1994; 56: 295–302.

47. Angeli, R.G., Masera, M.L. Sartori, et al. Modulation by cytokines of glucocorticoid action. *Ann. N.Y. Acad. Sci.* 1999; 876: 210–220.

48. Ziegler, R., and C. Kasperk. Glucocorticoid-induced osteoporosis: prevention and treatment. *Steroids* 1998; 63 (5–6): 344–348.

49. Lane, N.E., and B. Lukert. The science and therapy of glucocorticoid-induced bone loss. *Endocrinol. Metab. Clin. North Am.* 1998; 27 (2): 465–483.

50. Chrousos, G.P. The role of stress and the hypothalamic-pituitary-adrenal axis in the pathogenesis of the metabolic syndrome: neuroendocrine and target tissue-related causes. *Int. J. Obes. Relat. Metab. Disord.* 2000; 24 (Suppl. 2): S50–55.

51. Reid, I.R. Glucocorticoid osteoporosis— mechanisms and management. *Eur. J. Endocrinol.* 1997; 137 (3): 209–217.

52. Pearce, G., D.A. Tabensky, P.D. Delmas, et al. Corticosteroid-induced bone loss in men. *J. Clin. Endocrinol. Metab.* 1998; 83 (3): 801–806.

53. Scane, A.C., R.M. Francis, A.M. Sutcliffe, et al. Case-controlled study of the pathogenesis and sequelae of symptomatic vertebral fractures in men. *Osteoporos. Int.* 1999; 9 (1): 91–97.

54. Yen, S.S., and G.A. Laughlin. Aging and the adrenal cortex. *Exp. Gerontol.* 1998; 33 (7–8): 897–910.

55. Harper, A.J., J.E. Buster, and P.R. Casson. Changes in adrenocortical function with aging and therapeutic implications. *Semin. Reprod. Endocrinol.* 1999; 17 (4): 327–338.

56. Phillips, G.B. Relationship between serum dehydroepiandrosterone sulfate, androstenedione, and sex hormones in men and women. *Eur. J. Endocrinol.* 1999; 134 (2): 201–206.

57. Spratt, D.I., C. Longcope, P.M. Cox, et al. Differential changes in serum concentrations of androgens and estrogens (in relation to cortisol) in postmenopausal women with acute illness. *J. Clin. Endocrinol. Metab.* 1993; 76 (6): 1542–1547.

58. Castelo-Branco, C., E. Caslas, F. Figeruas, et al. Two-year prospective and comparative study on the effects of tibolone on lipid pattern, behavior of apolipoprotein A1 and B. *Menopause* 1999; 6 (2): 92–97.

59. Casson, P.R., K.E. Elkind, J.E. Buster, et al. Effect of postmenopausal

estrogen replacement on circulating androgens. *Obstet. Gynecol.* 1997; 90 (6): 995–998.

60. Simon, J., E. Klaiber, B. Witta, et al. Differential effects of estrogen-androgen and estrogen-only therapy on vasomotor symptoms, gonadotrophin secretion, and endogenous androgen bioavailability in postmenopausal women. *Menopause* 1999; 6 (2): 138–146.

61. Phillips, G.B. Relationship between serum dehydroepiandrosterone sulfate, androstenedione, and sex hormones in men and women. *Eur. J. Endocrinol.* 1996; 134 (2): 201–206.

62. Phillips, G.B. Relationship between serum dehydroepiandrosterone sulfate, androstenedione, and sex hormones in men and women. *Eur. J. Endocrinol.* 1996; 134 (2): 201–206.

63. Eakman, G.D., J.S. Dallas, S.W. Ponder, et al. The effects of testosterone and dihydrotestosterone on hypothalamic regulation of growth hormone secretion. *J. Clin. Endocrinol. Metab.* 1996; 81 (3): 1217–1223.

64. Genazzani, A.D., O. Gamba, L. Nappi, et al. Modulatory effects of a synthetic steroid (tibolone) and estradiol on spontaneous and GHRH-induced GH secretion in postmenopausal women. *Maturitas* 1997; 28 (1): 27–33.

65. Hobbs, C.J., S.R. Plymate, C.J. Rosen, et al. Testosterone administration and insulin-like growth factor-1 levels in normal men. *J. Clin. Endocrinol. Metab.* 1994; 78 (6): 1360–1367.

66. Morales, A.J., J.J. Nolan, J.C. Nelson, et al. Effects of replacement dose of dehydroepiandrosterone in men and women of advancing age. *J. Clin. Endocrinol. Metab.* 1994; 78 (6): 1360–1367.

67. Gelato, M.C., and R.A. Frost. IGFBP-3. Functional and structural implications in aging and wasting syndromes. *Endocrine* 1997; 7 (1): 81–85.

68. Casson, P.R., N. Santoro, K. Elkind-Hirsch, et al. Postmenopausal dehydroepiandrosterone administration increases free insulin-like growth factor-1 and decreases high-density lipoprotein: a six month trial. *Fertil. Steril.* 1998; 70 (1): 107–110.

69. Jorgensen, J.O., N. Vahl, T.B. Hansen, et al. Determinants of serum insulin-like growth factor 1 in growth hormone deficient adults as compared to healthy subjects. *Clin. Endocrinol.* 1998; *(Oxf.)* 48 (4): 479–486.

70. Morales, A.J., R.H. Haubrich, J.Y. Hwang, et al. The effects of six months treatment with 100mg daily dose of dehydroepiandrosterone (DHEA) on circulating sex steroids, body composition, and muscle strength in age-advanced men and women. *Clin. Endocrinol. (Oxf.)* 1998; 49 (4): 421–434.

71. Span, J.P., G.F. Pieters, C.G. Sweep, et al. Gender difference in insulin-like growth factor 1 response to growth hormone (GH) treatment and GH-deficient adults: role of sex hormone replacement. *J. Clin. Endocrinol. Metab.* 2000; 85 (3): 1121–1125.

72. Savine, R., and P. Sonksen. Growth hormone — hormone replacement for somatopause? *Horm. Res.* 2000; 53 (Suppl. S3): 37–41.

73. Ovesen, P., J. Moller, J.O. Jorgensen, et al. Effect of growth hormone administration on circulating levels of luteinizing hormone, follicle stimulating hormone and testosterone in normal healthy men. *Hum. Reprod.* 1993; 8 (11): 1869–1872.

74. Lee, P.D., S.K. Durham, V. Martinez, et al. Kinetics of insulin-like growth factor (IGF) and IGF-binding protein responses to a single dose of growth hormone. *J. Clin. Endocrinol. Metab.* 1997; 82 (7): 2266–2274.

75. Cuttica, C.M., L. Castoldi, G.P. Gorrini, et al. Effects of six-month administration of recombinant human growth hormone to healthy elderly subjects. *Aging (Milano)* 1997; 9 (3): 193–197.

76. Lemmey, A.B., J. Glassford, H.C. Flick-Smith, et al. Different regulation of

tissue insulin-like growth factor-binding protein (IGFBP)-3, IGF-1, and IGF type 1 receptor mRNA levels, and serum IGF-1 and IGFBP concentrations by growth hormone and IGF-1. *J. Endocrinol.* 1997; 154 (2): 319–328.

77. Nilsson, A., D. Swolin, S. Enerback, et al. Expression of functional growth hormone receptors in cultured human osteoblast-like cells. *J. Clin. Endocrinol. Metab.* 1995; 80 (12): 3483–3488.

78. Ghiron, L.J., J.L. Thompson, L. Holloway, et al. Effects of recombinant insulin-like growth factor-1 and growth hormone on bone turnover in elderly women. *J. Bone Miner. Res.* 1995; 10 (12): 1844–1852.

79. Baum, H.B., B.M. Miller, J.S. Finkelstein, et al. Effects of physiologic growth hormone therapy on bone density and body composition in patients with adult-onset growth hormone deficiency. A randomized, placebo-controlled trial. *Ann. Intern. Med.* 1996; 125 (11): 883–890.

80. Murphy, M.G., M.A. Bach, D. Plotkin, et al. Oral administration of the growth hormone secretagogue MK-677 increases markers of bone turnover in healthy and functionally impaired elderly adults. The MK-677 Study Group. *J. Bone Miner. Res.* 1999; 14 (7): 1182–1188.

81. Johansson, A.G., E. Lindh, W.F. Blum, et al. Effects of growth hormone and insulin-like growth factor 1 in men with idiopathic osteoporosis. *J. Clin. Endocrinol. Metab.* 1996; 81 (1): 44–48.

82. Isaksson, O.C., C. Ohlsson, B.A. Bengtsson, et al. GH and bone; experimental and clinical studies. *Endocr. J.* 2000; 47 (Suppl.): S9–16.

83. Ohlsson, C., J.O. Jansson, and O. Isaksson. Effects of growth hormone and insulin-like growth factor-1 on body growth and adult bone metabolism. *Curr. Opin. Rheumatol.* 2000; 12 (4): 246–348.

84. Borges, M.H., F.B. DiNinno, and A.M. Lengyel. Different effects of growth hormone releasing peptide (GHRP-6) and GH-releasing hormone on GH release in endogenous and exogenous hypercortisolism. *Clin. Endocrinol. (Oxf.)* 1997; 46 (6): 713–718.

85. Pereira, R.C., F. Blanquaert, and E. Canalis. Cortisol enhances the expression of mac25/insulin-like growth factor-binding protein-related protein-1 in cultured osteoblasts. *Endocrinology* 1999; 140 (1): 228–232.

86. Chrousos, G.P. The role of stress and the hypothalamic-pituitary-adrenal axis in the pathogenesis of the metabolic syndrome: neuroendocrine and target tissue-related causes. *Int. J. Obes. Relat. Metab. Discord.* 2000; 24 (Suppl. 2): S50–55.

87. Skrtic, S., and C. Ohlsson. Cortisol decreases hepatocyte growth factor levels in human osteoblast-like cells. *Calcific. Tissue Int.* 2000; 66 (2): 108–102.

88. McCarthy, T.L., C. Ji, Y. Chen, et al. Time- and dose-related interactions between glucocorticoid and cyclic adenosine 3', 5'-monophosphate on CCAAT/enhancer-binding protein-dependent insulin-like growth factor 1 expression by osteoblasts. *Endocrinology* 2000; 141 (1): 127–137.

89. Swolin, D., C. Brantsing, C. Matejka, et al. Cortisol decreases IGF-1 mRNA levels in human osteoblast cells. *J. Endocrinol.* 1996; 146: 397–403.

90. Angeli, A., R.G. Masera, M.L. Sartori, et al. Modulation of cytokines of glucocorticoid action. *Ann. N.Y. Acad. Sci.* 1999; 876: 210–220.

91. Swolin-Eide, D., and C. Ohlsson. Effects of cortisol on the expression of interleukin-6 and interleukin-1 beta in human osteoblast-like cells. *J. Endocrinol.* 1998; 156 (1): 107–114.

92. Suzuki, Y., Y. Ichikawa, E. Saito, et al. Importance of increased urinary calcium excretion in the development of secondary hyperparathyroidism of patients undergoing glucocorticoid therapy. *Metabolism* 1983; 32: 151–156.

93. Cosman, F., J. Nieves, J. Herbert, et al. High dose glucocorticoids in multiple sclerosis patients exert different effects on the kidney and skeleton. *J. Bone Miner. Res.* 1994; 9: 1097–1105.

94. Gordon, C.M., J. Glowacki, and M.S. LeBoff. DHEA and the skeleton (through the ages). *Endocrine* 1999; 11 (1): 1–11.

95. Lane, N.E., and B. Lukert. The science and therapy of glucocorticoid-induced bone loss. *Endocrinol. Metab. Clin. North Am.* 1998; 27 (2): 465–483.

96. Lems, W.F., J.W. Jacobs, J.C. Netelenbos, et al. [Pharmacological prevention of osteoporosis in patients on corticosteroid medication.] *Ned. Tijdschr. Geneeskd.* 1998; 142 (34): 1904–1908.

97. Gennari, C. Differential effects of glucocorticoids on calcium absorption on bone mass. *Br. J. Rheumatol.* 1993; 32 (Suppl. 2): 11–14.

98. Tomita, A. [Glucocorticoid-induced osteoporosis— mechanisms and preventions.] *Nippon Rinsho* 1998; 56 (6): 1574–1578.

99. Reid, I.R., and H.K. Ibbertson. Evidence of decreased tubular resorption of calcium in glucocorticoid-treated patients. *Horm. Res.* 1987; 27: 200–204.

100. Ziegler, R., and C. Kasperk. Glucocorticoid-induced osteoporosis: prevention and treatment. *Steroids* 1998; 63 (5–6): 344–348.

101. Brandli, D.W., G. Golde, M. Greenwald, et al. Corticosteroid-induced osteoporosis: a cross-sectional study. *Steroids* 1991; 56: 518–523.

102. Chappard, D., E. Legrand, M.F. Basle, et al. Altered trabecular architecture induced by corticosteroids: a bone histomorphometric study. *J. Bone Miner. Res.* 1996; 11: 676–685.

103. Erlichman, N., and T.V. Holohan. Bone densitometry: patients receiving prolonged steroid therapy. *Health Technol. Assess.* 1996; 9: 1–31.

104. Lukert, B.P., and L.G. Raisz. Glucocorticoid-induced osteoporosis: pathogenesis and management. *Ann. Intern. Med.* 1990; 112: 352–364.

105. Brochner-Mortensen, K., S. Gjorup, and J.H. Thaysen. The metabolic effect of new anabolic 19–nor-steroids: Metabolic studies on patients with chronic rheumatoid arthritis during combined therapy with Prednisone and anabolic steroid. *Act. Med. Scand.* 1959; 165 (3): 197–205.

106. Fruehan, A.E., and T.F. Frawley. Current status of anabolic steroids. *JAMA* 1963; 184 (7): 527–532.

107. Parsons, L., and S.C. Sommers. *Gynecology.* Philadelphia and London: W.B. Saunders Company, 1962, p. 1056.

108. Williams, R.H. *Textbook of Endocrinology.* Philadelphia and London: W.B. Saunders Company, 1962, p. 500.

109. Beeson, P.B., and W. McDermott. *Textbook of Medicine.* Philadelphia and London: W.B. Saunders Company, 1963, p. 1501.

110. Goodman, L.S., and A. Gilman. *The Pharmacological Basis of Therapeutics.* Toronto and London: The Macmillan Company, 1970, p. 1576.

111. Krusen, F.H. *Physical Medicine and Rehabilitation.* Philadelphia, London, and Toronto: W.B. Saunders Company, 1971, p. 563.

112. Revised package insert for Winstrol (stanozolol), Winthrop Laboratories, New York, 1965.

113. Revised package insert for Dianabol (methandrostendione), Ciba Laboratories, New York, 1980

114. Revised package insert for Winstrol (stanozolol), Winthrop Laboratories, New York, 1971.

115. Woodward, D. Treating of osteoporosis (letter). *N. Engl. J. Med.* 1984; 312 (10): 647.

116. Lockefeer, J.H. [Revision consensus osteoporosis.] *Ned. Tijdschr. Geneeskd.* 1992; 136 (25): 1204–1209.

117. Wilmore, D.H. Deterrents to the successful clinical use of growth factors that enhance protein anabolism. *Curr. Opin. Clin. Nutr. Metab. Care* 1999; 2 (1): 15–21.

118. Wilmore, D.H. Impediments to the successful use of anabolic agents in clinical care. *J. Parenter. Enteral Nutr.* 1999; 23 (6 Suppl.): S210–213.

119. Pollock, A.S., L. Legg, P. Langehorne, et al. Barriers to achieving evidence-based stroke rehabilitation. *Clin. Rehabil.* 2000; 14 (6): 611–617.

120. Garcia de Lorenzo, A., and J.M. Culebras. [Hormones, growth factors, and drugs in metabolism and nutrition.]. *Nutr. Hosp.* 1995; 10 (5): 297–305.

121. Adami, S., and M. Rossini. Anabolic steroids in corticosteroid-induced osteoporosis. *Wein. Med. Wochenschr.* 1993; 143 (14–15): 395–397.

122. Geusens, P. Nandrolone decanoate: pharmacological properties and therapeutic use in osteoporosis. *Clin. Rheumatol.* 1995; 14 (Suppl. 3): 32–39.

123. Bijlisma, J.W. Can we use steroid hormones to immunomodulate rheumatic diseases? Rheumatoid arthritis as an example. *Ann. N.Y. Acad. Sci.* 1999; 876: 366–376.

124. Khosla, S. The effects of androgens on osteoblast function in vitro. *Mayo Clin. Proc.* 2000; 75 (Suppl.): S51–54.

125. van Vollenhoven, R.F. Dehydroepiandrosterone in systemic lupus erythematosus. *Rheum. Dis. North. Am.* 2000; 26 (2): 349–362.

126. Cutolo, M. Sex hormone adjuvant therapy in rheumatoid arthritis. *Rheum. Dis. Clin. North Am.* 2000; 26 (4): 881–895.

127. Reid, I.R., D.J. Wattie, M.C. Evans, et al. Testosterone therapy in glucocorticoid-treated men. *Arch. Intern. Med.* 1996; 156 (11): 1173–1177.

128. Picado, C., and M. Luengo. Corticosteroid-induced bone loss. Prevention and management. *Drug Saf.* 1996; 15 (5): 347–359.

129. Reid, I.R. Glucocorticoid osteoporosis—mechanisms and management. *Eur. J. Endocrinol.* 1997; 137 (3): 209–217.

130. Adachi, J.D., W.G. Bensen, and A.B. Hodsman. Corticosteroid-induced osteoporosis. *Semin. Arthritis Rheum.* 1993; 22 (6): 375–384.

131. Adachi, J.D., W.P. Olszynski, D.A. Hanley, et al. Management of corticosteroid-induced osteoporosis. *Semin. Arthritis Rheum.* 2000; 29 (4): 228–251.

132. Zappa, D, and D.J. Jackson. Diagnosis and treatment of glucocorticoid-induced osteoporosis. *Cleveland Clin. J. Med.* 1999; 66 (4): 221–230.

133. Adami, S., and M. Rossini. Anabolic steroids in corticosteroid-induced osteoporosis. *Wien Med. Wochenschr.* 1993; 143 (14–15): 395–397.

134. Geusens, P. Nandrolone decanoate: pharmacologic properties and therapeutic use in osteoporosis. *Clin. Rheumatol.* 1995; 3: 32–39.

135. Reid, I.R., D.J. Wattie, M.C. Evans, et al. Testosterone therapy in glucocorticoid-treated men. *Arch. Intern. Med.* 1996; 156 (11): 1173–1177.

136. Hamdy, R.C., S.W. Moore, K.E. Whalen, et al. Nandrolone decanoate for men with osteoporosis. *Am. J. Ther.* 1998; 5 (2): 89–95.

137. van Vollenhoven, R.F., J.L. Park, M.C. Genovese, et al. A double-blind, placebo-controlled, clinical trial of dehydroepiandrosterone in severe systemic lupus erythematosus. *Lupus* 1999; 8 (3): 181–187.

138. Sinigaglia, L., A. Nervetti, Q. Mela, et al. A multicenter cross sectional study on bone mineral density in rheumatoid arthritis. Italian Study Group on Bone Mass in Rheumatoid Arthritis. *J. Rheumatol.* 2000; 27 (11): 2582–2589.

139. Morley, K.D., A. Parke, G.R.V. Hughes. Systemic lupus erythematosus: two patients treated with danazol. *Br. Med. J.* 1982; 284: 1431–1432.

140. van Vollenhoven, R.F., E.G. Engleman, and J. L. McGuire. An open study

of dehydroepiandrosterone in systemic lupus erythematosus. *Arthritis Rheum.* 1994; 37 (9): 1305–1310.

141. van Vollenhoven, R.F., E.G. Engleman, and J.L. McGuire. Dehydroepiandrosterone in systemic lupus erythematosus. Results of a double-blind, placebo-controlled, randomized clinical trial. *Arthritis Rheum.* 1995; 38 (12): 1826–1831.

142. van Vollenhoven, R.F., and J.L. McGuire. Studies of dehydroepiandrosterone (DHEA) as a therapeutic agent in systemic lupus erythematosus. *Ann. Med. Interne. (Paris)* 1996; 147 (4): 290–296.

143. Insiripong, S., T. Chanchairujira, and T. Bumpenboon. Danazol for thrombocytopenia in pregnancy with underlying systemic lupus erythematosus. *J. Med. Assoc. Thai.* 1996; 79 (5): 330–332.

144. Blanco, R., V.M. Martinez-Tamboada, V. Rodriguez-Valverde, et al. Successful therapy with danazol in refractory autoimmune thrombocytopenia associated with rheumatic diseases. *Br. J. Rheumatol.* 1997; 36 (10): 1095–1099.

145. van Vollenhoven, R.F., L.M. Morabito, E.G. Engelman, et al. Treatment of systemic lupus erythematosus with dehydroepiandrosterone: 50 patients treated up to 12 months. *J. Rheumatol.* 1998; 25 (2): 285–289.

146. Ferry, R.J., R.W. Cerri, and P. Cohen. Insulin-like growth factor binding proteins: new proteins, new functions. *Horm. Res.* 1999; 51 (2): 53–67.

147. Arvat, E., F. Broglio, and E. Ghigo. Insulin-like growth factor 1: implications in aging. *Drugs Aging.* 2000; 16 (1): 29–40.

148. Baum, H.B., B.M. Miller, J.S. Finkelstein, et al. Effects of physiologic growth hormone therapy on bone density and body composition in patients with adult-onset growth hormone deficiency. A randomized, placebo-controlled trial. *Ann. Intern. Med.* 1996; 125 (11): 883–890.

149. Johansson, A.G., E. Lindh, W.F. Blum, et al. Effects of growth hormone and insulin-like growth factor 1 in men with idiopathic osteoporosis. *J. Clin. Endocrinol. Metab.* 1996; 81 (1): 44–48.

150. Cuttia, C.M., L. Castoldi, G.P. Gorrini, et al. Effects of six-month administration of recombinant human growth hormone to healthy elderly adults. *Aging (Milano)* 1997; 9 (3): 193–197.

151. Murphy, M.G., M.A. Bach, D. Plotkin, et al. Oral administration of the growth hormone secretagogue MK-677 increases markers of bone turnover in healthy and functionally impaired elderly adults. The MK-677 Study Group. *J. Bone Miner. Res.* 1999; 14 (7): 1182–1188.

152. Buckley, L.M., M. Marquez, R. Feezor, et al. Prevention of corticosteroid-induced osteoporosis: results of a patient survey. *Arthritis Rheum.* 1999; 42 (8): 1736–1739.

153. Hougardy, D.M., G.M. Peterson, M.D. Bleasel, et al. Is enough attention being given to the adverse effects of corticosteroid therapy? *J. Clin. Pharm. Ther.* 2000; 25 (3): 227–234.

5

Rationale for Anabolic Therapy for Postmenopausal Osteoporosis and Hormone Replacement Therapy in Women

Introduction: Postmenopausal Androgen Deficiency and Underutilization of Androgen Therapy

Osteoporosis is the most common metabolic bone disease in the adult population and its prevalence rate will increase as our population grows older, unless the use of anabolic therapies become much more utilized. Despite the substantial amount of scientific, evidence-based material that has been accumulated over the past six decades on the efficacy of androgen therapy for osteoporosis, the clinical use of androgens remains markedly underutilized. The result of this phenomenon has been the osteoporosis epidemic, especially postmenopausal osteoporosis, in the United States.[1]

It has been shown that normal women become hypoandrogenic by three mechanisms that occur in phases associated with aging. These mechanisms and phases are:

(1) the perimenopausal phase that results in a progressive decrease in ovarian androgen production.[2, 3, 4]

(2) the menopausal phase that results in an abrupt and dramatic decrease in ovarian production of androgenic, estrogenic and progesterogenic steroids.[5]

(3) the postmenopausal phase that results in a progressive decrease

in adrenal androgen production and increased cortisol production that often results in an increased catabolic cortisol-androgen secretion ratios, especially in response to stress or disease conditions.[6, 7, 8, 9, 10]

These mechanisms and phases of decreased androgen production in women can result in *hypoandrogenemia and a concomitant hyposomatomedinemia* which are associated with the pathogenesis of reduced bone formation, accelerated loss of bone, and the development of postmenopausal osteoporosis.[11]

Statistics gathered on osteoporosis since 1995 and 1998 have indicated that[12, 13, 14]:

(1) osteoporosis affects nearly 30 million Americans, three-quarters of whom are postmenopausal women.

(2) over 1.5 million osteoporotic fractures occur annually.

(3) women older than 50 years have a 4 in 10 chance of incurring an osteoporosis-related fracture during their remaining lifetime.

(4) thirty percent of postmenopausal white women already have osteoporosis, and an additional 54 percent have low bone mineral density and may be developing osteoporosis.

(5) the cost of caring for patients with complications of osteoporosis exceeds $14 billion annually.

(6) one in five women who sustain a hip fracture and who do not die as an immediate consequence will require long-term nursing-home care while suffering a drastic decline in the quality of life, such as crippling pain, lasting disability, forced retirement, and permanent disfigurement.

(7) a woman's risk of an osteoporosis-related hip fracture is equal to her *combined* risk of developing breast, uterine and ovarian cancers.

The mechanisms by which the skeletal effects of sex steroids are mediated remain incompletely understood. However, in recent years there have been considerable advances in knowledge of how sex steroids, primarily estrogens and androgens, influence bone modeling and remodeling in health, aging, and disease conditions.[15] The development of osteoporosis depends on an individual's peak bone mass attained and bone mass loss after the peak. Estrogens and androgens have an impact on both of these processes.[16]

Many women, just before (perimenopause) and after menopause, may develop symptoms of androgen deficiency: unexplained fatigue, irregular menstrual periods, vasomotor symptoms, changes in mood and cognition, reduced sense of well-being, insomnia, and diminished libido.[17] In many cases, physicians do not recognize this constellation of symptoms as the well-accepted androgen deficiency.[18]

About a decade or so prior to actual menopause (perimenopause) a normal woman's ovaries may begin to diminish in their production of sex steroids. The class of sex steroids that diminishes earliest and most profoundly has been shown to be androgens, thus, the perimenopausal years have been called "andropause" by some authors. This relative androgen deficiency in perimenopausal women has been shown to manifest itself as impaired sexual function, reduced sense of well-being, loss of energy, and losses in BMD.[19, 20, 21] Since the absolute decline in androgen levels generally begins during the perimenopausal years, it is not surprising that many women experience these symptoms and conditions.[22] It has been shown that the perimenopause phenomenon differs from the sudden drop in estrogen and androgen levels that occurs during the menopausal transition.[23] If plasma levels of bioavailable testosterone are low, these symptoms have been shown to diminish by judicious androgen therapy. The addition of androgens to hormone replacement therapy (HRT) is becoming more widespread, and other uses include prevention and treatment of bone loss, treatment of spontaneous or iatrogenic androgen deficiency and the management of premenstrual syndrome.[24]

In postmenopausal women, the addition of androgens to HRT results in significant additional improvement in bone mineral density (BMD) compared to estrogen replacement alone. Accumulating evidence indicates that androgens play an important role in the health of bone; it also indicates the benefit of adding these agents to HRT.[25] Both historical data and evolving data support the use of estrogen-androgen replacement therapy in postmenopausal women.[26] Clinical studies have shown that estrogen-androgen replacement therapies prevent the development of osteoporosis, as determined by BMD determinations, bone marker analyses, and histomorphometric analyses of serial bone biopsies. Cross-sectional studies have shown that *bioavailable testosterone levels are a statistically significant, independent determinant of BMD in postmenopausal women.*[27] Addition of an androgen to HRT prevents bone loss and stimulates bone formation via a number of specific and systemic mechanisms.[28]

Androgen Deficiency Links Many Diseases in Postmenopausal Women

Androgens have some anabolic effect on virtually every tissue in the human body, and it is likely that adding androgens to HRT contributes to health maintenance in as yet undefined ways and that androgen deficiency in women may be responsible for significantly more morbidity and mortality than is currently known.[29] Androgen deficiency has become an increasingly well-recognized condition that is related to the pathogenesis of many diseases.

In postmenopausal women, hypoandrogenemia, and its associated hyposomatomedinemia, has been recently linked to many diseases and debilitating conditions including some conditions that have only recently become evident. For instance, postmenopausal women with osteoporosis without appropriate HRT have a greater incidence of adverse dental outcomes and significantly higher dental care costs than those on adequate HRT.[30] As a second example, recent studies have also correlated hypoandrogenemia in postmenopausal women with a significant increased risk for developing cognitive deficits, Alzheimer's disease, and senile dementia.[31, 32, 33] As a third example, recent studies have linked hypoandrogenemia and hyposomatomedinemia and related catabolic cytokine profiles with the pathogenesis of congestive heart failure (CHF) in postmenopausal women.[34, 35, 36] Correction of these catabolic conditions with anabolic hormones has been shown to improve cardiac function in both postmyocardial infarction and CHF patients by stimulating myocardial contractility, increasing ejection fraction, stroke volume, cardiac output, and promoting myocardial regeneration and remodeling.[37, 38]

Other recent studies have linked osteoporosis to several other diseases in women, including breast cancer, osteoarthritis, autoimmune diseases, rheumatic diseases, heart disease, stroke, heart attack, CHF, decreased pulmonary function, and others.[39] Several of these diseases are interrelated. For instance, low BMD and postmenopausal osteoporosis have been shown to be associated with a significantly increased risk for thromboembolic events.[40] A recent study has shown that postmenopausal women with BMD values in the lowest quartile have a greater risk (statistically significant) for incurring a first stroke.[41] Also, stroke patients have been shown to have a significantly increased risk for subsequent BMD loss and osteoporotic fractures.[42, 43, 44] A recent study has shown that stroke patients have a statistically significant four-fold increased risk of incurring an osteoporotic femoral neck fracture.[45] However, strokes do not cause postmenopausal osteoporosis, and postmenopausal osteoporosis does not cause strokes. However, stroke and postmenopausal osteoporosis share a common pathogenesis factor: androgen deficiency.

A growing body of evidence has shown that many diseases, including atherogenesis, some autoimmune diseases, rheumatic diseases, postmenopausal osteoporosis, some immunodeficiency wasting conditions, sarcopenia, accelerated aging, dementia, depression, and others are inextricably linked through a common pathogenesis or association: *androgen deficiency.* This is not such a surprising finding, since androgens provide the major anabolic stimulus throughout the body.

Barriers for Adequate Management of Postmenopausal Osteoporosis

Anabolic steroids (henceforth simply included with androgens as a class of steroids) were first developed in the 1950s to provide the anabolic advantages of androgens with less androgenic action. Throughout the following decades, androgens have been widely used in the treatment of osteoporosis, although their mechanisms of action have only recently been demonstrated with the advent of bone densitometry, serum bone markers, and advanced histological techniques.[46]

Despite the overwhelming evidence that has indicated that androgen therapy prevents and reverses losses in BMD, reduces fracture occurrence, and reduces the bone pain that accompanies osteoporotic states, there are barriers perceived by physicians and patients to both the diagnosis of osteoporosis and initiation of androgen therapy.[47] For instance, a recent study has shown that a substantial number of postmenopausal women patients with osteoporosis proven by DEXA received no therapy at all from their physicians.[48] Another recent study has shown that only 35 percent of women older than 50 years have had a documented osteoporosis risk assessment, and only 19 percent (of the 35 percent) of these women received an osteoporosis-related-specific intervention (such as calcium supplementation or counseling about HRT).[49] In a study published in December 2000, primary care providers providing health maintenance examinations for postmenopausal women were found to feel that osteoporosis is not as important an issue as tobacco smoking, cancer prevention, exercise, or diet.[50]

A major effort in curbing the osteoporosis epidemic and sarcopenia-induced frailty has been directed at attempts to deliver an anabolic stimulus to elderly adults on a mass scale.[51] This challenge (addressed by the National Institute on Aging) behooves physicians to create an improved dialogue between several areas of science and medicine and to utilize multidisciplinary approaches to make anabolic solutions available to patients.[52] American physicians have been slow to adopt the approach of prescribing anabolic agents in patients who have age-related or disease-related catabolic states that result in decreased musculoskeletal strength, bone mass, and activity levels.[53]

Adequate training and retraining of physicians and changes in the present approaches and attitudes in caring for patients may be the greatest obstacles to overcome if application of anabolic agents to patient care is to be realized.[54] Perceived barriers for initiation of anabolic agents in osteoporosis management include cost of therapy, patient or family reluctance to accept therapy, and time or expense involved with making the definitive diagnosis.[55]

Androgens have been shown to be safe, effective, currently available, and cost-effective in the anabolic treatment of postmenopausal osteoporosis. Also, it has been suggested that the use of anabolic agents can at the same time decrease loss of body proteins, muscle mass, and BMD as well as promote and accelerate recovery from disabling conditions, thereby shortening hospital stay and reducing rehabilitation and convalescence time.[56]

Androgen Therapy Mimics Ovarian Function

Androgen therapy for women patients began in the late 1930s.[57, 58] However, the concept of using estrogen-androgen cotherapy for postmenopausal women was pioneered in the early 1940s by Robert Greenblatt, M.D. at the Medical College of Georgia.[59, 60] Dr. Greenblatt, who was Boarded in both endocrinology and obstetrics and gynecology, published his views and results on the benefits of androgen therapy to women for five decades.[61, 62, 63, 64, 65, 66, 67, 68, 69, 70, 71, 72, 73, 74, 75, 76] A tribute to his pioneering, persistent, and influential work with androgen therapy for women has been published, as a memorial, by one of his many former residents and son-in-law, Anthony E. Karpas, M.D., an endocrinologist in Atlanta, GA.[77] In 1987, in one of Dr. Greenblatt's last publications published prior to his death, he stated:[78]

"Androgens are psychotropic drugs, participating in both physiologic and psychologic components of sexual behavior. They modulate the neurohumors of the brain and affect behavior. Androgens in nonvirilizing doses complement estrogens, are synergistic rather than contraphysiologic, and may be employed effectively by most women administered alone or in combination with an estrogen. The menopausal woman who has failed to experience the benefits of estrogen replacement should be offered a trial of estrogen-androgen combination. Androgens are helpful in many gynecologic and nongynecologic disorders. Their use has not been exploited fully."

It is well known that the functioning human ovaries synthesize three classes of sex steroids: androgenic, progesterogenic, and estrogenic steroids. When the ovaries are removed surgically, as with a total hysterectomy, or when the ovaries cease to produce sex steroids in adequate quantities, as in natural menopause, it makes sense to utilize a HRT regimen that includes some combination of these classes of ovarian sex steroids.[79, 80 81, 82]

It has been demonstrated that approximately 85 percent of circulating androgens are produced by the ovaries, with the remaining, smaller percentages secreted by the adrenal glands in normal premenopausal women.[83, 84] In normal ovulating women, the amount of androgens produced by the ovaries fluctuates according to the phases of the menstrual cycle.[85]

A transient elevation in androgen secretion, causing a transient hyperandrogenemia, occurs mainly in the early follicular phase of the menstrual cycle, in response to elevated levels of luteinizing hormone (LH).[86] This transient hyperandrogenemia has been shown to have an important regulatory role in bone formation and maintenance of normal BMD, as determined by serum osteoblast activity markers, in healthy eumenorrhoic women.[87, 88] Elevated serum androgen levels have been shown to correlate with increased BMD in women.[89]

It has been postulated that cyclical or periodic use of androgens, with estrogenic or progesterogenic steroid replacement, mimics normal, premenopausal ovarian function, and results in significant increases in BMD and lean body mass in postmenopausal women.[90] Furthermore, it has been suggested that, in the usual case of postmenopausal osteoporosis, the osteoblasts become somewhat dormant. Periodic stimulation of osteoblasts by androgen therapy may stimulate osteoblastic activities for a period of time, similar to that shown with the normal, physiologic transient hyperandrogenemia that occurs in premenopausal women.[91] Cyclical or periodic androgen therapy affords anabolic osteoblast effects while minimizing hepatic tolerance, virilization, and other adverse effects. Therefore, a short burst of androgen therapy (such as stanozolol, with a high therapeutic index,[92, 93] for 10 days each month) allows for appropriate osteoblast stimulation.[94]

Androgen Therapy Reverses BMD Deficits in Postmenopausal Osteoporosis

Several cross-sectional studies of postmenopausal women have shown that BMD is positively correlated with circulating androgen levels. A recent study has also indicated that elderly women with previous total hysterectomy have significantly lower androgen levels and BMDs than age-matched women who have undergone normal menopause.[95] Numerous studies have shown that androgen therapy increases BMD in postmenopausal women.[96, 97, 98, 99, 100, 101, 102, 103, 104, 105, 106, 107, 108, 109, 110, 111, 112, 113, 114, 115, 116, 117, 118, 119, 120, 121, 122, 123, 124, 125, 126, 127, 128, 129] Addition of androgen therapy to estrogenic steroid monotherapy has been shown to provide statistically significant increases in BMD over estrogen monotherapy.[130, 131] Androgen therapy has been recommended by several authors for the prevention and treatment of postmenopausal osteoporosis.[132, 133, 134, 135, 136, 137, 138, 139, 140, 141]

A few studies have shown that androgen therapy assists in maintaining BMD and reducing fracture risk even after such therapy has been discontinued.[142, 143] This effect results from two mechanisms. The first and short-term mechanism, is that androgen therapy has been shown to stimulate osteoblast activities that will continue (as exemplified by serum bone markers and histomorphometric studies) in the days and weeks after androgen therapy has been discontinued.[144, 145, 146, 147] The second and long-term mechanism, since osteoporosis and sarcopenia have a common pathogenesis (hypoandrogenemia), stems from the results of androgen therapy, which are that the therapy has been shown to increase overall anabolic reactions. These anabolic effects have been shown to enhance muscle mass and strength, and improve body composition and physical fitness. Such enhancements constitute a prolonged benefit of androgen therapy on BMD in postmenopausal women.[148, 149, 150, 151, 152, 153, 154, 155, 156] Therefore, it has been thoroughly proven that low-dose androgen therapy has both restorative and prolonged effects on bone formation and BMD.

Historical Highlights Regarding the Clinical Use of Androgen Therapy in Women

The clinical use of androgen therapy for postmenopausal women was widespread during the 1960s and early 1970s in the United States. By 1963, over a dozen androgens had been approved the U.S. Food and Drug Administration (FDA) for clinical use.[157] During this period, authors in several major medical textbooks recommended androgen therapy for osteoporosis and as a component of HRT in women. The following quotations illustrate these recommendations.

"In menopausal women estrogen-androgen combination improves physical, mental, and emotional status."— Parsons and Sommers, *Gynecology* (1962).[158]

"Endocrine therapy consists of administration of estrogen or estrogen plus androgen."— Williams, *Textbook of Endocrinology* (1962).[159]

"For osteoporosis, androgens or estrogen-androgen combination is the therapy of choice."—Cecil-Loeb, *Textbook of Medicine* (1963).[160]

"The current consensus seems to be that androgens and their various anabolic steroids are useful in the treatment of osteoporosis. In women, estrogen given concurrently with small doses of androgen minimizes virilization."—Goodman and Gilman, *The Pharmacological Basis of Therapeutics* (1970).[161]

"Although several medical approaches to treatment are recommended for osteoporosis, the most unanimously endorsed, as well as the most definitive, is the use of anabolic steroids."—Krusen, *Physical Medicine and Rehabilitation* (1971).[162]

These textbook recommendations were echoed by the information contained in the *Physician's Desk Reference (PDR)* and the package inserts regarding androgen therapy for osteoporosis that was approved by the FDA. Such information contained statements such as: "anabolic steroids are indicated for osteoporosis from corticosteroid therapy"[163] and "anabolic steroids are probably effective as for postmenopausal and senile osteoporosis.[164, 165]

In the mid–1970s medical politics began to override the evidence-based information and clinical use of androgen therapy in postmenopausal osteoporosis. Dogmatic and political statements contained in major medical textbooks discouraged androgen therapy by claiming that androgens were gender-specific male hormones and ineffective in women. The following quotations illustrate this point.

"In osteoporosis, testosterone preparations are useful in the treatment of men with gonadal deficiency, but there are no convincing reports of their efficacy in men with normal gonadal function. So-called anabolic steroids are weak androgens, and there is no advantage to their use in women. There is also no proved advantage to combinations of estrogens and androgens."—Harrison's *Principles of Internal Medicine* (1977).[166]

"Mild depression is not uncommon in menopausal women, its frequency tending to be inversely proportional to the patient's understanding of menopausal physiology. A 'menopausal syndrome' in a psychiatric sense appears to be non-existent. Psychological problems unrelated to the menopause per se are common in the 40- to 55-year-old group and relate to 'empty nest' syndrome; responsibility for the care of adolescent children and aging parents; ungratified sexuality; fears of obesity, cancer, and loss of sexual attractiveness; and the fear of having ultimately to depend on children or charity.... The attitude of many physicians as well as patients toward hormonal treatment is ambivalent.... Although testosterone is present in measurable amounts in the circulation of the female, the ovarian contribution is negligible." — Harrison's *Principles of Internal Medicine* (1977).[167]

These dogmatic and incorrect statements influenced federal policy-makers regarding androgen therapy for postmenopausal osteoporosis during the early 1980s. Two major federal actions directly impacted androgen therapy. The first was the enacting of generic drug laws that removed the patent protection of previously approved androgens. In effect, primarily for financial reasons, the pharmaceutical industry was much less likely to submit a new drug application (NDA) for newly discovered indications for older drugs. The second federal action was that the FDA was mandated to "clean up" all existing FDA-approved uses for prescription medications. As a consequence, in 1984, the FDA withdrew the osteoporosis indications for androgens. *These two federal actions, taken together, resulted in no new reapplications for the osteoporosis indications for androgens being submitted to the FDA.* The consequence of these actions essentially left no other approved medication for treating postmenopausal osteoporosis for nearly a decade.

Physicians who continued to prescribe androgens for their postmenopausal women patients with osteoporosis or as a component of HRT did so in an "off-label" fashion. Some physicians discontinued androgen therapy in their patients. In response to the FDA's action, in a letter to the editor, published in the *New England Journal of Medicine*, a prominent physician sharply condemned the FDA's decision:

"The recent decision of the FDA to withdraw approval for the use of anabolic steroids in treating osteoporosis appears counterproductive and unjustified by the available research."[168]

Other federal decisions also played a role in the prescribing habits of physicians regarding androgen therapy for postmenopausal women. Despite available scientific and clinical evidence to the contrary,[169, 170] the FDA published the italicized statement in the *PDR*: "*Warning: anabolic steroids do not enhance athletic ability.*" Coupled with the enactment of generic drug laws, these federal actions quickly became major building blocks for the construction of the anabolic steroid epidemic in the mid–1980s and 1990s.[171] A huge black market network for androgens, fueled by massive quantities illegally diverted by the generic pharmaceutical industry, made these steroids easily obtainable, without a prescription, for athletes and bodybuilders (over one million regular users in the United States).[172] Influential proposals for federal reclassification of androgens as controlled substances were published.[173, 174] As a result, congressional hearings were held, and androgens were reclassified as Schedule III controlled substances under federal law in November 1990.[175] As a consequence, many physicians, who were taught that androgens were ineffective as medical therapy and as athletic muscle-building drugs, refrained from prescribing androgen therapy for their patients. The medical antipathy for androgen therapy expanded due to the abuse of these steroids by athletes and bodybuilders and the prevailing lack of knowledge, by physicians, about the effects of androgens in clinical practice. This point can be illustrated by the following quotation.

"For a long period of time, physicians were skeptical about whether or not exogenous androgens had muscle-building effects, and endocrinologists were more skeptical than most. This belief was incorrect."—Geoffrey Redmond, M.D., President, Foundation for Developmental Endocrinology, *The Good News About Women's Hormones* (1995).[176]

These shortsighted decisions by the FDA have been suggested to be one of the primary reasons for the current osteoporosis epidemic in the United States.[177] Questions still remain as to why the FDA withdrew the previously approved indications for androgen therapy in osteoporosis. The FDA's decision was not supported by the scientific and clinical knowledge available at that time, and, despite dozens of publications exemplifying the beneficial effects of androgen therapy for postmenopausal osteoporosis and HRT in women, and the endorsement by many authors, remnants of these dogmatic, incorrect, and political positions persist. Much of this misinformation has been recycled and promulgated without appropriate review of the medical literature. This point can be illustrated by the following passage which, in its wording, essentially the same as it was 23 years previously.

"Testosterone preparations are useful in the treatment of osteoporotic men with gonadal insufficiency, but there is no evidence of efficiency in men with normal gonadal function. There is also no proven advantage to combinations of estrogens and androgens in either sex."— Harrison's *Principles of Internal Medicine* (2000).[178]

It is difficult to estimate the negative impact on patient care that this misinformation has had over the decades. One probable impact has been that American physicians have been slow to use anabolic therapies for the treatment of osteoporosis.[179] Harrison's *Principles of Internal Medicine* has been the most popular medical textbook and the primary text utilized for the education of the medical students and residents in the United States over the past three decades.

Unfortunately, the FDA's decision to withdraw the osteoporosis indications for androgens was made several years prior to the development of DEXA, updated serum osteoblast activity markers, and improvements in histomorphometric, bioassay, immunochemical, and bone cell receptor techniques. These advancements have proven many of the mechanisms that androgen therapy has on bone formation and homeostasis and ushered in a renewed interest in androgen therapy. For osteoporosis therapy, "anabolic steroids have recently made a comeback," especially outside the United States.[180]

Androgen therapy has been shown to be safe and effective treatment for elderly women patients.[181, 182] Low dose-androgen therapy does not create "superwomen" as seen with androgen abuse by bodybuilders.[183]

Androgens Directly and Indirectly Stimulate Normal Bone Formation

It is now well recognized that osteoblasts are bone-forming cells that are stimulated by androgens, growth hormone (GH), insulin-like growth factor-1 (IGF-1) and other anabolic agents and cytokines. Studies in osteoporotic men and women patients, utilizing serial bone biopsies and histomorphometric techniques prior to and after androgen therapy, have proven that androgens stimulate normal bone formation.[184, 185, 186]

In vitro studies have shown that androgens bind to osteoblast receptors, and this finding has stimulated renewed interest in androgen effects on bone, an interest that has been overshadowed by conventional wisdom's interest in estrogen-related bone effects.[187] Other in vitro studies have shown that the androgen-dependent osteoblast stimulating effects produced are locally mediated in bone tissue, in part, by androgen-dependent IGF-1 production, and systemically by androgen-dependent regulation of circulating IGFBPs.[188]

The anabolic effects of androgens on osteoblast bioactivities have been indicated by a number of specific molecules in the serum of patients.[189] These biochemical serum markers of bone formation and osteoblast activities include serum osteocalcin (Oc), bone-specific alkaline phosphatase (bAP), N- and C-terminal propeptide of type 1 procollagen (PINP and PICP respectively), and others.[190, 191, 192, 193, 194, 195, 196] These bone markers have been shown to indicate osteoblast activity that reflects formation of normal organic bone matrix.[197]

The discovery of these biochemical markers, along with improved imaging techniques, including dual-energy x-ray absorptiometry (DEXA), have provided updated methods to assess the pharmacological therapies that stimulate osteoblast activities and result in increases in BMD.[198, 199, 200] These developments have also allowed an improved understanding of the effects that endogenous and exogenous hormone interactions have on bone formulation and homeostasis.

Recent studies on postmenopausal women, utilizing serum bone markers, have shown that the androgen-induced effect on osteoblasts is both prolonged and restorative, and that osteoblast stimulation continues for a period of time after androgen therapy is discontinued.[201, 202, 203, 204, 205, 206, 207] Androgen therapy has been shown (by DEXA) to increase BMD),[208, 209, 210, 211, 212, 213, 214, 215, 216, 217] and to increase BMD over and above estrogen monotherapy in postmenopausal women.[218, 219, 220] Moreover, androgen therapy has been shown to reduce osteoporotic bone pain[221, 222] and reduce the occurrence and risk for osteoporotic fractures in postmenopausal women.[223, 224]

Androgen Therapy Corrects Hypoandrogenemia and Hyposomatomedinemia

It is well recognized that androgen therapy corrects hypoandrogenemia. Androgen therapy has also been shown to correct hyposomatomedinemia and normalize the GHRH-GH-IGF-IGFBP axis that plays a role in bone formation and homeostasis. Hypoandrogenemia can result in a depressed GHRH-GH-IGF-IGFBP axis and hyposomatomedinemia in postmenopausal women.

Androgens have been shown to directly stimulate the GHRH-GH-IGF-IGFBP axis at the hypothalamic level by a direct stimulatory effect that increases GHRH amplitudes.[225, 226] Such androgen stimulation has been shown to elevate circulating IGF-1, free IGF-1, and IGFBP-3 levels in normal, hypogonadal, hyposomatotrophic, and aging individuals.[227, 228, 229, 230, 231, 232, 233, 234] Thus, androgens have been shown to drive the GHRH-GH-IGF-IGFBP axis and result in an overall anabolic state that results in bone formation and musculoskeletal enhancement.

Therapy with other anabolic agents can normalize the GHRH-GH-IGF-IGFBP axis and correct hyposomatomedinemia in postmenopausal women. Administering GHRH or GH has been shown to elevate IGF-1, free IGF-1, and IGFBP-3 levels.[235, 236] Besides having a direct stimulatory effect on IGF-1 synthesis,[237] it has been shown that GH may have a direct stimulatory function on IGFBP-3 by enhancing its synthesis.[238]

Growth hormone has been shown to directly stimulate osteoblasts in vitro[239] and increase osteoblast activity in vivo as determined by serum markers of osteoblast activities.[240, 241, 242] Growth hormone increases bone formation via a direct interaction with GH receptors located on osteoblasts and via locally produced IGF-1 (autocrine/paracrine action).[243, 244] It has been shown that individuals with GH-deficient states have a reduction in osteoblast activities that often results in low BMD, osteoporosis, and fractures.[245] In postmenopausal women, therapy with recombinant GH or IGF-1 has shown both beneficial and differential osteoblast-stimulating effects as reflected by serum markers of bone markers.[246]

Androgen Therapy Improves Menopausal Vasomotor Symptoms, Elevates Mood, Increases Libido, Improves Quality of Life, and Modulates Anabolic Cytokines

It is now well recognized that cotherapy with estrogens and androgens, improves cytokine balance, improves menopausal vasomotor symptoms, elevates mood, increases libido and orgasmic response, increases sense of well-being and energy levels, and improves quality of life for postmenopausal women. Recent studies[247, 248, 249, 250, 251, 252, 253, 254, 255, 256, 257, 258, 259, 260, 261, 262, 263, 264] have confirmed earlier studies[265, 266, 267, 268, 269, 270, 271] on these issues. Several mechanisms have been shown to be involved with these subjective and objective postmenopausal conditions.

It has been recognized that adequate suppression of luteinizing hormone (LH) reduces vasomotor symptoms in postmenopausal women. It has been shown that estrogen-androgen therapy suppresses LH secretion significantly better than estrogen monotherapy, indicating that added androgen therapy results in a more pronounced negative feedback inhibition on the hypothalamic-pituitary axis.[272]

Another mechanistic advantage of an androgen component for HRT involves sex hormone binding globulin (SHBG) and bioavailable androgen levels. It has been shown that estrogen monotherapy for HRT results in profound reduction in free, bioavailable androgen levels, causing a significant hypoandrogenic state[273] by marked elevations in circulating sex hormone binding globulin (SHBG) levels.[274] Addition of androgen to estrogen monotherapy has been shown to normalize SHBG, increase the bioavailability of androgens, and reduce the required estrogen dose to achieve control of vasomotor symptoms.[275]

Some vasomotor symptoms have a central nervous system origin. In recent years investigations have shown that androgens belong to the group of neurosteroids that are synthesized and metabolized by a variety of brain tissues.[276] Androgens are also made available to the brain via the general circulation after they are synthesized by the endocrine system or introduced via exogenous routes. Androgens have been shown to exhibit neurosteroid, neuroprotective, and neuroregenerative properties in:

(1) evidence from cell culture experiments which has shown that androgens increase the survival, differentiation, and regeneration of neurons, glial cells, and Schwann cells, and that they can be synthesized from cholesterol within both central and peripheral nervous systems.[277, 278, 279, 280]

(2) evidence from immunochemistry which had shown that androgens serve as precursors for other steroids in biosynthetic pathways within oligodendrocytes and glial cells that stimulate myelin synthesis.[281, 282, 283]

(3) evidence indicating that androgens are synthesized by pyramidal neurons and stimulate the hippocampal neurons that play an important role in memory and learning. [284]

(4) evidence indicating that androgens exhibit neurotransmitter modulation effects via receptor-mediated binding to ligand-gated ion channels, which results in the repolarization of the plasma membrane and inhibits further neuronal firing. These androgen-mediated actions have been shown in GABA(A), NMDA, sigma, substance P, dopamine, serotonin, and opioid receptors, which in turn has been shown to result in neuroprotective, neuromodulatory, cognition-enhancing, memory-enhancing, anxiolytic, mood-elevating, and analgesic effects.[285, 286, 287, 288, 289, 290, 291, 292, 293, 294, 295, 296 297, 298, 299, 300, 301, 302, 303, 304, 305, 306, 307, 308, 309, 310, 311, 312]

(5) evidence that androgens increase the serum and tissue levels of a number of anabolic and neurotrophic polypeptide growth factors that play a role in the homeostasis, stimulation, neovascularization, and regeneration of central nervous system tissues.[313, 314]

(6) evidence that androgens promote anabolic influences on cytokines and modulate or correct inflammatory and autoimmune cytokine imbalances.[315, 316, 317, 318] Hypoandrogenemia has been found to play a role in the pathogenesis of several cytokine-mediated, immunity-related, diseases in women, such as stroke, myocardial infarction, atherosclerosis, rheumatoid arthritis, systemic lupus erythematosus, Sjogren's disease, scleroderma, multiple sclerosis, osteoporosis, fibromyalgia, chronic fatigue syndrome, depression, and dementia (see the sections on these specific diseases for a detailed discussion). Estrogen monotherapy as HRT as been shown to adversely alter cytokine and immune system parameters that may play a role in the course or pathogenesis of these diseases in women.[319]

Mimicking ovarian function by using estrogen-androgen cotherapy for postmenopausal osteoporosis and HRT has recently gained significant clinical attention. In May 1995, a scientific clinical symposium was held in San Francisco on this topic entitled "Emerging Role of Androgens in Menopausal Treatment." Some of the salient points made in this symposium were:

(1) Women who use combination sex steroid therapy (estrogen-androgen) in menopause lead better lives, as judged by most quality-of-life measures, and live longer as well. This type of HRT should be provided for all women who desire it, and should be continued indefinitely. Many women can expect to live nearly half of their lifespan suffering from the sequelae of ovarian involution. Menopause should be considered as a continuum rather than a passage.

(2) Androgens may be used to improve the quality of life without detracting from the cardiovascular benefits of estrogenic monotherapy alone. Androgens, when combined with estrogenic steroids, appear to be both safe and beneficial.

(3) By correlating perceived distress from menopausal symptoms with sexual drive, the physician can offer treatment and improve the potential for the patient's adherence to therapy for the other aspects, by using estrogen-androgen cotherapy. Estrogen-androgen cotherapy improves energy level and mood in menopausal women. Androgens are responsible for the sexual drive in women, and sexual drive has been shown to increase adherence to therapy in some women after estrogen-androgen cotherapy is instituted.

(4) Progesterogenic steroids can be added to the HRT regimen to help reduce the small risk of uterine cancer.

In 1997, at the 15th World Congress of Gynecology and Obstetrics meeting in Copenhagen, Denmark, a daylong symposium was presented entitled "The Emerging Role of Estrogen-Androgen Therapy in the Care of the Postmenopausal Patient." The important points of this scientific clinical symposium were:

(1) Adding small amounts of androgens to HRT can restore failing libido, resolve persistent hot flashes, and restore decreased BMD, which are all consequences of menopause that can affect the quality of life in postmenopausal women.

(2) Androgen, for some women, is the "missing hormone" of HRT. Estrogen-androgen cotherapy can be a significantly better option for some women than estrogen monotherapy or estrogen-progesterone therapy alone.

(3) Androgen production in women decreases gradually over the years leading up to menopause and for decades after menopause. As a result, clinical signs and symptoms of androgen deficiency are expected as the menopausal transition begins and will continue to persist during the postmenopausal years.

(4) Postmenopausal women who have received estrogen-androgen

cotherapy have been shown to have improvement in sexual desire, fantasy, frequency of intercourse, enhanced orgasmic response, and less vaginal dryness than those on estrogen monotherapy alone. Estrogen-androgen cotherapy is superior to estrogen monotherapy or estrogen-progesterone therapy in alleviating vasomotor symptoms and insomnia. Estrogen doses can be reduced when low-dose androgens are added. Estrogens and androgens work synergistically to inhibit LH secretion and reduce vasomotor symptoms.

(5) There is a growing body of research evidence in HRT that indicates that "one-size-doesn't-fit-all." Sex steroid replacement therapy should be tailored to each woman according to her postmenopausal symptoms and conditions.

(6) The addition of an androgen may reduce the risk of breast cancer when combined with a reduced estrogen dose for HRT. In women with a history of breast cancer, androgen therapy alone has been shown to be a valid alternative for HRT in postmenopausal women.

Impact of Estrogen-Androgen HRT on Lipids and Thromboembolic Event Risks

While estrogen-androgen cotherapy has been shown in numerous studies to be superior to estrogen monotherapy for controlling vasomotor symptoms, increasing BMD, and improving all quality-of-life factors, the effects of cotherapy on lipid profiles and cardiovascular risk factors are mixed.[320] Studies have shown no impact on lipid profiles,[321] or improved lipid profiles,[322] while others have shown a mixed[323, 324] or an atherogenic lipid pattern.[325] Cyclical androgen therapy, when combined with estrogen therapy, has been shown to have no impact on serum lipid profiles.[326]

Any deleterious impact on serum lipids, if any, must be weighed against the improvements in body composition, enhanced fibrinolytic activities, and improved cytokine profiles, especially when compared to the deleterious impacts on these parameters with estrogen monotherapy. Androgen therapy in women has been shown to reduce tissue plasminogen activator antigen, plasminogen activator inhibitor type 1 (PAI-1) and fibrinogen levels, and to increase fibrinolysis.[327, 328, 329] These profibrinolytic effects of androgens have been shown to be of particular interest with regards to the beneficial effects of HRT for decreasing atherogenesis and thromboembolism.[330, 331]

Estrogen monotherapy for HRT in postmenopausal women has been shown to elevate the risk for thromboembolic events despite the improvements in lipid and lipoprotein profiles. This apparent dichotomy has been attributed to the adverse impacts that estrogen therapy has on the fibrinolysis mechanisms. Recent studies have shown that estrogen monotherapy in postmenopausal women significantly elevates the risk of deep venous thrombosis (three fold),[332] ischemic cerebrovascular stroke,[333] and pulmonary thromboembolism.[334]

Overall, estrogen-androgen cotherapy probably reduces the atherogenesis process and the risk for thromboembolic events despite any mild adverse impact on serum lipids and lipoprotein profiles. Addition of an androgen component enhances fibrinolysis by several mechanisms that may prove beneficial over and above any detrimental impact on serum lipoprotein profiles. Estrogen-androgen cotherapy as HRT probably has a point-counterpoint balancing effect on fibrinolysis, serum lipids, and lipoprotein profiles. Since cyclical oral androgens come closest to mimicking ovarian function when combined with estrogens, this treatment regimen may provide the best overall balance of androgen and estrogen effects.

Summary

Androgens should be strongly considered as a routine part of HRT and for the prevention and treatment of postmenopausal osteoporosis, especially for women who are undergoing physical rehabilitation from illness or injury. Judicious use of androgens provides multifaceted beneficial effects that clearly outweigh any adverse effects for most women. Mimicking the function of endocrine glands that go through involution or produce inadequate levels of particular hormones has been common practice in medicine. Estrogen-androgen cotherapy, or estrogen-progesterone-androgen therapy mimics the classes of sex steroids that are normally produced by the functioning, healthy human ovaries. No other drugs or combination of drugs offers the wide range of benefits that have been demonstrated with estrogen-androgen cotherapy.

In this chapter, androgen therapy as a component of HRT and for the prevention and treatment of postmenopausal osteoporosis has been shown to have many beneficial effects. These beneficial effects are:

(1) increased osteoblast activities (reflected by DEXA, serum bone formation markers, bioassay studies, bone receptor studies, and histomorphometric studies) that have provided known mechanisms for the prevention and reversal of BMD losses and reduced risk for osteoporotic fractures.

(2) increased pain tolerance and an analgesic effect in patients with osteoporotic bone fractures.

(3) reduction in estrogen replacement dose requirements while providing improved control of vasomotor symptoms and more effective suppression of LH secretion.

(4) prevention and reversal of muscle mass losses and sarcopenia (see the chapter on sarcopenia for a detailed discussion).

(5) enhancement of fibrinolysis that counteracts the deleterious effects that estrogen monotherapy produces on parameters involved with the clotting cascade.

(6) improvements in all quality of life measurements, including improved libido and sexual satisfaction levels.

(7) improved modulation of cytokine profiles that favor anabolic and protective profiles in bone, brain, myocardium, skeletal muscle, immune system, and other tissues.

(8) enhanced anabolic capacities as reflected by improved GH secretion, elevated IGF-1, and increased IGF-1 bioavailability, both systemically and in local tissues (see the chapter on sarcopenia for a full discussion).

(9) improved modulation of cytokine profiles on the immune system parameters that are neuroprotective and immunoprotective against autoimmune diseases which are significantly more common in women than men (see the chapter on autoimmune disease for a full discussion).

(10) improved immune system function, especially in postmenopausal women with acquired immune deficiencies, such as AIDS and cytomegalovirus infections (see the chapter on immunodeficiency syndromes for a full discussion).

(11) improved mental health, including elevation in mood and cognition (see the chapter on Alzheimer's disease and dementia for a full discussion).

(12) normalized SHBG levels that increase the bioavailibity of androgens.

Androgens and estrogens were among the first true drugs synthesized from chemical reactions and have been clinically available for over six decades. It has taken nearly 50 years to gain a fuller understanding of the biochemical importance of these steroids, owing to the fact that it has taken that long for the technical advancements involved with their recent evaluations to be developed. Nonvirilizing doses of androgens represent a valid therapeutic option. It is time for physicians to reassess this matter, clear themselves of unfounded fears and reinforce the physiological and scientific foundations of our appropriate options for treating and preventing osteoporosis.[335]

Women who are androgen depleted develop physical and behavioral symptoms to a female androgen deficiency syndrome. Androgen replacement therapy is a much-neglected area of medical practice and further research is needed to identify all women who will benefit from it since studies in menopausal women have shown appropriate androgen therapy to be well tolerated and safe. Such therapy is underused and under-researched. Cosmetic side effects are rare if supraphysiologic doses are avoided.[336]

Postmenopausal women make up a substantial portion of the usual practice in physical medicine and rehabilitation. These patients should be evaluated and considered for androgen therapy or some other anabolic agent (such as stimulators to the GHRH-GH-IGF-IGFPB axis) to hasten and improve rehabilitative outcomes and to prevent and/or reverse postmenopausal osteoporosis. Most postmenopausal women who are not on anabolic therapy will have a substantial reduction in anabolic potentials to fully react to the conventional rehabilitative modalities. Thus, an appropriate pharmacologic, anabolic stimulus is necessary for maximal rehabilitative outcomes in postmenopausal women.

Notes

1. Taylor, W.N. *Osteoporosis: Medical Blunders and Treatment Strategies* Jefferson, N.C. McFarland & Company, Inc., Publishers, 1996.

2. Barnhart, K.T., E. Freeman, J.A. Grisso, et al. The effect of dehydroepiandrosterone supplementation to symptomatic perimenopausal women on serum endocrine profiles, lipid parameters, and health-related quality of life. *J. Clin. Endocrinol. Metab.* 1999; 84 (11): 3896–3902.

3. Rako, S. Testosterone supplemental therapy after hysterectomy with or without concomitant oophorectomy: estrogen alone is not enough? *J. Womens Health Gend. Based. Med.* 2000; 9 (8): 917–923.

4. Frackiewicz, E.J., and N.R. Cutler. Women's health care during the perimenopause. *J. Am. Pharm. Assoc. (Wash.)* 2000; 40 (6): 800–811.

5. Davis, S.R. Androgen treatment in women. *Med. J. Aust.* 1999; 170 (11): 545–549.

6. Spratt, D.I., C. Longcope, P.M. Cox, et al. Differential changes in serum concentrations of androgens and estrogens (in relation with cortisol) in postmenopausal women with acute illness. *J. Clin. Endocrinol. Metab.* 1993; 76 (6): 1542–1547.

7. Phillips, G.B. Relationship between serum dehydroepiandrosterone sulfate, androstenedione, and sex hormones in men and women. *Eur. J. Endocrinol.* 1996; 134 (2): 201–206.

8. Yen, S.S., and G.A. Laughlin. Aging and the adrenal cortex. *Exp. Gerontol.* 1998; 33 (7–8): 897–910.

9. Harper, A.J., J.E. Buster, and P.R. Casson. Changes in adrenocortical function with aging and therapeutic implications. *Semin. Reprod. Endocrinol.* 1999; 17 (4): 327–338.

10. Chrousos, G.P. The role of stress and the hypothalamic-pituitary-adrenal axis in the pathogenesis of the metabolic syndrome: neuroendocrine and target tissue-related causes. *Int. J. Obes. Relat. Metab. Disord.* 2000; 24 (Suppl. 2): S50–55.

11. Hansen, K.A., and S.P. Tho. Androgens and bone health. *Semin. Reprod. Endocrinol.* 1998; 16 (2): 129–134.

12. Shoupe, D. Androgens and bone: clinical implications for menopausal women. *Am. J. Obstet. Gynecol.* 1999; 180 (3): S329–333.

13. Lips, P. Epidemiology and predictors of fractures associated with osteoporosis. *Am. J. Med.* 1997; 103 (Suppl.): 3S–8S.

14. National Osteoporosis Foundation. Osteoporosis: review of the evidence for prevention, diagnosis and treatment and cost effectiveness analysis. *Osteoporos. Int.* 1998; 8: S1–S88.

15. Compston, J.E. Sex steroids and bone. *Physiol. Rev.* 2001; 81 (1): 419–447.

16. Adler, R.A. Sex steroids and osteoporosis. The role of estrogens and androgens. *Clin. Lab. Med.* 2000; 20 (3): 549–558.

17. Frackiewicz, E.J., and N.R. Cutler. Women's health care during the perimenopause. *J. Am. Pharm. Assoc. (Wash.)* 2000; 40 (6): 800–811.

18. Rako, S. Testosterone supplementation therapy after hysterectomy with or without concomitant oophorectomy: estrogens alone are not enough. *J. Womens Health Gend. Based Med.* 2000; 9 (8): 917–923.

19. Steinberg, K.K., L.W. Freni-Titulaer, E.G. Du Peuy, et al. Sex steroids and bone density in perimenopausal women. *J. Clin. Endocrinol. Metab.* 1989; 69: 533–539.

20. Frock, J., and J. Money. Sexuality and the menopause. *Psychother. Psychosom.* 1992; 57: 29–33.

21. Longcope, C., C. Franz, C. Morello, et al. Steroid and gonadotrophin levels in women during the peri-menopausal years. *Maturitas* 1996; 8: 189–196.

22. Zumoff, B., G.W. Strain, L.K. Miller, et al. Twenty-four hour mean plasma testosterone concentrations declines with age in normal premenopausal women. *J. Clin. Endocrinol. Metab.* 1995; 80: 3537–3545.

23. Rannevik, G.S., O. Jeppsson, O. Johnell, et al. A longitudinal study of the perimenopausal transition: altered profiles of steroid and pituitary hormones, SHBG and bone mineral density. *Maturitas* 1995; 21: 103–113.

24. Davis, S.R. Androgen treatment in women. *Med. J. Aust.* 1999; 170 (11): 545–549.

25. Hansen, K.A., and S.P. Tho. Androgens and bone health. *Semin. Reprod. Endocrinol.* 1998; 16 (2): 129–134.

26. Bachmann, G.A. Androgen cotherapy in menopause: evolving benefits and challenges. *Am. J .Obstet. Gynecol.* 1999; 180 (3): S308–311.

27. Zofkova, I. R., Bahbouh, and M. Hill. The pathophysiological implications of circulating androgens on bone mineral density in a normal female population. *Steroids* 2000; 65 (12): 857–861.

28. Shoupe, D. Androgens and bone: clinical implications for menopausal women. *Am. J. Obstet. Gynecol.* 1999; 180 (3): S329–333.

29. Rako, S. Testosterone supplemental therapy after hysterectomy with or without concomitant oophorectomy: estrogen alone is not enough. *J. Womens Health Gend. Based Med.* 2000; 9 (8): 917–923.

30. Allen, I.E., M. Monroe, J. Connelly, et al. Effect of postmenopausal hormone replacement therapy on dental outcomes: systematic review of the literature and pharmacoeconomic analysis. *Manag. Care Interface* 2000; 13 (4): 93–99.

31. Hillen, T., A. Lun, F.M. Reichies, et al. DHEA-S plasma levels and incidence of Alzheimer's disease. *Biol. Psychiatry* 2000; 47 (2): 161–163.

32. Drake, E.B., V.W. Henderson, F.Z. Stanczyk, et al. Associations between circulating sex steroid hormones and cognition in normal elderly women. *Neurology* 2000; 54 (3): 599–603.

33. Magri, F., F. Terenzi, T. Ricciardi, et al. Associations between changes in adrenal secretion and cerebral morphometric correlates in normal aging and senile dementia. *Dement. Geriatr. Cogn. Disord.* 2000; 11 (2): 90–99.

34. Niebauer, J., Pflaum, C.D., A.L. Clark, et al. Deficient insulin-like growth factor 1 in chronic heart failure predicts altered body composition, anabolic deficiency, cytokine and neurohormones activation. *J. Am. Coll. Cardiol.* 1998; 32 (2): 393–397.

35. Anker, S.D., P.P. Ponikowski, A.L. Clark, et al. Cytokines and neurohormones relating to body composition alterations in the wasting syndrome of chronic heart failure. *Eur. Heart J.* 1999; 20 (9): 683–693.

36. Moriyama, Y., H. Yasue, M. Yoskimura, et al. The plasma levels of dehydroepiandrosterone sulfate are decreased in patients with chronic heart failure in proportion to the severity. *J. Clin. Endocrinol. Metab.* 2000; 85 (5): 1843–1840.

37. Ren, J., W.K. Samson, and J.R. Sowers. Insulin-like growth factor 1 as a cardiac hormone: physiological and pathophysiological implications in heart disease. *J. Mol. Cell. Cardiol.* 1999; 31 (11): 2049–2061.

38. Osterziel, K.J., M.B. Ranke, O. Strohm, et al. The somatotrophic system in patients with dilated cardiomyopathy: relation of insulin-like growth factor-1 and its alterations during growth hormone therapy to cardiac function. *Clin. Endocrinol. (Oxf.)* 2000; 51 (1): 61–68.

39. Wolf, R.L., J.M. Zumda, K.L. Stone, et al. Update on the epidemiology of osteoporosis. *Curr. Rheumatol. Rep.* 2000; 2 (1): 74–86.

40. Browner, W.S., A.R. Pressman, M.C. Nevitt, et al. Association between bone density and stroke in elderly women. *Stroke* 1993; 24 (7): 940–946.

41. Jorgensen, L, T. Engstad, and B.K. Jacobsen. Bone mineral density in acute stroke patients: low bone mineral density may predict first stroke in women. *Stroke* 2001; 32 (1): 47–51.

42. Ramnemark, A., L. Nyberg, B. Borssen, et al. Fractures after stroke. *Osteoporos. Int.* 1998; 8 (1): 92–95.

43. Lui, M., T. Tsuji, Y. Higuchi, et al. Osteoporosis in hemiplegic stroke patients as studied with dual-energy X-ray absorptiometry. *Arch. Phys. Med. Rehabil.* 1999; 80 (10): 1219–1226.

44. Sato, Y. Abnormal bone and calcium metabolism in patients after stroke. *Arch. Phys. Med. Rehabil.* 2000; 81 (1): 117–121.

45. Ramnemark, A., M. Nilsson, B. Borssen, et al. Stroke, a major increasing risk factor for femoral neck fracture. *Stroke* 2000; 31 (7): 1572–1577.

46. Need, A.G., T.C. Durbridge, and B.E. Nordin. Anabolic steroids in postmenopausal osteoporosis. *Wien. Med. Wochenschr.* 1993; 143 (14–15): 392–395.

47. McKercher, H.G., R.G. Crilly, and M. Kloseck. Osteoporosis management in long-term care. Survey of Ontario physicians. *Can. Fam. Physician* 2000; 46: 2228–2235.

48. Economides, P.A., V.G. Kaklamani, I. Karavas, et al. Assessment of physician responses to abnormal results of bone densitometry studies. *Endocr. Pract.* 2000; 6 (5): 351–356.

49. Schrager, S., T. Kausch, and J.A. Bobula. Osteoporosis risk assessment by family practice faculty and residents: a chart review. *Wis. Med. J.* 1999; 98: 34–36.

50. Schrager, S., M.B. Plane, M.P. Mundt, et al. Osteoporosis prevention counseling during health maintenance examinations. *J. Fam. Pract.* 2000; 49 (12): 1099–1103.

51. Roubenoff, R. Sarcopenia: a major modifiable cause of frailty in the elderly. *J. Nutr. Health Aging* 2000; 4 (3): 140–142.

52. Dutta, C., and E.C. Hadley. The significance of sarcopenia in old age. *J. Gerontol. A. Biol. Sci. Med. Sci.* 1995; 50 (Spec. No.): 1–4.

53. Wilmore, D.W. Deterrents to the successful clinical use of growth factors that enhance protein anabolism. *Curr. Opin. Clin. Nutr. Metab. Care* 1999; 2 (1): 15–21.

54. Wilmore, D.W. Impediments to the successful use of anabolic agents in clinical care. *J. Parenter. Enteral. Nutr.* 1999; 2 (1): 15–21.

55. McKercher, H.G, R.G. Crilly, and M. Kloseck. Osteoporosis management in long-term care. Survey of Ontario physicians. *Can. Fam. Physician* 2000; 46: 2228–2235.

56. Garcia de Lorenzo, A., and J.M. Culebras. [Hormones, growth factors, and drugs in metabolism and nutrition.] *Nutr. Hosp.* 1995; 10 (5): 297–305.

57. Goldman, A. Androgen therapy in women. *J. Clin. Endocrinol.* 1942; 2: 750.

58. Salmon, U.J., and S.H. Geist. Effect of androgens upon libido in women. *J. Clin. Endocrinol. Metab.* 1943; 3: 235–238.

59. Greenblatt, R.B. Androgenic therapy in women. *J. Clin. Endocrinol. Metab.* 1942; 2: 65–66.

60. Greenblatt, R.B. Medical College of Georgia, Augusta. *Geratrics* 1976; 31 (7): 100–102.

61. Greenblatt, R.B., W.E. Barfield, and J.F. Garner, et al. Evaluation of an estrogen, androgen, estrogen-androgen combination, and a placebo on the treatment of the menopause. *J. Clin. Endocrinol. Metab.* 1950; 10: 1547–1558.

62. Greenblatt, R.B., and J.C. Emperaire. Changing concepts in the management of the menopause. *Med. Times* 1970; 98 (6): 153–164.

63. Greenblatt, R.B. and S. Dalla Pria. [Hormonal treatment of menopause.] *Minerva Ginecol.* 1972; 24 (1): 35–41.

64. Greenblatt, R.B., and J.J. Leng. Factors influencing sexual behavior. *J. Am. Geriatr. Soc.* 1972; 20 (2): 49–54.

65. Greenblatt, R.B. The psychogenic and endocrine aspects of sexual behavior. *J. Am. Geriat. Soc.* 1974; 22 (9): 393–396.

66. Greenblatt, R.B., M.L. Colle, and V.B. Mahesh. Ovarian and adrenal steroid production in the postmenopausal woman. *Obstet. Gynecol.* 1976; 47 (4): 383–387.

67. Greenblatt, R.B., M. Oettinger, and C.S. Bohler. Estrogen-androgen levels in aging men and women: therapeutic considerations. *J. Am. Geriat. Soc.* 1976; 24 (4): 173–178.

68. Asch, R.H., and R.B. Greenblatt. Steroidogenesis in the postmenopausal ovary. *Clin. Obstet. Gynaecol.* 1977; 4 (1): 85–106.

69. Greenblatt, R.B. Aging through the ages. *Geriatrics* 1977; 32 (6): 101–102.

70. Greenblatt, R.B. Update on the male and female climacteric. *Am. J. Geriatr. Soc.* 1979; 27 (11): 481–490.

71. Greenblatt, R.B. Hormone therapy for the menopause. *Geratrics* 1981; 36 (7): 53–61.

72. Greenblatt, R.B. Dwarfs, standing on the shoulders of giants, see further. *Prog. Clin. Biol. Res.* 1982; 112 (Pt.A.): 1–11.

73. Greenblatt, R.B. Extended view of the menopause. *Reproduction* 1982; 6 (2): 107–112.

74. Greenblatt, R.B., and A. Karpas. Hormone therapy for sexual dysfunction. The only "true aphrodisiac." *Postgrad. Med.* 1983; 74 (3): 78–80, 84–89.

75. Greenblatt, R.B. Is there a place for androgens in gynecological disorders? *Gynecol. Endocrinol.* 1987; 1 (2): 209–219.

76. Greenblatt, R.B. The use of androgens in the menopause and other gynecic disorders. *Obstet. Gynecol. N. America* 1987; 14 (1): 251.

77. Karpas, A.E. In memoriam Robert B. Greenblatt. *Int. J. Fertil.* 1988; 33 (2): 143.

78. Greenblatt, R.B. The use of androgens in the menopause and other gynecic disorders. *Obstet. Gynecol. N. America* 1987; 14 (1): 251.

79. Imparato, E., L. Marino, and A. Sallusto. [Use of estrogen-progesterone-testosterone combination in control of the menopausal syndrome. Double-blind clinical studies.] *Ann. Ostet. Ginecol. Med. Perinat.* 1973; 94 (5): 361–372.

80. Taylor, W.N., and C. Alanis. Triple sex steroid replacement therapy for osteoporosis after surgical menopause. *J. Neurol. Orthop. Med. Surg.* 1992; 13: 16–19.

81. Taylor, W.N., C. Alanis, and D.J. Wigley. Oral cyclical stanozolol and daily micronized 17–beta estradiol combination therapy for postmenopausal osteoporosis: a preliminary report. *J. Neurol. Orthop. Med. Surg.* 1994; 15: 25–29.

82. Taylor, W.N. *Anabolic Steroids and the Athlete* 2nd edition. Jefferson, N.C.: McFarland & Company, Inc., Publishers, 2001.

83. Judd, J.C., J.E. Judd, W.E. Lucas, et al. Endocrine function of the postmenopausal ovary: concentration of androgens and estrogens in ovaries and peripheral vein blood. *J. Clin. Endocrinol. Metab.* 1974; 1020–1030.

84. Loncope, C. Adrenal and gonadal androgen secretion in normal females. *J. Clin. Endocrinol. Metab.* 1986; 15: 213–218.

85. Judd, H.L., and S.S.C. Chen. Serum androstenedione and testosterone levels during the menstrual cycle. *J. Clin. Endocrinol. Metab.* 1973; 36: 475–481.

86. Martins, J.M., F. Carrieras, A. Afonso, et al. Transient hyperandrogenemia and its relation to ovulation. *Fertil. Steril.* 1998; 70 (4): 664–670.

87. Schlemmer, A., C. Hassager, J. Risteli, et al. Possible variation in bone resorption during the normal menstrual cycle. *Acta Endocrinol. (Copenh.)* 1993; 129 (5): 388–392.

88. Massafra, C., C. De Felice, D.P. Agunsdei, et al. Androgens and osteocalcin during the menstrual cycle. *J. Clin. Endocrinol. Metab.* 1999; 84 (3): 971–974.

89. Adami, S., N. Zamberlan, R. Casetllo, et al. Effects of hyperandrogenism and menstrual cycle abnormalities on bone mass and bone turnover in young women. *Clin Endocrinol. (Oxf.)* 1998; 48 (2): 169–173.

90. Taylor, W.N., and C. Alanis. Triple sex steroid replacement therapy for osteoporosis after surgical menopause. *J. Neurol. Orthop. Med. Surg.* 1992; 13: 16–19.

91. Taylor, W.N., C. Alanis, and D.J. Wigley. Oral cyclical stanozolol and daily micronized 17–beta estradiol combination therapy for postmenopausal osteoporosis: a preliminary report. *J. Neurol. Orthop. Med. Surg.* 1994; 15: 25–29.

92. Taylor, W.N. *Macho Medicine: A History of the Anabolic Steroid Epidemic.* Jefferson, N.C.: McFarland & Company, Inc., Publishers, 1991.

93. Taylor, W.N. *Anabolic Steroids and the Athlete*, 2nd edition. Jefferson, N.C.: McFarland & Company, Inc., Publishers, 2001.

94. Taylor, W.N. *Osteoporosis: Medical Blunders and Treatment Strategies.* Jefferson, N.C.: McFarland & Company, Inc, Publishers, 1996.

95. Laughlin, G.A., E. Barrett-Connor, D. Kritz-Siverstein, et al. Hysterectomy, oophorectomy, and endogenous sex hormone levels in older women: the Rancho Bernardo Study. *J. Clin. Endocrinol. Metab.* 2000; 85 (2): 645–651.

96. Hollo, I., J. Szucs, and K. Steczek. Effect of norandrostenolone-decanoate on calcium tolerance curves in patients with primary osteoporosis. Data on the mode of action of anabolic compounds in osteoporosis. *Endokrinologie* 1971; 58 (3): 326–330.

97. Robin, J.C., O.W. Suh, and J.L. Ambrus. Studies on osteoporosis VII. Effect

of 17 beta-hydroxy-4–estren-3–one 17–decanoate on experimental osteoporosis. *Steroids* 1982; 40 (2): 125–132.

98. Riggs, B.L., J. Jowsey, R.S. Goldsmith, et al. Short- and long-term effects of estrogen and synthetic anabolic hormone in postmenopausal osteoporosis. *J. Clin. Invest.* 1972; 51 (7): 1659–1663.

99. Lindsay, R., D. McKhart, and A. Kraszewski. Prospective double-blind trial of synthetic steroid (Org OD 14) for preventing postmenopausal osteoporosis. *Br. Med. J.* 1980; 5: 1207–1210.

100. Chesnut, C.H., J.L. Ivey, H.E. Gruber, et al. Stanozolol in postmenopausal osteoporosis: therapeutic efficacy and possible mechanisms of action. *Metabolism* 1983; 32 (6): 571–580.

101. Need, A.G., B.E. Chatterton, C.J. Walker, et al. Comparison of calcium, calcitrol, ovarian hormones and nandrolone in the treatment of osteoporosis. *Maturitas* 1986; 8 (4): 275–280.

102. Taylor, W.N., and C. Alanis. Triple sex steroid replacement therapy for osteoporosis after surgical menopause. *J. Neurol. Orthop. Med. Surg.* 1992; 13: 16–19.

103. Geusens. P., J. Dequeker, A. Versraeten, et al. Bone mineral content, cortical thickness and fracture rate in osteoporotic women after withdrawal of treatment with nandrolone decanoate, I-alpha hydroxyvitamin D3, or intermittent calcium infusions. *Maturitas* 1986; 8 (4): 281–289.

104. Need, A.G., M. Horowitz, C.J. Walker, et al. Cross-over study of fat-corrected forearm mineral content during nandrolone decanoate therapy for osteoporosis. *Bone* 1989; 10 (1): 3–6.

105. Johansen, J.S., C. Hassager, J. Podenphant, et al. Treatment of postmenopausal osteoporosis: is the anabolic steroid nandrolone decanoate a candidate? *Bone Miner.* 1989; 6 (1): 77–86.

106. Gennari, C., D. Agnus Dei, S. Gonnelli, et al. Effects of nandrolone decanoate therapy on bone mass and calcium metabolism in women with established postmenopausal osteoporosis: a double-blind placebo-controlled study. *Maturitas* 1989; 11 (3): 187–197.

107. Hassager, C., B.J. Riis, J. Podenphant, et al. Nandrolone decanoate treatment of post-menopausal osteoporosis for 2 years and effects of withdrawal. *Maturitas* 1989; 11 (4): 305–317.

108. Need, A.G., M. Horowitz, A. Bridges, et al. Effects of nandrolone decanoate and antiresorportive therapy on vertebral density in osteoporotic postmenopausal women. *Arch. Intern. Med.* 1989; 149 (1): 57–60.

109. Szucs, J., E. Horvath, E. Kollin, et al. [Treatment of postmenopausal osteoporosis with low doses of calcitonin and calcitonin-anabolic combination.] *Orv. Hetil.* 1992; 133 (23): 1414–1418.

110. Hassager, C., and C. Christiansen. Epidemiology, biochemistry and some results with treatment of postmenopausal osteoporosis. *Wein. Med. Wochenscher.* 1993; 143 (14–15): 389–395.

111. Need, A.G., T.C. Durbridge, and B.E. Nordin. Anabolic steroids in postmenopausal osteoporosis. *Wien. Med. Wochenschr.* 1993; 143 (14–15): 392–395.

112. Passeri, M. M. Pedrazzoni, G. Pioli, et al. Effects of nandrolone decanoate on bone mass in established osteoporosis. *Maturitas* 1993; 17 (3): 211–219.

113. Taylor, W.N., C. Alanis, and D.J. Wigley. Oral cyclical stanozolol and daily micronized 17–beta estradiol combination therapy for postmenopausal osteoporosis. *J. Neurol. Orthop. Med. Surg.* 1994; 15: 25–29.

114. Lyritis, G.P., C. Androulakis, B. Magiasis, et al. Effect of nandrolone

decanoate and 1–alpha-hydroxy-calciferol on patients with vertebral osteoporotic collapse. A double-blind clinical trial. *Bone Miner.* 1994; 27 (4): 209–217.

115. Erdsieck, R.J., H.A. Pols, C. van Kuijk, et al. Course of bone mass during and after hormonal replacement therapy with and without addition of nandrolone decanoate. *J. Bone Miner. Res.* 1994; 9 (2): 277–283.

116. Di Renzo, G.C., G. Coata, E.V. Cosmi, et al. Management of postmenopausal osteoporosis. *Eur. J. Obstet. Gynecol. Reprod. Biol.* 1994; 56 (1): 47–53.

117. Watts, N.B., M. Notelovitgs, M.C. Timmons, et al. Comparison of oral estrogens and estrogens plus androgen on bone mineral density, menopausal symptoms, and lipid-lipoprotein profiles in surgical menopause. *Obstet. Gynecol.* 1995; 85 (4): 529–537.

118. Lyritis, G.P., S. Karpathios, K. Basdekis, et al. Prevention of post-oophorectomy bone loss with tibolone. *Maturitas* 1995; 22 (3): 247–253.

119. Raisz, L.G., B. Wiita, A. Artis, et al. Comparison of the effects of estrogen alone and estrogen plus androgen on biochemical markers of bone formation and resorption in postmenopausal women. *J. Clin. Endocrinol. Metab.* 1996; 81 (1): 37–43.

120. Bjarnason, N. H., K. Bjarnason, J. Haarbo, et al. Tibolone: Prevention of bone loss in late postmenopausal women. *J. Clin. Endocrinol. Metab.* 1996; 81 (7): 2419–2422.

121. Berning, B., C.V. Kuijk, J.W. Kuiper, et al. Effects of two doses of tibolone on trabecular and cortical bone loss in early postmenopausal women: a two-year randomized, placebo-controlled study. *Bone* 1996; 19 (4): 395–399.

122. Bjarnason, N.H., K. Bjarnason, J. Haarbo, et al. Tibolone: prevention of bone loss in late postmenopausal women. *J. Clin. Endocrinol. Metab.* 1996; 81 (7): 2419–2422.

123. Labrie, F., P. Diamond, L. Cusan, et al. Effect of 12–month dehydroepiandrosterone replacement therapy on bone, vagina, and endometrium in postmenopausal women. *J. Clin. Endocrinol. Metab.* 1997; 82 (10): 3498–3505.

124. Flicker, L., J.L. Hopper, R.G. Larkins, et al. Nandrolone decanoate and intranasal calcitonin as therapy for established osteoporosis. *Osteoporos. Int.* 1997; 7 (1): 29–35.

125. Bjarnason, N.H., K. Bjarnason, C. Hassager, et al. The response in spinal bone mass to tibolone treatment is related to bone turnover in elderly women. *Bone* 1997; 20 (2): 151–155.

126. Phillips, E., and C. Bauman. Safety surveillance of esterified estrogens-methyltestosterone (Estratest and Estratest HS) replacement therapy in the United States. *Clin. Ther.* 1997; 19 (5): 1070–1084.

127. Studd, J., Arnala, I., P.M. Kicovic et al. A randomized study of tibolone on bone mineral density in osteoporotic postmenopausal women with previous fractures. *Obstet. Gynecol.* 1998; 92 (4): 547–549.

128. Reginster, J.Y., V. Halkin, Y. Henrotin, et al. Treatment of osteoporosis: role of bone-forming agents. *Osteoporosis Int.* 1999; 9 (Suppl. 2): 291–96.

129. Castelo-Branco, C., J.J. Vicente, F. Figueras, et al. Comparative effects of estrogens plus androgens and tibolone on bone, lipid pattern and sexuality in postmenopausal women. *Maturitas* 2000; 34 (2): 161–168.

130. Barrett-Conner, E., R. Young, M. Notelovitz, et al. A two-year, double-blind comparison of estrogen-androgen and conjugated estrogens in surgically menopausal women. Effects on bone mineral density, symptoms and lipid profiles. *J. Reprod. Med.* 1999; 44 (12): 1012–1020.

131. Castelo-Branco, C., J.J. Vincent, F. Figueras, et al. Comparative effects of estrogens plus androgens and tibolone on bone, lipid pattern and sexuality in postmenopausal women. *Maturitas* 2000; 34 (2): 161–168.

132. Lyritis, G.P., S. Karpathios, K. Basdekis, et al. Prevention of post-oophorectomy bone loss with tibolone. *Maturitas* 1995; 22 (3): 247–253.

133. Adachi, J.D. Current treatment options for osteoporosis. *J. Rheumatol. Suppl.* 1996; 45: 11–14.

134. Riggs, B.L. Editorial: Tibolone as an alternative to estrogen for the prevention of postmenopausal osteoporosis in selected postmenopausal women. *J. Clin. Endocrinol. Metab.* 1996; 81 (7): 2417–2418.

135. Albertazzi, P., R. Di Micco, and E. Zanardi. Tibolone: a review. *Maturitas* 1998; 30 (3): 295–305.

136. Rako, S. Testosterone supplemental therapy after hysterectomy with or without concomitant oophorectomy: estrogen alone is not enough. *J. Womens Health Gend. Based Med.* 2000; 9 (8): 917–923.

137. Frackiewicz, E.J., and N.R. Cutler. Women's heath care during the perimenopause. *J. Am. Pharm. Assoc. (Wash.)* 2000; 40 (6): 800–811.

138. Wimalawansa, S.J. Prevention and treatment of osteoporosis: efficacy of combination of hormone replacement therapy with other antiresorptive agents. *J. Clin. Densitom.* 2000; 3 (2): 197–201.

139. Martin-Du Pan, R.C., and F. Luzuy. [What's new in hormone replacement therapy for postmenopausal women? I. Advantages of hormone replacement therapy.] *Rev. Med. Suisse Romande* 2000; 120 (6): 515–521.

140. Baulieu, E.E., G. Thomas, S. Legrain, et al. Dehyroepiandrosterone (DHEA), DHEA sulfate, and aging: contribution of the DHEAage Study to a sociobiomedical issue. *Proc. Natl. Acad. Sci. USA* 2000; 11 (97-8): 4279–4284.

141. Floter, A., K. Carlstrom, B. von Schoultz, et al. Administration of testosterone undecanoate in postmenopausal women: effects on androgens, estradiol, and gonadotrophins. *Menopause* 2000; 7 (4): 251–256.

142. Geusens, P., J. Dequeker, A. Verstraeten, et al. Bone mineral content, cortical thickness and fracture rate in osteoporotic women after withdrawal of treatment with nandrolone decanoate, 1–alpha hydroxyvitamin D3, or intermittent calcium infusions. *Maturitas* 1986; 8 (4): 281–289.

143. Erdtsieck, R.J., H.A. Pols, C. Kuijk, et al. Course of bone mass during and after hormonal replacement therapy with and without addition of nandrolone decanoate. *J. Bone Miner. Res.* 1994; 9 (2): 227–283.

144. Couch, M., F.E. Preston, R.G. Malia, et al. Changes in plasma osteocalcin concentrations following treatment with stanozolol. *Clin. Chim. Acta* 1986; 158: 43–47.

145. Vaischnav, R., J.N. Beresford, J.A. Gallagher, et al. Effects of anabolic steroid stanozolol on cells derived from human bone. *Clin. Sci.* 1988; 74: 455–460.

146. Gennari, C. D. Agnus Dei, S. Gonnelli, et al. Effects of nandrolone decanoate therapy on bone mass and calcium metabolism in women with established postmenopausal osteoporosis: a double-blind placebo-controlled study. *Maturitas* 1989; 11 (3): 187–197.

147. Beneton, M.N.C., A.J. P. Yates, S. Rogers, et al. Stanozolol stimulates remodeling of trabecular bone and net bone formation of bone at the endocortical surface. *Clin. Sci.* 1991; 81: 543–549.

148. Johansen, J.S., C. Hassager, J. Podenphant, et al. Treatment of postmenopausal osteoporosis: is the anabolic steroid nandrolone decanoate a candidate? *Bone Miner.* 1989; 6 (1): 77–86.

149. Erdtsieck, R.J., H.A. Pols, C. van Kuijk, et al. Course of bone mass during and after hormonal replacement therapy with and without addition of nandrolone decanoate. *J. Bone Miner. Res.* 1994; 9 (2): 277–283.

150. Lovejoy, J.C., G.A. Bray, M.O. Bourgeois, et al. Exogenous androgens

influence body composition and regional body fat distribution in obese postmenopausal women's clinical research center study. *J. Clin. Endocrinol. Metab.* 1996; 81 (6): 2198–2203.

151. Bonnefoy, M., T. Kostka, M. C. Patricot, et al. Physical activity and dehydroepiandrosterone sulfate, insulin-like growth factor 1 and testosterone in healthy active elderly people. *Age Aging* 1998; 27 (6): 745–751.

152. De Lorenzo, A., S. Lello, A. Andreoli, et al. Body composition and androgen pattern in the early period of postmenopause. *Gynecol. Endocrinol.* 1998; 12 (3): 171–177.

153. Casson, P.R., N. Santoro, K. Elkind-Hirsch, et al. Postmenopausal dehydroepidandrosterone administration increases free insulin-like growth factor-1 and decreases high-density lipoprotein: a six-month trial. *Fertil. Steril.* 1998; 70 (1): 107–110.

154. Dionne, I.J, K.A. Kinaman, and E.T. Poehlman. Sarcopenia and muscle function during menopause and hormone-replacement therapy. *J. Nutr. Health Aging* 2000; 4 (3): 156–161.

155. Kostka, T., L. M. Arsac, M.C. Patricot, et al. Leg extensor power and dehydroepiandrosterone sulfate, insulin-like growth factor-1 and testosterone in healthy active elderly people. *Eur. J. Appl. Physiol.* 2000; 82 (1–2): 83–90.

156. Taaffe, D.R., and R. Marcus. Musculoskeletal health and the older adult. *J. Rehabil. Res. Dev.* 2000; 37 (2): 245–254.

157. Fruehan, A.E., and T.F. Frawley. Current status of anabolic steroids. *JAMA* 1963; 184 (7): 527–532.

158. Parson, L., and S.C. Sommers. *Gynecology.* Philadelphia and London: W.B. Saunders Company, 1962, p. 1056.

159. Williams, R.H. *Textbook of Endocrinology.* Philadelphia and London: W.B. Saunders Company, 1962, p. 500.

160. Beeson, P.B., and W. McDermott. *Textbook of Medicine.* Philadelphia and London: W.B. Saunders Company, 1963, p. 1501.

161. Goodman, L.S., and A. Gilman. *The Pharmacological Basis of Therapeutics.* Toronto and London: The Macmillian Company, 1970, p. 1576.

162. Krusen, F.H. *Physical Medicine and Rehabilitation.* Philadelphia, London, and Toronto: W.B. Saunders Company, 1971, p. 563.

163. Revised package insert for Winstrol (stanozolol), Winthrop Laboratories, New York, 1965.

164. Revised package insert for Winstrol (stanozolol), Winthrop Laboratories, New York, 1971.

165. Revised package insert for Dianabol (menandrostenedione), Ciba Laboratories, New York, 1980.

166. Harrison, T.R. *Principles of Internal Medicine* (eighth edition). New York: McGraw-Hill Book Company, 1977, p. 2032.

167. Harrison, T.R. *Principles of Internal Medicine* (eighth edition). New York: McGraw-Hill Book Company, 1977, pp. 606–612.

168. Woodward, D. Treating of osteoporosis (letter). *N. Engl. J. Med.* 1984; 312 (10): 647.

169. Taylor, W.N. *Anabolic Steroids and the Athlete.* Jefferson, N.C.: McFarland & Company, Inc., Publishers, 1982.

170. Haupt, H.A., and G.D. Rovere. Anabolic steroids: a review of the literature. *Am.J. Sports Med.* 1984; 12 (6): 469–484.

171. Taylor, W.N. *Macho Medicine: A History of the Anabolic Steroid Epidemic.* Jefferson, N.C.: McFarland & Company, Inc., Publishers, 1991.

172. Taylor, W.N. *Hormonal Manipulation: A New Era of Monstrous Athletes* Jefferson, N.C.: McFarland & Company, Inc., Publishers, 1985.

173. Taylor, W.N. Synthetic anabolic-androgenic steroids: A plea for controlled substance status. *Physician Sportsmed.* 1987; 15 (5): 140–150.

174. Taylor, W.N. Drug issues in sports medicine, part 1: Steroid abuse and non-steroidal anti-inflammatory (NSAID) selection in athletic/active patients. *J. Neurol. Orthop. Med. Surg.* 1988; 992): 159–164.

175. Taylor, W.N. *Anabolic Steroids and the Athlete* (2nd edition). Jefferson, N.C.: McFarland & Company, Inc., Publishers, 2001.

176. Redmond, G. *The Good News About Women's Hormones.* New York: Warner Books, Inc. 1995, p. 63.

177. Taylor, W.N. *Osteoporosis: Medical Blunders and Treatment Strategies.* Jefferson, N.C.: McFarland & Company, Inc., Publishers, 1996.

178. Harrison, T.R, II, and A.S. Fauci. *Principles of Internal Medicine* (14th Platinum edition) New York, McGraw-Hill Health Professions Division, 2000, p. 2252.

179. Wilmore, D.H. Impediments to the successful use of anabolic agents in clinical care. *J. Parenter, Enteral Nutr.* 1999; 23 (6 Suppl.): S210–213.

180. Lockefeer, J.H. [Revision consensus osteoporosis.] *Ned. Tijdschr. Geneeskd.* 1992; 136 (25): 1204–1209.

181. Casson, P.R., N. Santoro, K. Eldind-Hirsch, et al. Postmenopausal dehydroepiandrosterone administration increases free insulin-like growth factor-1 and decreases high-density h lipoprotein: a six month trial. *Fertil. Steril.* 1998; 70 (1): 107–110.

182. Legrain, S., C. Massien, N. Lahlou, et al. Dehydroepiandrosterone replacement administration: pharmacokinetic and pharmacodynamic studies in healthy elderly subjects. *J. Clin. Endocrinol. Metab.* 2000; 85 (9): 3208–3217.

183. Baulieu, E.E., G. Thomas, S. Legrain, et al. Dehydroepiandrosterone (DHEA), DHEA sulfate, and aging: contribution of the DHEAage Study to a socio-biomedical issue. *Proc. Natl. Acad. Sci. USA* 2000; 97 (8): 4279–4284.

184. Chesnut, C.H., J.L. Ivey, H.E. Gruber, et al. Stanozolol in postmenopausal osteoporosis: therapeutic efficacy and possible mechanisms of action. *Metabolism* 1983; 32 (6): 571–580.

185. Gennari, C., D. Agnus Dei, S. Gonnelli, et al. Effects of nandrolone decanoate therapy on bone mass and calcium metabolism in women with established postmenopausal osteoporosis: a double-blind placebo-controlled study. *Maturitas* 1988; 11 (3): 187–197.

186. Beneton, M.N.C., A.J.P. Yates, S. Rogers, et al. Stanozolol stimulates remodeling of trabecular bone and net formation of bone at the endocortical surface. *Clin. Sci.* 1991; 543–549.

187. Khosla, S. The effects of androgens on osteoblast function in vitro. *Mayo Clin. Proc.* 2000; 75 (Suppl.): S51–54.

188. Gori, F., L.C. Hofbauer, C.A. Conover, et al. Effects of androgens on the insulin-like growth factor system in an androgen-responsive human osteoblast cell line. *Endocrinology* 1999; 149 (12): 5579–5586.

189. Labrie, F., A. Belanger, V. Luu-The, et al. DHEA and the intracrine formation of androgens and estrogens in peripheral target tissues: its role during aging. *Steroids* 1998; 63 (5–6): 322–328.

190. Cosman, F., J. Nieves, C. Wilkinson, et al. Bone density change and biochemical indices of skeletal turnover. *Calcif. Tissue Int.* 1996; 58 (4): 236–243.

191. Dresner-Pollak, R., R.A. Parker, M. Poku, et al. Biochemical markers of bone turnover reflect femoral bone loss in elderly women. *Calcif. Tissue Int.* 1996; 59 (5): 328–333.

192. Ganero, P., and P.D. Delmas. New developments in biochemical markers for osteoporosis. *Calcif. Tissue Int.* 1996; 59 (7): 2–9.

193. Russell, R.G. The assessment of bone metabolism in vivo using biochemical approaches. *Horm. Metab. Res.* 1997; 29 (3): 138–144.

194. Eyre, D.R. Bone biomarkers as tools in osteoporosis management. *Spine* 1997; 22 (24 Suppl.): 17S–24S.

195. Ganero, P., and P.D. Delmas. Biochemical markers of bone turnover. Applications for osteoporosis. *Endocrinol. Metab. Clin. North Am.* 1998; 27 (2): 303–323.

196. Fink, E., C. Cornier, P. Steinmetz, et al. Differences in the capacity of several biochemical bone markers to assess high bone turnover in early menopause and response to alendronate therapy. *Osteoporos. Int.* 2000; 11 (4): 295–303.

197. Christenson, R.H. Biochemical markers of bone metabolism: an overview. *Clin. Biochem.* 1997; 30 (8): 573–593.

198. Adachi, J.D. The correlation of bone mineral density and biochemical markers to fracture risk. *Calcif. Tissue Int.* 1996; 59 (7): 16–19.

199. Seibel, M.J., and H.W. Woitge. Basic principles and clinical applications of biochemical markers of bone metabolism: biochemical and technical aspects. *J. Clin. Densitom.* 1999; 2 (3): 299–321.

200. Hunter, D.J., and P.N. Sambrook. Bone loss: Epidemology of bone loss. *Arthritis Res.* 2000; 2 (6): 441–445.

201. Couch, M., F.E. Preston, R.G. Malia, et al. Changes in plasma osteocalcin concentrations following treatment with stanozolol. *Clin. Chim. Acta* 1986; 158: 43–47.

202. Gennari, C., D. Agnus Dei, S. Gonnelli, et al. Effects of nandrolone decanoate therapy on bone mass and calcium metabolism in women with established postmenopausal osteoporosis: a double-blind placebo-controlled study. *Maturitas* 1989; 11 (3): 187–197.

203. Bjarnason, N.K., K. Bjarnason, J. Haarbo, et al. Tibolone: Prevention of bone loss in late postmenopausal women. *J. Clin. Endocrinol. Metab.* 1996; 81 (7): 2419–2422.

204. Raisz, L.G., B. Wiita, A. Artis, et al. Comparison of the effects of estrogen alone and estrogen plus androgen on biochemical markers of bone formation and resorption in postmenopausal women. *J. Clin. Endocrinol. Metab.* 1996; 81 (1): 37–43.

205. Bjarnason, N.H., K. Bjarnason, C. Hassager, et al. The response in spinal bone mass to tibolone treatment is related to bone turnover in elderly women. *Bone* 1997; 20 (2): 151–155.

206. Labrie, F., P. Diamond, L. Cusan, et al. Effect of 12–month dehydroepiandrosterone replacement therapy on bone, vagina, and endometrium in postmenopausal women. *J. Clin. Endocrinol. Metab.* 1997; 82 (10): 3498–3505.

207. Albertazzi, P., R. Di Micco, and E. Zanardi. Tibolone: a review. *Maturitas* 1998; 30 (3): 295–305.

208. Taylor, W.N., and C. Alanis. Triple sex steroid replacement therapy for osteoporosis after surgical menopause. *J. Neurol. Orthop. Med. Surg.* 1992; 13: 16–19.

209. Passeri, M., M. Pedrazzoni, G. Pioli, et al. Effects of nandrolone decanoate on bone mass in established osteoporosis. *Maturitas* 1993; 17 (3): 211–219.

210. Taylor, W.N., C. Alanis, and D.J. Wigley. Oral cyclical stanozolol and daily micronized 17–beta estradiol combination therapy for postmenopausal osteoporosis: A preliminary report. *J. Neurol. Orthop. Med. Surg.* 1994; 15: 25–29.

211. Di Renzo, G.C., G. Coata, E.V. Cosmi, et al. Management of postmenopausal osteoporosis. *Eur. J. Obstet. Gynecol. Reprod. Biol.* 1994; 56 (1): 47–53.

212. Lyritis, G.P., C. Androulakis, B. Magiasis, et al. Effect of nandrolone decanoate and 1–alpha-hydroxy-calciferol on patients with vertebral osteoporotic collapse. A double-blind clinical trial. *Bone Miner.* 1994; 27 (3): 209–217.

213. Labrie, F., P. Diamond, L. Cusan, et al. Effect of 12-month dehydroepiandrosterone replacement therapy on bone, vagina, and endometrium in postmenopausal women. *J. Clin. Endocrinol. Metab.* 1997; 82 (10): 3498–3505.

214. Flicker, L., J.L. Hopper, R.G. Larkins, et al. Nandrolone decanoate and intranasal calcitonin as therapy in established osteoporosis. *Osteoporos. Int.* 1997; 7 (1): 29–35.

215. Studd, J., I. Arnala, P.M. Kicovic, et al. A randomized study of tibolone on bone mineral density in osteoporotic postmenopausal women with previous fractures. *Obstet. Gynecol.* 1998; 92 (4): 574–579.

216. Beardsworth, S.A., C.E. Kearney, and D.W. Purdie. Prevention of postmenopausal bone loss at lumbar spine and upper femur with tibolone: a two-year randomized controlled trial. *Br. J. Obstet.Gynaecol.* 1999; 106 (7): 678–683.

217. Pavolv, P.W., J. Ginsburg, P.M. Kicovic, et al. Double-blind, placebo-controlled study of the effects of tibolone on bone mineral density in postmenopausal osteoporotic women with and without previous fractures. *Gynecol. Endocrinol.* 1999; 13 (4): 230–237.

218. Raisz, L.G., B. Wiita, A. Artis, et al. Comparison of the effects of estrogen alone and estrogen plus androgen on biochemical markers of bone formation and resorption in postmenopausal women. *J. Clin. Endocrinol. Metab.* 1996; 81 (1): 37–43.

219. Barrett-Conner, E., R. Young, M. Notelovitz, et al. A two-year, double-blind comparison of estrogen-androgen and conjugated estrogens in surgically menopausal women. Effects on bone mineral density, symptoms, and lipid profiles. *J. Reprod. Med.* 1999; 44 (12): 1012–1020.

220. Castelo-Branco, C., J.J. Vicente, F. Figueras, et al. Comparative effects of estrogens plus androgens and tibolone on bone, lipid pattern and sexuality in postmenopausal women. *Maturitas* 2000; 34 (2): 161–168.

221. Passeri, M., M. Pedrazzoni, G. Pioli, et al. Effects of nandrolone decanoate on bone mass in established osteoporosis. *Maturitas* 1993; 17 (3): 211–219.

222. Lyritis, G.P., C. Androulakis, B. Magiasis, et al. Effect of nandrolone decanoate and 1-alpha-hyeroxy-calciferol on patients with vertebral osteoporotic collapse. A double-blind clinical trial. *Bone Miner.* 1994; 27 (3): 209–217.

223. Chesnut, C.H., J.L. Ivey, H.E. Gruber, et al. Stanozolol in postmenopausal osteoporosis: therapeutic efficacy and possible mechanisms of action. *Metabolism* 1983; 32 (6): 571–580.

224. Geusens. P., J. Dequeker, A. Verstaeten, et al. Bone mineral content, cortical thickness and fracture rate in osteoporotic women after withdrawal of treatment with nandrolone decanoate, 1-alpha hydroxyvitamin D3, or intermittent calcium infusions. *Maturitas* 1986; 8 (4): 281–289.

225. Eakman, G.D., J.S. Dallas, S.W. Ponder, et al. The effects of testosterone and dihydrotestosterone on hypothalamic regulation of growth hormone secretion. *J. Clin. Endocrinol. Metab.* 1996; 81 (3): 1217–1223.

226. Genazzani, A.D., O. Gamba, L. Nappi, et al. Modulatory effects of synthetic steroid (tibolone) and estradiol on spontaneous and GHRH-induced GH secretion in postmenopausal women. *Maturitas* 1997; 28 (1): 27–33.

227. Hobbs, C.J., S.R. Plymate, C.J. Rosen, et al. Testosterone administration increases insulin-like growth factor-1 levels in normal men. *J. Clin. Endocrinol. Metab.* 1994; 78 (6): 1360–1367.

228. Morales, A.J., J.J. Nolan, J.C. Nelson, et al. Effects of replacement dose of dehydroepiandrosterone in men and women of advancing age. *J. Clin. Endocrinol. Metab.* 1994; 78 (6): 1360–1367.

229. Gelato, M.C., and R.A. Frost. IGFBP-3. Functional and structural implications in aging and wasting syndromes. *Endocrine* 1997; 7 (1): 81–85.

230. Casson, P.R., N. Santoro, K. Elkind-Hirsch, et al. Postmenopausal dehydroepiandrosterone administration increases free insulin-like growth factor-1 and decreases high-density lipoprotein: a six month trial. *Fertil. Steril.* 1998; 70 (1): 107–110.

231. Jorgensen, J.O., N. Vahl, T.B. Hansen, et al. Determinants of serum insulin-like growth factor 1 in growth hormone deficient adults as compared to healthy subjects. *Clin. Endocrinol. (Oxf.)* 1998; 48 (4): 479–486.

232. Morales, A.J., R.H. Haubrich, J.Y. Hwang, et al. The effects of six months treatment with 100mg daily dose of dehydroepiandrosterone (DHEA) on circulating sex steroids, body composition, and muscle strength in age-advanced men and women. *Clin. Endocrinol. (Oxf.)* 1998; 49 (4): 421–434.

233. Span, J.P., G.F. Pieters, C.G. Sweep, et al. Gender difference in insulin-like growth factor-1 response to growth hormone (GH) treatment and GH-deficient adults: role of sex hormone replacement. *J. Clin. Endocrinol. Metab.* 2000; 85 (3): 1121–1125.

234. Savine, R., and P. Sonksen. Growth hormone — hormone replacement for somatopause? *Horm. Res.* 2000; 53 (Suppl. 3): 37–41.

235. Ovesen, P., J. Moller, J.O. Jorgensen, et al. Effect of growth hormone administration on circulating levels of luteinizing hormone, follicle stimulating hormone, and testosterone in normal healthy men. *Hum. Reprod.* 1993; 8 (11): 1869–1872.

236. Lee, P.D., S.K. Durham, V. Martinez, et al. Kinetics of insulin-like growth factor (IGF) and IGF-binding protein responses to a single dose of growth hormone. *J. Clin. Endocrinol. Metab.* 1997; 82 (7): 2266–2274.

237. Cuttica, C.M., L. Castoldi, G.P. Gorrini, et al. Effects of six-month administration of recombinant human growth hormone to healthy elderly adults. *Aging (Milano)* 1997; 9 (3): 193–197.

238. Lemmey, A.B., J. Glassford, H.C. Flick-Smith, et al. Different regulation of tissue insulin-like growth factor-binding protein (IGFBP)-3, IGF-1, and IGF type 1 receptor mRNA levels, serum IGF-1 and IGFBP concentrations by growth hormone and IGF-1. *J. Endocrinol.* 1997; 154 (2): 319–328.

239. Nilsson, A., D. Swolin, S. Enerback, et al. Expression of functional growth hormone receptors in cultured human osteoblast-like cells. *J. Clin. Endocrinol. Metab.* 1995; 80 (12): 3483–3488.

240. Ghiron, L.J., J.L. Thompson, L. Holloway, et al. Effects of recombinant insulin-like growth factor-1 and growth hormone on bone turnover in elderly women. *J. Bone Miner. Res.* 1995; 10 (12): 1844–1852.

241. Baum, H.B., B.M. Miller, J.S. Finkelstein, et al. Effects of physiologic growth hormone therapy on bone density and body composition in patients with adult-onset growth hormone deficiency. A randomized, placebo-controlled trial. *Ann. Intern. Med.* 1996; 125 (11): 883–890.

242. Murphy, M.G., M.A. Bach, D. Plotkin, et al. Oral administration of the growth hormone secretagogue MK-677 increases markers of bone turnover in healthy and functionally impaired elderly adults. The MK-677 Study Group. *J. Bone Miner. Res.* 1999; 14 (7): 1182–1188.

243. Johansson, A.G., E. Lindh, W.F. Blum, et al. Effects of growth hormone and insulin-like growth factor-1 in men with idiopathic osteoporosis. *J. Clin. Endocrinol. Metab.* 1996; 81 (1): 44–48.

244. Isaksson, O.C., C. Ohisson, B.A. Bengsston, et al. GH and boneùexperimental and clinical studies. *Endocr. J.* 2000; 47 (Suppl.): S9–S16.

245. Ohlsson, C., J.O. Jansson, and O. Isaksson. Effects of growth hormone and insulin-like growth factor-1 on body growth and adult bone metabolism. *Curr. Opin. Rheumatol.* 2000; 12 (4): 246–248.

246. Ghiron, L.J., J.L. Thompson, L. Holloway, et al. Effects of recombinant

insulin-like growth factor-1 and growth hormone on bone turnover in elderly women. *J. Bone Miner. Res.* 1995; 10 (12): 1844–1852.

247. Sherwin, B.B., and M.M. Gelfand. Effects of parenteral administration of estrogen and androgen on plasma hormone levels and hot flushes in the surgical menopause. *Am. J. Obstet. Gynecol.* 1984; 148: 552–556.

248. Burger, H.G., J. Hailes, M. Melelaus, et al. The management of persistent symptoms with estradiol-testosterone implants: clinical, lipid and hormonal results. *Maturitas* 1984; 6: 351–358.

249. Sherwin, B.B., and M.M. Gelfand. Sex steroids and their effect in the surgical menopause: A double-blind, cross-over study. *Psychoneuroendocrinol.* 1985; 10 (3): 325–335.

250. Foster, G.V., H.A. Zacur, and J.A. Rock. Hot flashes in postmenopausal women ameliorated by danazol. *Fertil. Steril.* 1985; 43 (3): 401–404.

251. Sherwin, B.B., and M.M. Gelfand. Differential symptom response to parenteral estrogen and/or androgen administration in the surgical menopause. *Am. J. Obstet. Gynecol.* 1985; 151 (2): 153–160.

252. Burger, H.G., J. Hailes, J. Nelson, et al. Effect of combined implants of estradiol and testosterone on libido in postmenopausal women. *Br. Med. J.* 1987; 294: 936–937.

253. Sherwin, B.B., and M.M. Gelfand. The role of androgen in the maintenance of sexual functioning in oophorectomized women. *Psychosom. Med.* 1987; 49: 397–402.

254. Taylor, W.N., and C. Alanis. Triple sex steroid replacement therapy for osteoporosis after surgical menopause. *J. Neurol. Orthop. Med. Surg.* 1992; 13: 16–19.

255. Palacios, S., C. Menendez, and A.R. Jurado. Changes in sex behavior after menopause: effects of tibolone. *Maturitas* 1995; 22 (2): 155–161.

256. Raisz, L.G., B. Wiita, A. Artis, et al. Comparison of the effects of estrogen alone and estrogen plus androgen on biochemical markers of bone formation and resorption in postmenopausal women. *J. Clin. Endocrinol. Metab.* 1996; 81 (1): 37–43.

257. Argyroudis, E.M., G. Iatrakis, A. Kourkoubas, et al. Tibolone in the treatment of psychosomatic symptoms in menopause. *Clin. Exp. Obstet. Gynecol.* 1997; 24 (3): 167–168.

258. Nathorst-Boos, and M. Hammar. Effect of sexual life — a comparison between tibolone and a continuous estradiol-norethisterone acetate regimen. *Maturitas* 1997; 26 (1): 15–20.

259. Warnock, J.K., J.C. Bundren, and D.W. Morris. Female hypoactive sexual desire disorder due to androgen deficiency: clinical and psychometric issues. *Psycholpharmacol. Bull.* 1997; 33 (4): 761–766.

260. Sarrel, P., B. Dobay, and B. Witta. Estrogen and estrogen-androgen replacement in postmenopausal women dissatisfied with estrogen-only therapy. Sexual behavior and neuroendocrine responses. *J. Reprod. Med.* 1998; 43 (10): 847–856.

261. Hammar, M., S. Chrisau, J. Nathosrt-Boos, et al. A double-blind, randomized trial of comparing the effects of tibolone and continuous combined hormone replacement therapy in postmenopausal women with menopausal symptoms. *Br. J. Obstet. Gynaecol.* 1998; 105 (8): 904–911.

262. Ross, L.A., E.M. Alder, E.H. Cawood, et al. Psychological effects of hormone replacement therapy: a comparison of tibolone and sequential estrogen therapy. *J. Psychosom. Obstet. Gynaecol.* 1999; 20 (2): 88–96.

263. Barrett-Conner, E., R. Young, M. Notelovitz, et al. A two-year, double-blind comparison of estrogen-androgen and conjugated estrogens in surgically menopausal women. Effects on bone mineral density, symptoms and lipid profiles. *J. Reprod. Med.* 1999; 44 (12): 1012–1020.

264. Rako, S. Testosterone supplementation therapy after hysterectomy with or without concomitant oophorectomy: estrogen alone is not enough. *J. Womens Health Gend. Based Med.* 2000; 9 (8): 917–923.

265. Greenblatt, R.B. Androgenic therapy in women. *J. Clin. Endocrinol. Metab.* 1942; 2: 65–66.

266. Goldman, A. Androgen therapy in women. *J. Clin. Endocrinol. Metab.* 1942; 2: 750.

267. Salmon, U.J., and S.H. Geist. Effect of androgens upon libido in women. *J. Clin. Endocrinol. Metab.* 1943; 3: 235–238.

268. Greenblatt, R.B., W.E. Barfield, J.F. Garner, et al. Evaluation of an estrogen, androgen, estrogen-androgen combination, and a placebo in the treatment of the menopause. *J. Clin. Endocrinol. Metab.* 1950; 10: 1547–1558.

269. Masters, W.H., and D.T. Magallon. Androgen administration in the postmenopausal woman. *J. Clin. Endocrinol. Metab.* 1950; 10: 348–358.

270. Glass, S.J. The advantages of combined estrogen-androgen therapy in the menopause. *J. Clin. Endocrinol. Metab.* 1950; 10: 1611–1617.

271. Henneman, P.H., and S. Wallach. The use of androgens and estrogens and their metabolic effects: A review of prolonged use of estrogens and androgens in postmenopausal and senile osteoporosis. *Arch. Intern. Med.* 1957; 100: 715–723.

272. Simon, J., E. Klaiber, B. Wiita, et al. Differential effects of estrogen-androgen and estrogen-only therapy on vasomotor symptoms, gonadotrophin secretion, and endogenous androgen bioavailability in postmenopausal women. *Menopause* 1999; 6 (2): 138–146.

273. Castelo-Branco, C., E. Caslas, F. Figeruas, et al. Two-year prospective and comparative study on the effects of tibolone on lipid pattern, behavior of apolipoprotein A1 and B. *Menopause* 1999; 6 (2): 92–97.

274. Casson, P.R., K.E. Elkind, J.E. Buster, et al. Effect of postmenopausal estrogen replacement on circulating androgens. *Obstet. Gynecol.* 1997; 90 (6): 995–998.

275. Simon, J., E. Klaiber, B. Wiita, et al. Differential effects of estrogen-androgen and estrogen-only therapy on vasomotor symptoms, gonadotrophin secretion, and endogenous androgen bioavailability in postmenopausal women. *Menopause* 1999; 6 (2): 138–146.

276. Kleinrok, Z., and M. Siekulka-Dziuba. [Androgens and the brain.] *Gienkol. Pol.* 1994; 65 (1): 45–50.

277. Schumacher, M., P. Robel, E.E. Baulieu, et al. Development and regeneration of the nervous system: role for neurosteroids. *Dev. Neurosci.* 1996; 18 (1–2): 6–21.

278. Schumacher, M., F. Robert, and E.E. Baulieu. [Neurosteroids: trophic effects in the nervous system.] *J. Soc. Biol.* 1999; 193 (3): 285–292.

279. Jordan, C.L. Glia as mediators of steroid hormone action on the nervous system: an overview. *J. Neurobiol.* 1999; 40 (4): 434–445.

280. Zwain, I.H., and S.S. Yen. Dehydroepiandrosterone: biosynthesis and function. *Endocrinology* 1999; 140 (2): 880–887.

281. Robel, P., and E.E. Baulieu. Neurosteroids: biosynthesis and function. *Crit. Rev. Neurobiol.* 1995; 9 (4): 383–394.

282. Baulieu, E.E., and R. Robel. Neurosteroids: a new brain function? *J. Steroid Biochem. Mol. Biol.* 1990; 37 (3): 395–403.

283. Celotti, F., P. Negri-Cesi, and A. Poletti. Steroid metabolism in the mammalian brain: 5alpha-reduction and aromatization. *Brain. Bull.* 1997; 44 (4): 365–375.

284. Tsutsui, K., K. Ukena, M. Usui, et al. Novel brain function: biosynthesis and actions of neurosteroids in neurons. *Neurosci. Res.* 2000; 36 (4): 261–273.

285. Su, T.P., M. Pagliaro, P.J. Schmidt, et al. Neuropsychiatric effects of anabolic steroids in male normal volunteers. *JAMA* 269 (21): 2760–2764.

286. Janne, O.A., J.J. Palvimo, P. Kallio, et al. Androgen receptor and mechanism of androgen action. *Ann. Med.* 1993; 25 (1): 83–89.

287. Rubinow, D.R., and P.J. Schmidt. Androgens, brain, and behavior. *Am. J. Psychiatry* 1996; 153 (8): 974–984.

288. Frye, C.A., K.R. Van Keuren, P.N. Rao, et al. Analgesic effects of the neurosteroid 3 alpha-androstanediol. *Brain. Res.* 1996; 709 (1): 1–9.

289. Lambert, J.J., D. Belelli, C. Hill-Venning, et al. Neurosteroid modulation of native and recombinant GABA (A) receptors. *Cell. Mol. Neurobiol.* 1996; 16 (2): 155–174.

290. Spindler, K.D. Interactions between steroid hormones and the nervous system. *Neurotoxicology* 1997; 18 (3): 745–754.

291. Zinder, O., and D.E. Dar. Neuroactive steroids: their mechanism of action and their function in the stress response. *Acta Physiol. Scand.* 1999; 167 (3): 181–188.

292. Park-Chung, M., A. Malyev, R.H. Purdy, et al. Sulfated and unsulfated steroids modulate gama-aminobutyric acid A receptor function through distinct sites. *Brain Res.* 1999; 830 (1): 72–87.

293. Maurice, T., V.L. Phan, A. Urani, et al. Neuroactive neurosteroids as endogenous effectors for the sigma 1 (sigma 1) receptor: pharmacological evidence and therapeutic opportunities. *JPn. J. Pharmacol.* 1999; 81 (2): 125–155.

294. Green, A.R., A.H. Hainsworth, and D.M. Jackson. GABA potentiation: a logical pharmacological approach for the treatment of acute ischaemic stroke. *Neuropharmacology* 2000; 39 (9): 1483–1494.

295. Baulieu, E.E. Neurosteroids: of the nervous system, by the nervous system, for the nervous system. *Recent. Prog. Horm. Res.* 1997; 52: 1–32.

296. Wolf, O.T., Neumann, O., D.H. Hellhammer, et al. Effects of a two-week physiological dehydroepiandrosterone substitution on cognitive performance and well-being in healthy elderly women and men. *J. Clin. Endocrinol. Metab.* 1997; 82 (7): 2363–2367.

297. Wolkowitz, O.M., V.I. Reus, E. Roberts, et al. Dehydroepiandrosterone (DHEA) treatment of depression. *Boil. Psychiatry* 1997; 41 (3): 311–318.

298. Rubino, S. M. Stomati, C. Bersi, et al. Neuroendocrine effect of a short-term treatment with DHEA in postmenopausal women. *Maturitas* 1998; 28 (3): 251–257.

299. Gasior, M., R.B. Carter, and J.M. Witkin. Neuroactive steroids: potential therapeutic use in neurological and psychiatric disorders. *Trends Pharmacol. Sci.* 1999; 22 (9): 20 (3): 107–112.

300. Van Honk, J., A. Tuiten, R. Verbaten, et al. Correlations among salivary testosterone, mood, and selective attention to threat in humans. *Horm. Behav.* 1999; 36 (1): 17–24.

301. Rupprecht, R., and F. Holsboer. Neuroactive steroids: mechanisms of action and neuropsychopharmacological perspectives. *Trends Neurosci.* 1999; 22 (9): 410–416.

302. Stomati, M., S. Rubino, A. Spinetti, et al. Endocrine, neuroendocrine and behavioral effects of oral dehydroepiandrosterone sulfate supplementation in postmenopausal women. *Gyencol. Endocrinol.* 1999; 13 (1): 15–25.

303. Lapchak, P.A., D.F. Chapman, S.Y. Nunez, et al. Dehydroepiandrosterone sulfate is neuroprotective in a reversible spinal cord ischemia model: a possible involvement of GABA (A) receptors. *Stroke* 2001; 31 (8): 1953–1957.

304. Yang, L.Y., and A.P. Arnold. Interaction of BDNF and testosterone in the regulation of adult perineal motoneurons. *J. Neurobiol.* 2000; 44 (3): 308–319.

305. Morrison, M.F., E. Redei, T. TenHave, et al. Dehydroepiandrosterone sulfate and psychiatric measures in a frail, elderly residential care population. *Biol. Pschiatry* 2000; 47 (2): 144–150.

306. Barbaccia, M.L., S. Lello, T. Sidiropoulou, et al. Plasma 5alpha-androstane-3alpha, 17betadiol, an endogenous steroid that positively modulates GABA (A) receptor function and anxiety: a study in menopausal women. *Psychoneuroendocrinology* 2000; 25 (7): 659–675.

307. Genazzani, A.R., F. Bernardi, P. Monteleone, et al. Neuropeptides, neurotransmitters, neurosteroids, and the onset of puberty. *Ann. N.Y. Acad. Sci.* 2000; 900: 1–9.

308. Johansson, P., A. Lindqvist, F. Nyberg, et al. Anabolic androgenic steroids affect alcohol intake, defensive behaviors and brain opioid peptides in the rat. *Pharmacol. Biochem. Behav.* 2000; 67 (2): 271–279.

309. Hillen, T., A. Lun, F.M. Reishies, et al. DHEA-S plasma levels and incidence of Alzheimer's disease. *Biol. Psychiatry* 2000; 47 (2): 161–163.

310. Drake, E.B., V.W. Henderson, F.Z. Stanczyk, et al. Associations between circulating sex steroid hormones and cognition in normal elderly women. *Neurology* 2000; 54 (3): 599–603.

311. Magri, F., F. Terenzi, T. Ricaciardi, et al. Associations between changes in adrenal secretion and cerebral morphometric correlates in normal aging and senile dementia. *Dement. Geriatr. Cogn. Disord.* 2000; 11 (2): 90–99.

312. Harlan, R.E., H.E. Brown, C.S. Lynch, et al. Androgenic-anabolic steroids blunt morphine-enduced c-fos expression in the rat striatum: possible role of beta-endorphin. *Brain. Res.* 2000; 853 (1): 99–104.

313. Semkova, I., and J. Krieglstein. Neuroprotection mediated via neurotrophic factors and induction of neurotrophic factors. *Brain Res. Brain Res. Rev.* 1999; 30 (2): 176–188.

314. Cardounel, A., W. Regelson, and M. Kalimi. Dehydroepiandrosterone protects hippocampal neurons against neurotoxic-induced cell death: mechanism of action. *Proc. Soc. Biol. Med.* 1999; 222 (2): 145–149.

315. Fox, H.S. Sex steroids and the immune system. *Ciba. Found. Symp.* 1995; 191: 203–211.

316. Loria, R.M., D.A. Padgett, and P.N. Huynh. Regulation of the immune system by dehydroepiandrosterone and its metabolites. *J. Endocrinol.* 1996; 150 (Suppl): S209–220.

317. Bebo, B.F., J.C. Schuster, A.A. Vanderbark, et al. Androgens alter the cytokine profile and reduce encephalogenicity in myelin-reactive T-cells. *J. Immunol.* 1999; 162 (1): 35–40.

318. Verthelyi, D., and D.M. Klinman. Sex hormone levels correlate with the activity of cytokine-secreting cells in vivo. *Immunology* 2000; 100 (3): 384–390.

319. Fahlman, M.M., D. Boardley, M.G. Flynn, et al. Effects of hormone replacement therapy on selected indices of immune function in postmenopausal women. *Gynecol. Obstet. Invest.* 2000; 50 (3): 189–193.

320. Hassager, C., B.J. Riis, J. Podephant, et al. Nandrolone decanoate treatment of post-menopausal osteoporosis for 2 years and effects of withdrawal. *Maturitas* 1994; 11 (4): 305–317.

321. Lyritis, G.P., C. Androulakis, B. Magiasis, et al. Effect of nandrolone and I-alpha-hydroxy-calciferol on patients with vertebral osteoporotic collapse. A double-blind clinical trial. *Bone Miner.* 1994; 27 (3): 209–217.

322. Albertazzi, P., R. Di Micco, and E. Zanardi. Tibolone: a review. *Maturitas* 1998; 30 (3): 295–305.

323. Raisz, L.G., B. Wiita, A. Artis, et al. Comparison of the effects of estrogen alone and estrogen plus androgen on biochemical markers of bone formation and resorption in postmenopausal women. *J. Clin. Endocrinol. Metab.* 1996; 81 (1): 37–43.

324. Barrett-Conner, E., R. Young, M. Notelovitz, et al. A two-year, double-blind comparison of estrogen-androgen and conjugated estrogens in surgically menopausal women. Effects on bone mineral density, symptoms and lipid profiles. *J. Reprod. Med.* 1999; 44 (12): 1012–1020.

325. Castelo-Branco, C., Vicente, J.J., F. Figueras, et al. Comparative effects of estrogens plus androgens and tibolone on bone, lipid pattern and sexuality in post-menopausal women. *Maturitas* 2000; 34 (2): 161–168.

326. Taylor, W.N., and C. Alanis. Triple sex steroid replacement therapy for osteoporosis after surgical menopause. *J. Neurol. Orthop, Med. Surg.* 1992; 13: 16–19.

327. Van Wersch, J.W., J.M. Ubachs, A. van den Ende, et al. The effects of two regimens of hormone replacement therapy on the haemostatic profile in postmenopausal women. *Eur. J. Clin. Chem. Biochem.* 1994; 32 (6): 449–453.

328. Glueck, C.J., R. Freiberg, H.I. Gleuck, et al. Idiopathic osteonecrosis, hypofibrinolysis, high plasminogen activator inhibitor, high lipoprotein (a), and therapy with stanozolol. *Am. J. Hematol.* 1995; 48 (4): 213–220.

329. Winkler, U.H., R. Altkemper, B. Kwee, et al. Effects of tibolone and continuous combined hormone replacement therapy on parameters in the clotting cascade: a multicenter, double-blind, randomized study. *Fertil. Steril.* 2000; 74 (1): 10–19.

330. Winkler, U.H. Effects of androgens on haemostasis. *Maturitas* 1996; 24 (3): 147–155.

331. Bjarnason, N.H., K. Bjarnason, J. Haarbo, et al. Tibolone: inffifluence on markers of cardiovascular disease. *J. Clin. Endocrinol. Metab.* 1997; 82 (6): 1752–1756.

332. Martin-Du, R.C. Pan, and F. Luzuy. [What's new in hormone replacement therapy of postmenopausal women? II. Risks of hormone replacement therapy.] *Rev. Med. Suisse Romande.* 2000; 120 (6): 523–527.

333. Oger, E., and P.Y. Scarabin. [Hormone replacement therapy in menopause and the risk of cerebrovascular accident.] *Ann. Endocrinol. (Paris)* 1999; 60 (3): 232–241.

334. Tavani, A., and C. La Vecchia. The adverse effects of hormone replacement therapy. *Drugs Aging* 1999; 14 (5): 347–357.

335. da Silva, J.A. and A. Porto. [Sex hormones and osteoporosis: a physiological perspective for prevention and therapy.] *Acta Med. Port.* 1997; 10 (10): 689–695.

336. Sands, R., and J. Studd. Exogenous androgens in postmenopausal women. *Am. J. Med.* 1995; 98 (1A): 76S–79S.

6

Rationale for Anabolic Therapy for Osteoporosis and Andropause in Men

Introduction: Andropause Contributes to Osteoporosis and Other Diseases in Men

Osteoporosis remains a substantial problem in aging men. Twenty-five to 30 percent of all hip fractures occur among older men,[1] and those who sustain a hip fracture have a higher mortality rate following the fracture than do women.[2] Hypoandrogenemia (low serum androgen level) is a major risk factor for osteoporosis in men.[3]

It has been well recognized that androgen production in men decreases progressively with a concomitant increase in luteinizing hormone (LH) levels with age after early adulthood.[4, 5] It is also well-recognized that hypoandrogenemia in men is associated with the pathogenesis of a number of diseases and conditions (such as osteoporosis, Type II diabetes, heart disease, stroke, and autoimmune diseases), adverse alterations in the neuroimmune system, and the genesis of andropause, sarcopenia, erectile dysfunction, and frailty. However, hypoandrogenemia in aging men and the associated disease conditions are often greatly underrecognized entities by clinicians.[6]

Several studies have reconfirmed that androgen levels are reduced in aging men.[7, 8, 9, 10] Some of the recently published statistics have quantified the rates and incidence of the age-related decline in androgen production in aging men. These studies have indicated:

(1) that in a large population-based cross-sectional study of men aged 39 to 70 (the Massachusetts Male Aging Study) it has been shown

that free testosterone declines by 1.2 percent per year, androstenedione declines by 1.3 percent per year, and dehydroepiandrosterone (DHEA) declines by 3.1 percent per year.[11]

(2) that approximately 7 percent of normal men aged 40 to 60 have been shown to have plasma testosterone levels below the normal limit.[12]

(3) that 13 percent of nondiabetic men and 21 percent of men with Type II diabetes (aged 40 to 79 years) have been shown to have hypoandrogenemia with plasma testosterone levels below the categorically defined level for hypogonadism of 3,500 pg/dl.[13]

(4) that 20 percent of men aged 60 to 80 years have been shown to have serum androgen levels below the lower limit of normal.[14]

(5) that after men are 50 years old, testosterone levels dwindle quickly to become approximately 50 percent of the peak level by age 80 years.[15]

(6) that by age 70 years, more than 25 percent of men have been shown to have hypogonadal testosterone levels as reflected by strict laboratory values, and the majority have hypoandrogenemia when compared to peak testosterone levels.[16]

(7) that by age 75 years, mean plasma testosterone levels in men have been shown to be only 65 percent of levels in young adults, with over 25 percent of these men having bioavailable testosterone levels below the normal limit.[17]

(8) that the most definitive longitudinal study (the Baltimore Longitudinal Study of Aging from Johns Hopkins University School of Medicine) published to date has illustrated that hypoandrogenemia occurs, in otherwise healthy men, in a progressive age-related manner:[18]

    a) as measured as total serum testosterone levels in their 50s, 60s, 70s, and 80s at 12 percent, 19 percent, 28 percent, and 49 percent rates respectively; and,

    b) as measured as "free" serum testosterone levels in their 50s, 60s, 70s and 80s at 9 percent, 34 percent, 68 percent, and 91 percent rates respectively.

Numerous studies have linked hypoandrogenemia or low free androgen index in men with low bone mineral density (BMD), osteoporosis, and osteoporotic fracture risk.[19, 20, 21, 22, 23, 24, 25, 26, 27] Hypoandrogenemia has been shown to be associated (statistically significant) with low BMD and femoral neck fractures in men.[28] It has been shown that androgen action is crucial for the maintenance of bone mass in men, and that androgen therapy is necessary for men with osteoporosis and hypoandrogenemia.[29] These findings and recommendations have been recently supported by several authors[30, 31, 32, 33, 34, 35, 36, 37] and confirm the earlier findings and recommendations.[38, 39] However, other authors have recommended that androgen therapy should await the findings obtained from large, long-term, well-controlled studies.[40, 41, 42]

Redefining Andropause in Men

Numerous recent studies have linked hypoandrogenemia with the climacteric, andropause symptoms, and clinical findings in men. These studies are supported by findings that were published decades ago when androgen therapy was used empirically for and effectively treated andropause in men.[43, 44, 45, 46, 47, 48, 49]

Andropause in men has been recently redefined by a medley of signs and symptoms. Men with hypoandrogenemia and andropause have been shown to have[50, 51, 52, 53, 54, 55, 56, 57, 58, 59]:

(1) decreased libido, height, muscle strength, sense of well-being, energy, virility, body hair, hematocrit, fertility, and depressed GHRH-GH-IGF-IGFBP axis activity.

(2) increased erectile dysfunction, abdominal fat, fatigability, depression, dyslipidemias, cognitive deficits, asthenia, anxiety, insomnia, irritability, and insulin resistance.

(3) accelerated osteoporosis, sarcopenia, atherosclerosis, and physical frailty. However, while recent authors have redefined the signs and symptoms of male andropause, other authors have denounced the existence of it.[60, 61, 62] Whether or not andropause exists or not has been a debate that has gone on for decades.[63, 64, 65]

Meanwhile, other authors have recently proposed that andropause is a misnomer for a true clinical entity that should be called androgen decline in the aging male (ADAM).[66, 67, 68]

Historical Highlights of Androgen Therapy for Andropause in Men

By 1940, a considerable amount of knowledge had accumulated regarding andropause and the endocrinology of androgens in men. This is perhaps best illustrated by quotations taken from a review article that points about the role of androgen deficiency in and androgen therapy for andropause in aging men.[69]

(1) "Chemically the androgens and estrogens are intimately related to cholesterol from which they are prepared synthetically.... Both are hormones which are found in both men and women.... The normal predominance of the respective hormone in each sex determines the orientations in both the physiological and psychological spheres."

(2) "The production of testosterone in males follows a parabolic curve with its ascent started between the ages of 10 and 14, and continued gradually up to the age of 22 or 25. Then it remains almost at the same level for 5 to 10 years, and then starts a gradual decline, almost insensible at first, at the ages of 32 to 35. This decline will be rapidly accentuated between 40 and 50, and at the age of 55 to 60, in most men, the activity of the Leydig cells (testosterone producing cells) is about the same as that before puberty."

(3) "The number of Leydig cells is known to decrease in the interstitial tissue along with the passing years, and in old age there is a reversal to a state of that of early childhood, with the Leydig cells reduced to a minimum in the senile atrophied testicles."

(4) "The prostate, on the contrary, usually starts a process of fibrous hypertrophy about 40, in some cases slowly, in others rapidly, reaching a large size and interfering with the free elimination of urine under the influence of increased impulses of the gonadotrophic pituitary hormone."

(5) "Proved effects of testosterone propionate therapy in men past 40 are:

    a) definite improvement of the usually depressed and melancholic psychics with marked improvement in concentration and memory and ability to perform mental work.

    b) rapid established euphoria and renewed ambition with apparent increase in 'pep' and general bodily vigor.

    c) reduction of prostatism and nocturia.

    d) in climacteric men whose testes have not suffered too extensive degeneration, sexual powers and libido can be restored in a moderate degree, bringing in many cases peace and renewed marital happiness to them.

    e) because of advances of the last half century [1890–1940] of medical progress, his span of life is being prolonged far beyond his fifties, and we can also make those added years happier and more comfortable, creating with this addition of our armamentarium, a new weapon of incalculable possibilities."

Physicians in the 1940s–1960s treated andropause and osteoporosis in men empirically with androgen therapy. However, by the mid–1970s, the prevailing medical belief was that testosterone production *did not* decline in aging men. This belief can be demonstrated by the following quotation.

"Since this disorder [involutional melancholia and osteoporosis] occurs in conjunction with either the menopause or the male climacteric, endocrine depletion has been thought to play a role in its genesis. However, since there is no specific accompanying endocrinologic abnormality, and since its course has never been influenced by hormone replacement, such does not seem to be the case." Harrison's *Principles of Internal Medicine* (1977).[70]

The medical establishment went through a lengthy period of denial regarding the acceptance of declining androgen levels in normal aging men. Textbooks published during this period begrudgingly contained a paragraph or two regarding involutional melancholia and andropause symptoms in aging men, but the authors of such textbooks tended to minimize the hormonal cause of such a condition. During the mid–1970s and the decade that followed, it was if these textbook authors really didn't believe the results and conclusions of the earlier studies. In short, they espoused the fact that there was no biochemical explanation for andropause and osteoporosis in men and so there was no need for androgen therapy.

Androgens Directly and Indirectly Stimulate Normal Bone Formation

It is now well recognized that osteoblasts are bone-forming cells that are stimulated by androgens, growth hormone (GH), insulin-like growth factor-1 (IGF-1), and other anabolic agents and cytokines. Studies with osteoporotic men and women patients, utilizing serial bone biopsies and histomorphometric techniques prior to and after androgen therapy, have proven that androgens stimulate normal bone formation.[71, 72, 73]

In vitro studies have shown that androgens bind to osteoblast receptors, and this finding has stimulated renewed interest in androgen effects on bone.[74] Other in vitro studies have shown that the androgen-dependent osteoblast stimulating effects produced are locally mediated in bone tissue, in part, by androgen-dependent IGF-1 production, and systemically by androgen-dependent regulation of circulating IGFBPs.[75]

The anabolic effects of androgens on osteoblast activities have been indicated by a number of specific molecules found in the serum of patients.[76] These serum markers of bone formation and osteoblast activities include serum osteocalcin (Oc), bone-specific alkaline phosphatase (bAP),

N- and C-terminal propetide of type 1 procollagen (PINP and PICP respectively), and others.[77, 78, 79, 80, 81, 82, 83] These bone markers have been shown to indicate osteoblast activity that reflects formation of normal organic bone matrix.[84]

The discoveries of serum bone markers and DEXA have allowed for an improved understanding of the effects that endogenous and exogenous hormone interactions have on bone formation and homeostasis. These updated methods have allowed the ability to assess the pharmacological therapies that stimulate osteoblast activities and result in increases in BMD.[85, 86, 87]

Recent studies with elderly patients, utilizing serum bone markers, have shown that the androgen-induced effect on osteoblasts is both prolonged and restorative, and that once stimulated, osteoblast activities continue for a period after androgen therapy is discontinued.[88, 89, 90, 91] Androgen therapy has been shown to increase BMD in elderly individuals, while reducing fracture risk and osteoporotic bone pain.[92, 93, 94, 95, 96]

Androgen Therapy Corrects Hypoandrogenemia and Hyposomatomedinemia

It is well recognized that androgen therapy corrects hypoandrogenemia. Androgen therapy has also been shown to correct hyposomatomedinemia by stimulating the GHRH-GH-IGF-IGFBP axis. This axis plays a role in bone formation and homeostasis. Hypoandrogenemia can result in a depressed GHRH-GH-IGF-IGFBP axis in elderly men.

Androgens have been shown to directly stimulate the GHRH-GH-IGF-IGFBP axis at the hypothalamic level by a direct stimulatory effect that increases GHRH amplitudes.[97, 98] Also, androgen receptors have been identified in GH secreting cells in the anterior pituitary gland.[99] Androgen stimulation has been shown to elevate circulating IGF-1, free IGF-1, and IGFBP-3 levels in normal, hypogonadal, hyposomatotrophic, and aging individuals.[100, 101, 102, 103, 104, 105, 106] Thusly, androgens have been shown to drive the GHRH-GH-IGF-IGFBP axis (at the hypothalamic level, pituitary level, and local tissue sites) and result in an overall anabolic state that results in bone formation and anabolic effects on the musculoskeletal system.

Normalizing GH secretory patterns associated with androgen therapy or by administering GHRH, GHRH analogues, or GH, has been shown to elevate circulating IGF-1, free IGF-1, and IGFBP-3 levels.[107, 108] Besides having a direct stimulatory effect on IGF-1 synthesis,[109] it has been shown that GH may have a direct stimulatory function on IGFBP-3 by enhancing its synthesis.[110]

Growth hormone has been shown to directly stimulate osteoblasts in vitro[111] and increase osteoblast activity in vivo as determined by serum markers of osteoblast activities.[112, 113, 114] GH increases bone formation via a direct interaction with GH receptors located on osteoblasts and via local bone tissue production of IGF-1 (autocrine/paracrine) action.[115, 116] It has been shown that individuals with GH-deficient states have a reduction in circulating IGF-1 levels and in osteoblast activities which often results in low BMD, osteoporosis, and fractures.[117]

Therefore, androgen therapy stimulates osteoblast activities via direct and indirect mechanisms. First, androgen therapy corrects hypoandrogenemia and directly stimulates osteoblast activities. Second, androgen therapy corrects hyposomatomedinemia and promotes GH effects by stimulating the GRHR-GH-IGF-IGFBP axis at multiple sites, which results in elevated osteoblast activities.

Hypoandrogenemia, Androgen Therapy, and Risk for Prostate Cancer and Benign Prostatic Hypertrophy

Androgen dose-response relationships are central to the issue of androgen replacement therapy, within the context of both hypogonadal men and older men with declining androgen levels. A major critical issue is whether increased anabolic functions can be achieved with androgen doses that will not adversely affect lipid profile, cardiovascular risk, and the prostate.[118] Androgen replacement therapy is usually lifelong and is contraindicated in patients with prostate cancer.[119]

Carcinoma of the prostate is the most frequently diagnosed malignancy and second only to lung cancer as the leading cause of cancer-related deaths in men in the United States and many other Western countries.[120] Notwithstanding the importance of this malignancy, little is understood about its specific causes. It now appears that elevated androgen levels are not associated with prostate carcinogenesis. The epidemiology of prostate cancer strongly suggests that environmental factors, particularly diet and nutrition, are involved in its genesis. Moreover, a growing body of evidence is mounting to support important genetic risk factors for prostate cancer, including mutant androgen receptors and polymorphic genes that encode for steroid hormone receptors and enzymes involved with the metabolism and action of steroid hormones.[121, 122, 123, 124, 125]

It has been a long-held belief by many physicians that elevated endogenous androgen levels or exogenous androgen therapy plays a major role in the genesis of prostate cancer. However, many recent studies have refuted this theory. In fact, low circulating androgen levels and high luteinizing hormone (LH) secretion rates may be major culprits. Some physicians now believe that low circulating androgen levels and concomitant high levels of LH, that occur in aging men, are likely contributors to prostate cancer.[126] Several recent reports have indicated that genetic changes within the prostate, both androgen-dependent and androgen-independent, cause the cancer, especially in men with hypoandrogenic states. In addition, the possible involvement of estrogenic hormones may be suspect, but this is not entirely clear.[127]

Androgenic steroids are required to maintain the prostate gland in the adult state. Consistent with this requirement, hypoandrogenemic states typically induce a regression of mature prostate tissue that is accompanied by the extensive loss of prostate cells through a programmed cell death process referred to as apoptosis.[128] Genes regulated by androgens are of critical importance for the normal physiological function of the prostate gland, and they contribute to the etiology, development, and progression of prostate carcinoma.[129] Androgens, by activation of the androgen receptors in the prostate, control the differentiation of prostate cells.[130, 131] Prostatic cells, including carcinogenic ones, have been shown to possess mechanisms of adaptation to hypoandrogenic states, including mutations of the androgen receptors.[132, 133]

Several epidemiological studies have shown that there is no correlation between endogenous androgen levels and the development of prostate cancer[134, 135, 136, 137, 138, 139, 140] while other studies suggest that there may be a correlation.[141, 142] It has been recently been postulated that low androgen levels (with high LH secretion) cause prostate cancer and that androgen therapy for men with hypoandrogenemia may be protective against prostate cancer genesis.[143] Some studies have linked hypoandrogenemia, low free androgen levels, and elevated LH levels with prostatic pathology in older men.[144, 145]

Prostate cancer in African-Americans is more aggressive and common than in any other racial group. A long-held belief has cited an endocrine mechanism to account for this racial difference. A recent study has refuted this concept by reporting that, among elderly men, there are no racial differences in androgen levels, and that androgen levels were not different between healthy men and those with prostatic cancer.[146] Black men have been found to have higher circulating testosterone levels from birth to about age 35 to 40 years, but the racial differences in prostate cancer have been shown to stem from within the androgen/androgen receptor pathways, including genetic polymorphisms and androgen receptor mutations.[147] Similar findings regarding androgen receptor gene polymorphism and mutations with increased 5alpha-reductase enzyme activities have recently been made in men from other racial and ethnic groups.[148, 149]

Several studies have shown that long-term androgen therapy in hypogonadal men is not associated with an increase prevalence of prostate cancer or symptomatic benign prostatic hypertrophy, BPH.[150, 151, 152] These recent reports echo similar findings published in the 1930s and 1940s.[153, 154, 155, 156 157] Other recent studies have shown that genetic alterations, including upregulation and wild type mutations, in prostatic androgen receptors may play important pathogenic roles in prostate cancer development especially seen in hypoandrogenemic states and androgen ablation therapy.[158, 159, 160, 161] Prostate cancer cells may acquire the ability to survive and grow in hypoandrogenemic states by activating the androgen receptor pathways using growth factors, cytokines, and steroids other than androgens.[162] Therefore, it may be that hypoandrogenemia plays a pathogenic role within the prostate by encouraging androgen receptor mutation at an accelerated rate.

It now appears that low rather than high circulating androgen levels are involved in the pathogenesis of prostate cancer. Therefore, androgen replacement therapy may reduce the risk of developing prostate cancer by limiting the occurrence and expression of mutant androgen receptors. Since these mutant receptors have been shown to enhance the activity of reduction enzymes that convert testosterone to weak androgens, it could be suggested that androgen therapy should utilize androgens that have a steric hindrance to the action of 5alpha-reductase activity.

Enlargement of the prostate gland is a common condition in aging men. Long-held theories have postulated that benign prostate hypertrophy (BPH) is the result of elevated circulating androgen levels or exposure to circulating androgens for several decades. However, if elevated androgen levels are the culprit, then why does BPH occur in aging men with normal or low circulating androgen levels and not in younger men with high androgen levels? Results from the earliest studies have shown that androgen therapy *reduces* BPH and prostatism.

Therefore, it is more reasonable to suggest that elevated LH levels, and not elevated androgen levels, are involved in the genesis of BPH. Some recent studies, cited above, have linked BPH with low circulating androgen levels and elevated LH secretion. Androgen therapy for men with low androgen levels may prevent or reverse BPH by normalizing LH secretion.

Androgen therapy for these patients may also prevent prostatic carcinoma by limiting androgen receptor mutations that occur in an accelerated fashion in hypoandrogenic states. Further studies regarding androgen therapy on the pathogenesis of BPH and prostate cancer are warranted to completely unravel this apparent dichotomy.

Hypoandrogenemia, Androgen Therapy, and Cardiovascular Risk Factors

The association between circulating endogenous androgen levels and cardiovascular risk factors in men remains a topic of debate. The long-held traditional view has been that increased circulating androgen levels promote atherogenic lipid profiles, atherogenesis, and cardiovascular disease. This certainly has been shown for athletes who use huge supratherapeutic doses of androgens for bodybuilding. However, in regards to androgen therapy to promote physiologically normal androgen levels, this view has been refuted. In fact, recent studies have shown that men with hypoandrogenemia have atherogenic lipid profiles and increased risk for coronary artery disease and stroke which are corrected by androgen therapy.

In perhaps the best investigation, a recent nested case-control study of healthy men (matched by age and ethnic origin), showed that men who had low plasma total testosterone levels, compared to normal levels, had significantly increased risks for cardiovascular disease as indicated by:[163]

(1) higher body mass index (P< 0.01).

(2) higher waist/hip ratio (P< 0.001).

(3) higher systolic blood pressure (P< 0.05).

(4) higher fasting and 2-hour plasma glucose levels (P< 0.04 and P<0.02 respectively).

(5) higher serum triglyceride levels (P< 0.001).

(6) higher total cholesterol levels (P< 0.04).

(7) higher low density lipoprotein cholesterol levels (P< 0.01).

(8) higher apolipoprotein B levels (P< 0.01).

(9) higher fasting and 2-hour plasma insulin levels (P< 0.0001).

(10) lower serum high density lipoprotein cholesterol levels (P< 0.01).

(11) lower apolipoprotein A1 levels (P< 0.05).

(12) markedly lower SHBG levels (P< 0.0001).

A consensus of studies utilizing androgen therapy in men with hypoandrogenemia has shown that increasing androgen levels to midnormal range, results in decreased total cholesterol and LDL cholesterol, while increasing HDL cholesterol levels.[164] Thus, androgen therapy in men with hypoandrogenemia results in normalized lipid profiles and beneficial effects on serum lipoprotein profiles which reflect less atherogenic patterns.

Besides beneficial lipid-lowering effects, androgens have been shown to have beneficial effects on the clotting system and fibrinolysis that can significantly reduce cardiovascular and thromboembolic risks. Circulating testosterone levels have been shown to correlate positively with the major stimulator of fibrinolysis, tissue plasminogen activator activity (p=0.02), and inversely with two independent CAD risk factors, plasminogen activator inhibitor activity, the major fibrinolysis inhibitor (p=0.01), and fibrinogen levels (p=0.004).[165]

An extensive review of the relationship of endogenous circulating androgens to coronary heart disease (CHD) in men, including one intervention, eight cohort, and 30 cross-sectional studies, has concluded that serum androgens (testosterone and DHEA) had a favorable or neutral effect on coronary heart disease in men. In 18 of the 30 cross-sectional studies, reduced levels of testosterone and/or DHEA was associated with an increased risk in patients with CHD as compared to normal controls. In 11 of these 30 studies, similar circulating levels of androgens were found in CHD patients and normal controls. Only one of these cross-sectional studies found elevated androgen levels (DHEA) in CHD patients as compared to age-matched controls.[166]

Androgen administration, as potential cardiovascular drug therapy in aging men, has recently made a comeback. The earliest studies (from the 1930s and 1940s) had indicated that androgen therapy in aging men had a powerful effect on reducing the pain of angina pectoris, reducing hypertension, increasing exercise tolerance, improving abnormal ECG findings, and improving cardiac rehabilitation.[167, 168, 169, 170, 171, 172, 173, 174, 175, 176, 177, 178, 179] More recent studies have reconfirmed these beneficial antianginal, lipid lowering, and cardiac function effects,[180, 181, 182, 183] and that testosterone administration in physiological concentrations (intracoronary) induces coronary artery dilatation and increases coronary blood flow in men with established coronary artery disease.[184] Of particular importance, androgen receptors have recently been found in the smooth muscle cells of arterioles.[185]

Androgen receptors have been located within the myocardium of both men and women and androgen binding to these receptors probably plays a role in optimum cardiac functioning.[186, 187, 188, 189] Surprisingly, it has been found that androgen concentrations and androgen receptors are higher in normal myocardium than in skeletal muscle. It has also been shown that androgen concentrations and androgen receptors in cardiac and pulmonary tissues declines (statistically significant) with age.[190] It follows that age-related decreases in circulating androgen concentrations reflect reduced myocardial androgen and androgen receptor concentrations which results in decreased myocardial function. Moreover, androgen therapy may reverse and/or correct the age-related reduction in cardiac function that is associated with hypoandrogenemia in men.

In summary, androgen therapy in men with hypoandrogenemia as replacement treatment has been shown to benefit cardiovascular health by:

(1) beneficial impact on serum lipid, lipoprotein, glucose, and insulin levels, which promotes less atherogenic patterns.

(2) beneficial antianginal and antihypertension effects, via androgen receptor binding to myocardial and arteriolar muscle cells, to increase myocardial function, coronary blood flow, and reduced peripheral resistance.

(3) beneficial effects on the clotting system that results in a net increase in fibrinolysis and reduction of independent, clotting system-related risk factors for CHD and thromboembolic events.

(4) beneficial effects on body composition and muscle strength, which reduces CHD risk factors and improves physical fitness, stamina, and sense of well-being.

Androgen Therapy and Its Neurosteroid, Neuroprotective, and Neuroimmune Benefits

Circulating androgens are a major contributor to the mental health of men, especially aging men who gradually and progressively become androgen deficient in their later decades of life. In the past ten years or so, a substantial and growing body of evidence has accumulated that supports the subjective findings that androgen therapy improves mental health, sense of well-being, energy level, libido, and cognition of aging men.

In recent years investigations have shown that androgens belong to the group of neurosteroids that are synthesized and metabolized by a variety of brain tissues. Androgens are also made available to the brain via the general circulation after they are synthesized by the endocrine system or introduced via exogenous routes. Androgens have been shown to exhibit neurosteroid, neuroprotective, and neuroregenerative properties in:

(1) evidence from cell culture experiments that have shown that androgens increase the survival, differentiation, and regeneration of neurons, glial cells, and Schwann cells, and that they can be synthesized from cholesterol within both the central and peripheral nervous systems.[191, 192, 193, 194]

(2) evidence from immunochemistry that has shown that androgens serve as precursors for other neurosteroids in biosynthetic pathways within oligodendrocytes and glial cells that stimulate myelin synthesis.[195, 196, 197]

(3) evidence indicating that androgens are synthesized by pyramidal neurons and stimulate the hippocampal neurons that play an important role in memory and learning.[198]

(4) evidence indicating that androgens are direct neurotransmitters and exhibit neurotransmitter modulation effects via receptor mediated binding to several neuroreceptors. Androgen-mediated actions have been shown in GABA(A), NMDA, sigma, substance P, dopamine, serotonin, and opioid receptors that result in neuroprotective, neuromodulatory, cognition-enhancing, memory-enhancing, anxiolytic, mood-elevating, and analgesic effects.[199, 200, 201, 202, 203, 204, 205, 206, 207, 208, 209, 210, 211, 212, 213, 214, 215, 216, 217, 218, 219, 220, 221, 222, 223]

(5) evidence that androgens increase the serum and tissue levels of a number of anabolic and neurotrophic polypeptide growth factors that play a role in the homeostasis, stimulation, neovascularization, and regeneration of central nervous system tissues.[224, 225]

(6) evidence that androgens promote anabolic influences on cytokines and modulate or correct inflammatory and autoimmune cytokine imbalances.[226, 227 228, 229] Hypoandrogenemia has been found to play a role in the pathogenesis of several cytokine-mediated diseases in men, including stroke, myocardial infarction, atherosclerosis, rheumatoid arthritis, systemic lupus erythematosus, multiple sclerosis, osteoporosis, sarcopenia, fibromyalgia, chronic fatigue syndrome, depression, and dementia.

Summary

Androgen therapy for men with hypoandrogenemia should be a routine choice for physicians, especially physiatrists. Men with hypoandrogenemia make up a significant portion of the practice in physical medicine and rehabilitation. It has been shown that androgen therapy improves the rehabilitation outcomes in older men with a variety of illnesses.[230, 231]

Androgen therapy in older men has been associated with anabolic effects that reverse osteoporotic, anemic, and sarcopenic states by increasing BMD, lean body mass, muscle mass, neuromuscular strength, and the erythropoietic stimulus.[232, 233, 234, 235, 236, 237, 238, 239, 240] The anabolic effects of androgen replacement have been shown to be of particular importance for reversing the osteoporotic and sarcopenic effects induced both by corticosteroid therapy and Type II diabetes which promote hypoandrogenemic states in older men[241, 242, 243, 244, 245] (these specific conditions will be discussed in detail in other chapters in this book). These accumulating findings have provided the physiological evidence that androgen therapy should be considered as a pharmacological intervention against losses in BMD and lean body mass associated with age, disease, trauma, and burn injury.[246]

Physicians in the United States have been slow to utilize anabolic agents for osteoporosis and other catabolic, disabling diseases.[247] A number of barriers for prescribing anabolic therapy for patients have recently been identified, including inadequate training of physicians, poor coordination between medical specialties, improper and prevailing physician attitudes, third-party reimbursement practices, concerns regarding "off-label" use of anabolic agents, and others.[248, 249] However, use of anabolic agents may decrease catabolic states, promote and accelerate recovery, shorten hospital stay, and reduce the convalescence time associated with disabling diseases and conditions.[250]

A major facet of preventing musculoskeletal frailty should be delivering an anabolic stimulus to elderly adults on a mass scale.[251] This imperative (addressed by the National Institute on Aging) behooves physicians to create an improved dialogue between several areas of science and medicine, including endocrinology, neuroendocrinology, immunology, exercise physiology, clinical nutrition, and clinicians in order to use multidisciplinary approaches to make solutions available to patients.[252]

In this chapter, an appropriate rationale for androgen therapy as the solution for men with hypoandrogenemia has been provided. It has been shown that androgen therapy for men with hypoandrogenemia:

(1) provides an appropriate anabolic stimulus to the musculoskeletal system and hematological system that can prevent and/or reverse osteoporotic, sarcopenic, and anemic conditions.

(2) provides correction for both hypoandrogenemia and hyposomatomedinemia in a cost-effective, safe, and physiologically correct manner.

(3) provides a physiologically correct, multifaceted anabolic stimulus, via neurosteroid actions, to both the central and peripheral nervous

systems resulting in enhanced neurotransmitter, neuroprotective, and neuroregenerative actions. These actions may prevent and treat many of the subjective and objective findings associated with andropause, such as erectile dysfunction, depression, and disturbances in well-being and cognition.

(4) provides a physiologically correct anabolic and vasodilatation stimuli to the cardiovascular system that improves angina, hypertension, cardiac function, coronary artery blood flow, and exercise tolerance. Androgen therapy also stimulates erythropoiesis and corrects low-grade anemic states that can improve aerobic capacity and cardiac rehabilitation.

(5) provides a significant, multifaceted reduction in risk factors for CAD, atherogenesis, and thromboembolism by improving lipid, lipoprotein, fibrinolysis, and body composition profiles.

(6) provides an endocrine correction that improves insulin sensitivity and lowers serum glucose and insulin levels.

(7) provides a neuroendocrine and neuroimmune correction of cytokine balance that reduces the catabolic and autoimmune potentiating cytokine imbalances and hypercortisolemia that are associated with many diseases.

(8) provides a physiologically correct blunting to LH that may reduce BPH and risk for prostate cancer.

(9) provides an appropriate anabolic stimulus to hasten the recovery and rehabilitation outcomes of disabling diseases and conditions.

(10) provides stimuli for overall improvement in quality of life parameters and probable enhancement of longevity.

Before starting any androgen therapy, the presence of prostatic carcinoma should be excluded by rectal examination and prostate-specific antigen (PSA) measurement, and when in doubt, these tests should be complemented by transrectal echography or other modalities. The presence of prostatic carcinoma is an absolute contraindication for androgen therapy.[253, 254, 255]

Long-term androgen therapy has been associated with only mild, nonpathogenic increases in PSA.[256] So far, there have been no indications that androgen therapy stimulates the evolution of subclinical prostatic carcinoma to clinical carcinoma.[257] Declining rather than high levels of androgens probably contribute more to prostate carcinogenesis, and androgen therapy probably reduces the incidence of the disease.[258]

Androgen therapy for patients with hypoandrogenemia seems a correct way for patients to achieve the full benefits of the physical medicine and rehabilitation modalities. Prescribing the appropriate anabolic stimulus for patients with hypoandrogenemia should be inherent and obvious for patients with low androgen levels. Without supplying appropriate pharmacologic anabolic stimuli, it is doubtful that the practice of most physiatrists will progress beyond the palliative measures that are offered currently. It is time that physicians prescribed anabolic therapies for their patients who are aging with signs and symptoms of andropause, osteoporosis, and other catabolic illnesses.

Notes

1. Kenny, A.M., J.C. Gallagher, K.M. Prestwood, et al. Bone density, bone turnover, and hormone levels in men over age 75. *J. Gerontol. A. Biol. Sci. Med. Sci.* 1998; 53 (6): M419–425.

2. Kenny, A.M., K.M. Prestwood, K.M. Marcello, et al. Determinants of bone density in healthy older men with low testosterone levels. *J. Gerontol. A. Biol. Sci. Med. Sci.* 2000; 55 (9): M492–497.

3. Katznelson, L. Therapeutic role of androgens in the treatment of osteoporosis in men. *Baillieres Clin. Endocrinol. Metab.* 1998; 12 (3): 453–470.

4. Simon, D., P. Preziosi, E. Barrett-Conner, et al. Interrelation between plasma testosterone and plasma insulin in healthy adult men: The Telecom Study. *Diabetologia* 1992; 35 (2): 173–177.

5. Morley, J.E., F.E. Kaiser, H.M. Perry et al. Longitudinal changes in testosterone, luteinizing hormone, and follicle-stimulating hormone in healthy older men. *Metabolism* 1997; 46 (4): 410–413.

6. Tenover, J.L. Male hormone replacement therapy including "andropause." *Endocrinol. Metab. Clin. North Am.* 1998; 27 (4): 969–987.

7. Szarvas, F. [The male climacteric from the practical viewpoint.] *Wein. Med. Wochenschr.* 1992; 142 (5–6): 100–103.

8. Swerdloff, R.S., and C. Wang. Androgen deficiency and aging in men. *West. J. Med.* 1993; 159 (5): 579–585.

9. Morley, J.E., and H.M. Perry. Androgen deficiency in aging men. *Med. Clin. North Am.* 1999; 83 (5): 1279–1289.

10. Hermann, M., and P. Berger. Hormone replacement in the aging male? *Exp. Gerontol.* 1999; 34 (8): 923–933.

11. Gray, A., H.A. Feldman, J.B. McKinlay, et al. Age, disease, and changing sex hormone levels in middle-aged men: results of the Massachusetts Male Aging Study. *J. Clin. Endocrinol. Metab.* 1991; 73 (5): 1016–1025.

12. Vermeulen, A., and J.M. Kaufman. Ageing of the hypothalamo-pituitary-testicular axis in men. *Horm. Res.* 1995; 43 (1–3): 25–28.

13. Barrett-Connor, E., K.T. Khaw, and S.S. Yen. Endogenous sex hormone levels in older adult men with diabetes mellitus. *Am. J. Epidemiol.* 1990; 132 (5): 895–901.

14. Lund, B.C., K.A. Bever-Stille, and P.J. Perry. Testosterone and andropause: the feasibility of testosterone replacement therapy in elderly men. *Pharmacotherapy* 1999; 19 (8): 951–956.

15. Wu, C.Y., T.J. Yu, and M.J. Chen. Age related testosterone level changes and male andropause syndrome. *Chang. Keng I. Hsueeh. Tsa. Chih.* 2000; 23 (6): 348–353.

16. Vermeulen, A. [Senile hypogonadism in man and hormone replacement therapy.] *Acta Med. Austriaca* 2000; 27 (1): 11–17.

17. Vermeulen, A. Andropause. *Maturitas* 2000; 34 (1): 5–15.

18. Mitchell, S., E. Harman, E.J. Metter, et al. Longitudinal effects of aging on serum and free testosterone levels in healthy men. *J. Clin. Endocrinol. Metab.* 2001; 86 (2): 724–731.

19. Katznelson, L. Therapeutic role of androgens in the treatment of osteoporosis in men. *Baillieres Clin. Endocrinol. Metab.* 1998; 12 (3): 453–470.

20. Rapado, A., F. Hawkins, L. Sobrinho, et al. Bone mineral density and androgen levels in elderly males. *Calcif. Tissue Int.* 1999; 65 (6): 417–421.

21. Kenny, A.M., J.C. Gallagher, K.M. Prestwood, et al. Bone density, bone turnover, and hormone levels in men over age 75. *J. Gerontol. A. Biol. Sci. Med. Sci.* 1998; 53 (6): M419–425.

22. Francis, R.M. The effects of testosterone on osteoporosis in men. *Clin. Endocrinol. (Oxf.)* 1999; 50 (4): 411–414.

23. Winters, S.L. Current status of testosterone replacement therapy in men. *Arch. Fam. Med.* 1999; 8 (3): 257–263.

24. Scane, A.C., R.M. Francis, A.M. Sutcliffe, et al. Case-control study of pathogenesis and sequelae of symptomatic vertebral fractures in men. *Osteoporos. Int.* 1999; 9 (1): 91–97.

25. Vanderschueren, D., and L. Vandeput. Androgens and osteoporosis. *Andrologia* 2000; 32 (3): 125–130.

26. Allolio, B., M. Dambacher, R. Dreher, et al. [Osteoporosis in the male.] *Med. Klin.* 2000; 95 (6): 327–338.

27. Zarate, A., L. Basurto, and G. Fanghanel. [Osteoporosis in males is a frequently overlooked risk.] *Gac. Med. Mex.* 2000; 136 (1): 83–86.

28. Kenny, A.M., K.M. Prestwood, K.M. Marcello, et al. Determinants of bone density in healthy older men with low testosterone levels. *J. Gerontol. A. Biol. Sci. Med. Sci.* 2000; 5 (9): M497–497.

29. Vanderschueren, D., and L. Vandenput. Androgens and osteoporosis. *Andrologia* 2000; 32 (3): 125–130.

30. Rabijewski, M., M. Adamkiewicz, and S. Zgliczynski. [The influence of testosterone replacement therapy on well-being, bone mineral density and lipids in elderly men.] *Pol. Arch. Med. Wewn.* 1998; 100 (3): 212–221.

31. Katznelson, L. Therapeutic role of androgens in the treatment of osteoporosis in men. *Baillieres Clin. Endocrinol. Metab.* 1998; 12 (3): 453–470.

32. Winters, S.J. Current status of testosterone replacement therapy in men. *Arch. Fam. Med.* 1999; 8 (3): 257–263.

33. Basaria, S., and A.S. Dobs. Risks versus benefits of testosterone therapy in elderly men. *Drugs Aging* 1999; 15 (2): 131–142.

34. Zarate, A., L. Basurto, and G. Fanghanel. [Osteoporosis in males is a frequently overlooked risk.] *Gac. Med. Mex.* 2000; 136 (1): 83–86.

35. Allolio, B., M. Dambacher, R. Dreher, et al. [Osteoporosis in the male.] *Med. Klin.* 2000; 95 (6): 327–338.

36. Morley, J.E. Andropause, testosterone therapy, and quality of life in aging men. *Cleve. Clin. J. Med.* 2000; 67 (12): 880–882.

37. Legros, J.J. [Towards a consensus regarding androgen substitution therapy for andropause.] *Rev. Med. Liège.* 2000; 55 (5): 449–453.

38. Baronti, G., and G.P. Zucchelli. [19–Nortestosterone in the therapy of senile osteoporosis.] *Clin. Ter.* 1970; 52 (2): 155–161.

39. Cantatore, F.P., M. Carrozzo, M. D'Amore, et al. Serum osteocalcin in the treatment of senile osteoporosis with anabolic steroids. Further evidences for a new marker of bone formation. *Clin. Rheumatol.* 1986; 5 (4): 535–536.

40. Lund, B.C., K.A. Bever-Stille, and P.J. Perry. Testosterone and andropause: the feasibility of testosterone replacement therapy in elderly men. *Pharmacotherapy* 1999; 19 (8): 951–956.

41. Hermann, M., and P. Berger. Hormone replacement for the aging male? *Exp. Gerontol.* 34 (8): 923–933.

42. Vermeulen, A. Andropause. *Maturitas* 2000; 34 (1): 5–15.

43. Turner, H.H. The clinical use of synthetic male sex hormone. *Endocrinol.* 1939; 24 (6): 763–773.

44. Thomas, H.B., and R.T. Hill. Testosterone propionate and the male climacteric. *Endocrinol.* 1941; 26: 953–953.

45. Goldman, S.F., and M.J. Markham. Clinical use of testosterone in the male climacteric. *J. Clin. Endocrinol.* 1942; 2: 237–242.

46. Samuels, E., A.F. Austin, F. Henschel, et al. Influence of methyl testosterone on muscular work and creatine metabolism in normal men. *J. Clin. Endocrinol.* 1942; 2: 649–654.

47. Davidoff, E., and G.L. Goodstone. Use of testosterone propionate in treatment of involutional psychosis in the male. *Arch. Neuro. Psych.* 1942; 48: 811–817.

48. Danziger, L., and H.R. Blank. Androgen therapy in agitated depressions in the male. *Med. Ann. Dist. Columbia* 1942; 11 (5): 181–183.

49. Werner, A.A. The male climacteric: additional observations of thirty-seven patients. *J. Urology* 1943; 49; 872–882.

50. Swerdloff, R.S., and C. Wang. Androgen deficiency and aging in men. *West. J. Med.* 1993; 159 (5): 579–585.

51. Tenover, J.L. Male hormone replacement therapy including "andropause." *Endocrinol. Metab. Clin. North Am.* 1998; 27 (4): 969–987.

52. Sternbach, H. Age-associated testosterone decline in men: clinical issues for psychiatry. *Am. J. Pyschiatry* 1998; 155 (10): 1310–1318.

53. Lund, B.C., K.A. Bever-Stille, and P.J. Perry. Testosterone and andropause: the feasibility of testosterone replacement therapy in elderly men. *Pharmacotherapy* 1999; 19 (8): 951–956.

54. Hermann, M., and P. Berger. Hormone replacement in the aging male? *Exp. Gerontol.* 1999; 34 (8): 923–933.

55. Winters, S.J. Current status of testosterone replacement therapy in men. *Arch. Fam. Med.* 1999; 8 (3): 257–263.

56. Tan, R.S. Managing the andropause in aging men. *Clin. Geratrics* 1999; 7 (8): 63–68.

57. Morley, J.E., and H.M. Perry. Androgen deficiency in aging men. *Med. Clin. North Am.* 1999; 83 (5): 1279–1289.

58. Vermeulen, A. [Senile hypogonadism in man and hormone replacement therapy.] *Acta Med. Austriaca* 2000; 27 (1): 11–17.

59. Wu, C.Y., T.J. Yu, and M.J. Chen. Age related testosterone level changes and male andropause syndrome. *Chang. Keng. I. Hsueh Tsa Chih.* 2000; 23 (6): 348–353.

60. McKinlay, J.B., C. Longcope, and A. Gray. The questionable physiologic and epidemiologic basis for a male climacteric syndrome: preliminary results from the Massachusetts Male Aging Study. *Maturitas* 1989; 11 (2): 103–115.

61. Tomer, Y., B. Lunenfeld, and M. Berezin. *Harefuah* 1995; 128 (12): 785–788.

62. Burns-Cox, N., and C. Gingell. The andropause: fact or fiction. *Postgrad. Med. J.* 1997; 73: 553–556.

63. Vignalou, J., and J.P. Bouchon. [Is there an andropause?] *Rev. Prat.* 1965; 15 (15): 2065–2070.

64. Franchimont, P. [The andropause: slander or calumny? The andropause.] *Rev. Med. Liège.* 1975; 30 (12): 393–396.

65. Rollet, J. [Does the "andropause" exist?] *Rev. Prat.* 1987; 37 (7): 357–361.

66. Morales, A., J.P. Heaton, and C.C. Carson. Andropause: a misnomer for a true clinical entity. *J. Urol.* 2000; 163 (3): 705–712.

67. Tan, R. Re: andropause: a misnomer for a true clinical entity. *J. Urol.* 2000; 164 (4): 1319.

68. Basson, R. Re: andropause: a misnomer for a true clinical entity. *J. Urol.* 2000; 164 (4): 1319.

69. Lamar, C.P. Clinical endocrinology of the male with special reference to the male climacteric. *J. Florida Med. Assoc.* 1940; 26 (8): 398–404.

70. Harrison, T.R. *Principles of Internal Medicine.* New York: McGraw-Hill, Inc., 1977, p. 1961.

71. Chesnut, C.H., J.L. Ivey, H.E. Gruber, et al. Stanozolol in postmenopausal osteoporosis: therapeutic efficacy and possible mechanisms of action. *Metabolism* 1983; 32 (6): 571–580.

72. Gennari, C., D. Agnus Dei, S. Gonnelli, et al. Effects of nandrolone decanoate on bone mass and calcium metabolism in women with established postmenopausal osteoporosis: a double-blind placebo-controlled study. *Maturitas* 1988; 11 (3): 187–197.

73. Beneton, M.N.C., A.J.P. Yates, S. Rogers, et al. Stanozolol stimulates remodeling of trabecular bone and net formation of bone at the endocortical surface. *Clin. Sci.* 1991; 81: 543–549.

74. Khosla, S. The effects of androgens on osteoblast function in vitro. *Mayo Clin. Proc.* 2000; 75 (Suppl.): S51–54.

75. Gori, F., L.C. Hofbauer, C.A. Conover, et al. Effects of androgens on the insulin-like growth factor system in an androgen-responsive human osteoblast cell line. *Endocrinology* 1999; 149 (12): 5579–5586.

76. Labie, F., A. Belanger, V. Wilkinson, et al. DHEA and the intracrine formation of androgens and estrogens in peripheral target tissues: its role during aging. *Steroids* 1998; 63 (5–6): 322–328.

77. Cosman, F., J. Nieves, C. Wilkinson, et al. Bone density change and biochemical indices of skeletal turnover. *Calcif. Tissue Int.* 1996; 58 (4): 236–243.

78. Dresner-Pollak, R., R.A. Parker, M. Poku, et al. Biochemical markers of bone turnover reflect femoral bone loss in elderly women. *Calcif. Tissue Int.* 1996; 59 (5): 328–333.

79. Ganero, P., and P.D. Delmas. New developments in biochemical markers for osteoporosis. *Calcif. Tissue Int.* 1996; 59 (7): 2–9.

80. Russell, R.G. The assessment of bone metabolism in vivo using biochemical approaches. *Horm. Metab. Res.* 1997; 29 (3): 138–144.

81. Eyre, D.R. Bone biomarkers as tools in osteoporosis management. *Spine* 1997; 22 (24 Suppl.): 17S–24S.

82. Ganero, P., and P.D. Delmas. Biochemical markers of bone turnover. Applications for osteoporosis. *Endocrinol. Metab. Clin. North Am.* 1998; 27 (2): 303–323.

83. Fink, E., C. Cornier, P. Steinmetz, et al. Differences in the capacity of several biochemical bone markers to assess high bone turnover in early menopause and response to alendronate therapy. *Osteoporos. Int.* 2000; 11 (4): 295–303.

84. Christenson, R.H. Biochemical markers of bone metabolism: an overview. *Clin. Biochem.* 1997; 30 (8): 573–593.

85. Adachi, J.D. The correlation of bone mineral density and biochemical markers to fracture risk. *Calcif. Tissue Int.* 1996; 59 (7): 16–19.

86. Seibel, M.J., and H.W. Woitge. Basic principles and clinical applications of

biochemical markers of bone metabolism: biochemical and technical aspects. *J. Clin. Densitom.* 1999; 2 (3): 299–321.

87. Hunter, D.J., and P.N. Sambrook. Bone loss: Epidemiology of bone loss. *Arthritis Res.* 2000; 2 (6): 441–445.

88. Cantatore, F.P., M. Carrozzo, M. D'Amore, et al. Serum osteocalcin in the treatment of senile osteoporosis with anabolic steroids. Further evidences for a new marker of bone formation. *Clin. Rheumatol.* 1986; 5 (4): 535–536.

89. Couch, M., F.E. Preston R.G. Malia, et al. Changes in plasma osteocalcin concentrations following treatment with stanozolol. *Clin. Chem. Acta* 1986; 158: 43–47.

90. Gennari, C., D. Agnus Dei, S. Gonnelli, et al. Effects of nandrolone decanoate therapy on bone mass and calcium metabolism in women with established postmenopausal osteoporosis: a double-blind placebo-controlled study. *Maturitas* 1989; 11 (3): 187–197.

91. Raisz, L.G., B. Wiita, A. Artis, et al. Comparison of the effects of estrogen alone and estrogen plus androgen on biochemical markers of bone formation and resorption in postmenopausal women. *J. Clin. Endocrinol. Metab.* 1996; 81 (1): 37–43.

92. Passeri, M., M. Pedrazzoni, G. Pioli, et al. Effects of nandrolone decanoate on bone mass in established osteoporosis. *Maturitas* 1993; 17 (4): 211–219.

93. Lyritis, G.P., C. Androulakis, B. Magiasis, et al. Effect of nandrolone decanoate and 1–alpha-hydroxy-calciferol on patients with vertebral osteoporotic collapse. A double-blind clinical trial. *Bone Miner.* 1994; 27 (3): 209–217.

94. Katznelson, L. Therapeutic role of androgens in the treatment of osteoporosis in men. *Baillieres. Clin. Endocrinol. Metab.* 1998; 12 (3): 453–470.

95. Hamby, R.C., S.W. Moore, K.E. Whalen, et al. Nandrolone decanoate for men with osteoporosis. *Am. J. Ther.* 1998; 5 (2): 89–95.

96. Rabijewski, M., M. Adamkiewicz, and S. Zglizcynski. [The influence of testosterone replacement therapy on well-being, bone mineral density and lipids in elderly men.] *Pol. Arch. Med. Wewn.* 1998; 100 (3): 212–221.

97. Eakman, G.D., J.S. Dallas, S.W. Ponder, et al. The effects of testosterone and dihydrotestosterone on hypothalamic regulation of growth hormone secretion. *J. Clin. Endocrinol. Metab.* 1996; 81 (3): 1217–1223.

98. Genazzani, A.D., O. Gamba, L. Nappi, et al. Modulatory effects of synthetic steroid (tibolone) and estradiol on spontaneous and GHRH-induced GH secretion in postmenopausal women. *Maturitas* 1997; 28 (1): 27–33.

99. Kimura, N., A. Mizokami, T. Oonuma, et al. Immunocytochemical localization of androgen receptor with polyclonal antibody in paraffin-embedded human tissue. *J. Histochem. Cytochem.* 1993; 41 (5): 671–678.

100. Hobbs, C.J., S.R. Plymate, C.J. Rosen, et al. Testosterone administration increases insulin-like growth factor-1 levels in normal men. *J. Clin. Endocrinol. Metab.* 1993; 77 (3): 776–779.

101. Morales, A.J., J.J. Nolen, J.C. Nelson, et al. Effects of replacement dose of dehydroepiandrosterone in men and women of advancing age. *J. Clin. Endocrinol. Metab.* 1994; 78 (6): 1360–1367.

102. Gelato, M.C., and R.A. Frost. IGFBP-3. Functional and structural implications in aging and wasting syndromes. *Endocrine* 1997; 7 (1): 81–85.

103. Casson, P.R., N. Santoro, K. Elkin-Hirsch, et al. Postmenopausal dehydroepiandrosterone administration increases free insulin-like growth factor-1 and decreases high-density lipoprotein: a six month trial. *Fertil. Steril.* 1998; 70 (1): 107–110.

104. Jorgensen, J.O., N. Vahl, T.B. Hansen, et al. Determinants of serum insulin-like growth factor 1 in growth hormone deficient adults as compared to healthy subjects. *Clin. Endocrinol. (Oxf.)* 1998; 48 (4): 479–486.

105. Morales, A.J., R.H. Haubrich, J.Y. Hwang, et al. The effects of six months treatment with 100mg daily dose of dehydroepiandrosterone (DHEA) on circulating sex steroids, body composition, and muscle strength in age-advanced men and women. *Clin. Endocrinol. (Oxf.)* 1998; 49 (4): 421–434.

106. Span, J.P., G.F. Pieters, C.G. Sweep, et al. Gender difference in insulin-like growth factor-1 response to growth hormone (GH) treatment and GH-deficient adults: role of sex hormone replacement. *J. Clin. Endocrinol. Metab.* 2000; 85 (3): 1121–1125.

107. Ovesen, P., J. Moller, J.O. Jorgensen, et al. Effect of growth hormone administration on circulating levels of luteinizing hormone, follicle stimulating hormone, and testosterone in normal healthy men. *Hum. Reprod.* 1993; 8 (11): 1869–1872.

108. Lee, P.D., S.K. Durham, V. Martinez, et al. Kinetics of insulin-like growth factor (IGF) and IGF-binding protein response to a single dose of growth hormone. *J. Clin. Endocrinol. Metab.* 1997; 82 (7): 2266–2274.

109. Cuttica, C.M., L. Castoldi, G.P. Gorrini, et al. Effect of six-month administration of recombinant human growth hormone to healthy elderly adults. *Aging (Milano)* 1997; 9 (3): 193–197.

110. Lemmey, A.B., J. Glassford, H.C. Flick-Smith, et al. Different regulation of tissue insulin-like growth factor-1 and IGFBP concentrations by growth hormone and IGF-1. *J. Endocrinol.* 1997; 154 (2): 319–328.

111. Nilsson, A., D. Swolin, S. Enerback, et al. Expression of functional growth hormone receptors in cultured human osteoblast-like cells. *J. Clin. Endocrinol. Metab.* 1995; 80 (12): 3483–3488.

112. Ghiron, L.J., J.L. Thompson, L. Holloway, et al. Effects of recombinant insulin-like growth factor-1 and growth hormone on bone turnover in elderly women. *J. Bone Miner. Res.* 1995; 19 (10): 1844–1852.

113. Baum, H.B., B.M. Miller, J.S. Finkelstein, et al. Effects of physiologic growth hormone therapy on bone mineral density and body composition in patients with adult-onset growth hormone deficiency. A randomized, placebo-controlled trial. *Ann. Intern. Med.* 1996; 81 (1): 883–890.

114. Murphy, M.G., M.A. Bach, D. Plotkin, et al. Oral administration of the growth hormone secretagogue MK-677 increases markers of bone turnover in healthy and functionally impaired elderly adults. The MK-677 Study Group. *J. Bone Miner. Res.* 1999; 14 (7): 1182–1188.

115. Johansson, A.G., E. Lindh, W.F. Blum, et al. Effects of growth hormone and insulin-like growth factor-1 in men with idiopathic osteoporosis. *J. Clin. Endocrinol. Metab.* 1996; 81 (1): 44–48.

116. Isaksson, O.C., C. Ohisson, B.A. Bengsston, et al. GH and bone-experimental and clinical studies. *Endocr. J.* 2000; 47 (Suppl.): S9–S16.

117. Ohlsson, C., J.O. Jansson, and O. Isaksson. Effects of growth hormone and insulin-like growth factor-1 on body growth and adult bone metabolism. *Curr. Opin. Rheumatol.* 2000; 12 (4): 246–248.

118. Bhasin, S. The dose-dependent effects of testosterone on sexual function and on muscle mass and function. *Mayo Clin. Proc.* 2000; 75 (Suppl.): S70–S76.

119. Conway, A.J., D.L. Handelsman, D.W. Lording, et al. Use, misuse and abuse of androgens. The Endocrine Society of Australia consensus guidelines for androgen prescribing. *Med. J. Aust.* 2000; 172 (5): 220–224.

120. Cook, T., and W.P. Sheridan. Development of GnRH antagonists for prostate cancer: new approaches to treatment. *Oncologist* 2000; 5 (2): 162–168.

121. Bosland, M.C. The role of steroid hormones in prostate carcinogenesis. *J. Natl. Cancer Inst. Monogr.* 2000; 27: 39–43.

122. Culig, Z., A. Hobish, G. Bartsch, et al. Expression and function of androgen receptor in carcinoma of the prostate. *Microsc. Res. Tech.* 2000; 51 (5): 447–455.

123. Bartsch, G., R.S. Rittmaster, and H. Klocker. Dihydrotestosterone and the concept of 5alpha-reductase inhibition in human benign prostatic hyperplasia. *Eur. Urol.* 2000; 37 (4): 367–380.

124. Matias, P.M., P. Donner, R. Coelho, et al. Structural evidence for ligand specificity in the binding domain of the human androgen receptor. Implications for pathogenic gene mutations. *J. Biol. Chem.* 2000; 275 (34): 26164–26171.

125. Reichardt, J.K. Prostatic steroid 5 alpha-reductase, and androgen metabolic gene. *Mayo Clin. Proc.* 2000; 75 (Suppl.): S36–S39.

126. Prehn, R.T. On the prevention and therapy of prostate cancer by androgen administration. *Cancer Res.* 1999; 59 (17): 4164–4164.

127. Farnsworth, W.E. Estrogen in the etiopathogenesis of BPH. *Prostate* 1999; 41 (4): 263–274.

128. Buttyan, R., M.A. Ghafar, and A. Shabisgh. The effects of androgen deprivation on the prostate gland: cell death mediated by vascular regression. *Curr. Opin. Urol.* 2000; 10 (5): 415–420.

129. Lin, B., J.T. White, C. Ferguson, et al. Part-1: a novel human prostate-specific, androgen-regulated gene that maps to chromosome 5q12. *Cancer Res.* 2000; 60 (4): 858–863.

130. Tindall, D.L. Androgen receptors in prostate and skeletal muscle. *Mayo Clin. Proc.* 2000; 75 (Suppl.): S26–S30.

131. Prins, G.S. Molecular biology of the androgen receptor. *Mayo Clin. Proc.* 2000; 75 (Suppl.): S32–S35.

132. Culig, Z., A. Hobisch, G. Bartsch, et al. Androgen receptorùan update of mechanisms of action in prostate cancer. *Urol. Res.* 2000; 28 (4): 211–219.

133. Yong, E.L., J. Lim, W. Qi, et al. Molecular basis of androgen receptor diseases. *Ann. Med.* 2000; 32 (1): 15–22.

134. Eaton, N.E., G.K. Reeves, P.N. Appleby, et al. Endogenous sex hormones and prostate cancer: a quantitative review of prospective studies. *Br. J. Cancer* 1999; 80 (7): 930–934.

135. Heikkila, R., K. Aho, M. Heliovaara, et al. Serum testosterone and sex hormone-binding globulin concentrations and the risk of prostate carcinoma: a longitudinal study. *Cancer* 1999; 86 (2): 312–315.

136. Kubricht, W.S., B.J. Williams, T. Whatley, et al. Serum testosterone levels in African-American and white men undergoing prostate biopsy. *Urology* 1999; 54 (6): 1035–1038.

137. Schatzl, G., R.W. Reiter, T. Thurridl, et al. Endocrine patterns in patients with benign and malignant prostatic diseases. *Prostate* 2000; 44 (3): 219–224.

138. Asbell, S.O., K.C. Raimane, A.T. Montesano, et al. Prostate-specific antigen and androgens in African-American and white normal subjects and prostate cancer patients. *J. Natl. Med. Assoc.* 2000; 92 (9): 445–449.

139. Hayami, S., I. Sasagawa, and T. Nakada. Influence of sex hormones on prostatic volume in men on hemodialysis. *J. Androl.* 2000; 21 (2): 258–261.

140. Colao, A., S. Spiezia, C. Di Somma, et al. Effect of GH and/or testosterone deficiency on the prostate: an ultrasonographic and endocrine study in GH-deficient adult patients. *Eur. J. Endocrinol.* 2000; 143 (1): 61–69.

141. Gann, P.H., C.H. Hennekens, J. Ma, et al. Prospective study of sex hormone levels and risk of prostate cancer. *J. Natl. Cancer Inst.* 1996; 88 (16): 1118–1126.

142. Demark-Wahnfried, W., S.M. Lesko, M.R. Conaway, et al. Serum androgens: associations with prostate cancer and hair patterning. *J. Androl.* 1997; 18 (5): 494–500.

143. Prehn, R.T. On the prevention and therapy of prostate cancer by androgen administration. *Cancer Res.* 1999; 59 (17): 4161–4164.

144. Schatzl, G., C. Brossner, S. Schmid, et al. Endocrine status in elderly men with lower urinary tract symptoms: a correlation of age, hormone status, and lower urinary tract function. The Prostate Study Group of the Austrian Society of Urology. *Urology* 2000; 55 (3): 397–402.

145. Hoffman, M.A., W.C. DeWolf, and A. Morgentaler, et al. Is low serum free testosterone a marker for high grade prostate cancer? *J. Urol.* 2000; 163 (3): 824–827.

146. Asbell, S.O., K.C. Raimane, A.T. Montesano, et al. Prostate-specific antigen and androgens in African-American and white normal subjects and prostate cancer. *J. Natl. Med. Assoc.* 2000; 92 (9): 445–449.

147. Pettaway, C.A. Racial differences in the androgen/androgen receptor pathway in prostate cancer. *J. Natl. Med. Assoc.* 1999; 91 (12): 653–660.

148. Wu, A.H., A.S. Whittemore, L.N. Kolonel, et al. Serum androgens and sex hormone-binding globulins in relation to lifestyle factors in older African-American, white, and Asian men in the United States and Canada. *Cancer Epidemiol. Biomarkers Prev.* 1995; 4 (7): 735–741.

149. Jin, B., J. Beilin, J. Zajac, et al. Androgen receptor gene polymorphism and prostate zonal volumes in Australian and Chinese men. *J. Androl.* 2000; 21 (1): 91–98.

150. Behre, H.M., S. von Eckardstein, S. Kliesch, et al. Long-term substitution therapy of hypogonadal men with transscrotal testosterone over 7–10 years. *Clin. Endocrinol. (Oxf.)* 1999; 50 (5): 629–635.

151. Nieschlag, E., D. Buchter, S. Von Eckardstein, et al. Repeated intramuscular injections of testosterone undecanoate for substitution therapy in hypogonadal men. *Clin. Endocrinol. (Oxf.)* 1999; 51 (6): 757–763.

152. Snyder, P.J., H. Peachey, J.A. Berlin, et al. Effects of testosterone replacement in hypogonadal men. *J. Clin. Endocrinol. Metab.* 2000; 85 (8): 2670–2677.

153. Turner, H.H. The clinical use of synthetic male sex hormone. *Endocrinology* 1939; 24 (6): 763–777.

154. Lamar, C.P. Clinical endocrinology of the male with special reference to the male climacteric. *J. Florida Med. Assoc.* 1940; 26 (8): 398–404.

155. Thomas, H.B., and R.T. Hill. Testosterone propionate and the male climacteric. *Endocrinology* 1941; 26: 953–954.

156. Goldman, S.F., and M.J. Markham. Clinical uses of testosterone in the male climacteric. *J. Clin. Endocrinol. Metab.* 1942; 2: 237–242.

157. Werner, A.A. The male climacteric: additional observations of thirty-seven patients. *J. Urology* 1943; 49: 872–882.

158. Jenster, G. The role of the androgen receptor in the development and progression of prostatic cancer. *Semin. Oncol.* 1999; 26 (4): 407–421.

159. Sadar, M.D., and M.E. Gleave. Ligand-independent activation of the androgen receptor by the differentiation agent butyrate in human prostate cancer cells. *Cancer Res.* 2000; 60 (20): 5825–5831.

160. Palmberg, C., P. Koivisto, L. Kakkola, et al. Androgen receptor gene amplification at primary progression predicts response to combined androgen blockage as second line therapy for advanced prostate cancer. *J. Urol.* 2000; 164 (6): 1992–1995.

161. Zhao, X.Y., P.J. Malloy, A.V. Krishnan, et al. Glucocorticoids can promote androgen-independent growth of prostate cancer cells through a mutated androgen receptor. *Nat. Med.* 2000; 6 (6): 703–706.

162. Jenster, G. Ligand-independent activation of the androgen receptor in prostate cancer by growth factors and cytokines. *J. Pathol.* 2000; 191 (3): 227–228.

163. Simon, D., M.A. Charles, K. Nahoul, et al. Association between plasma total testosterone and cardiovascular risk factors in healthy adult men: The Telecom Study. *J. Clin. Endocrinol. Metab.* 1997; 82 (2): 682–685.

164. Shapiro, J., J. Christiana, and W.H. Frishman. Testosterone and other anabolic steroids as cardiovascular drugs. *Am. J. Ther.* 1999; 6 (3): 167–174.

165. Glueck, C.J., H.I. Glueck, D. Stroop, et al. Endogenous testosterone, fibrinolysis, and coronary heart disease in hyperlipidemic men. *J. Lab. Clin. Med.* 1993; 122 (4): 412–420.

166. Alexanderson, P., J. Haarbo, and C. Christiansen. The relationship of natural androgens to coronary heart disease in males: a review. *Atherosclerosis* 1996; 125 (1): 1–13.

167. Edwards, E.A., J.B. Hamilton, and S.Q. Duntley. Testosterone propionate as a therapeutic agent in patients with organic disease of the peripheral vessels: a preliminary report. *N. Engl. J. Med.* 1939; 220: 865–870.

168. Bonnell, R.W., C.P. Prichett, and T.E. Rardin. Treatment of angina pectoris and coronary artery disease with sex hormones. *Ohio State Med. J.* 1940; 37 (6): 554–556.

169. Lesser, M.A. The treatment of angina pectoris with testosterone propionate. *N. Engl. J. Med.* 1942; 226 (2): 51–54.

170. Hamm, L. Testosterone propionate in the treatment of angina pectoris. *J. Clin. Endocrinol.* 1942; 2: 325–328.

171. Walker, T.C. The use of testosterone propionate and estrogenic substance in the treatment of essential hypertension, angina pectoris and peripheral vascular disease. *J. Clin. Endocrinol.* 1942; 2: 560–568.

172. Lesser, M.A. The treatment of angina pectoris with testosterone propionate: further observations. *N. Engl. J. Med.* 1943; 228 (6): 185–188.

173. Levine, S.A., and W.B. Likoff. The therapeutic value of testosterone propionate in angina pectoris. *N. Engl. J. Med.* 1943; 229: 770–772.

174. McGavack, T.H. Angina-like pain; a manifestation of the male climacterium. *J. Clin. Endocrinol.* 1943; 3: 71–80.

175. Opit, L. The treatment of angina pectoris and essential hypertension by testosterone propionate. *Med. J. Australia* 1943; 1: 546.

176. Sigler, L.H., and J. Tulgan. Treatment of angina pectoris by testosterone. *New York State J. Med.* 1943; 43: 1424–1428.

177. Opit, L. The treatment of angina pectoris and peripheral vascular disease by testosterone propionate. *Med. J. Australia* 1943; 2: 173.

178. Strong, G.F., and A.W. Wallace. Treatment of angina pectoris and peripheral vascular disease with sex hormones. *Canad. Med. Assoc. J.* 1944; 50: 30–33.

179. Waldman, S. The treatment of angina pectoris with testosterone propionate. *J. Clin. Endocrinol.* 1945; 5: 305–317.

180. Wu, S.Z., X.Z. Weng, and X.X. Yao. [Antianginal and lipid lower effects of oral androgenic preparation (Andriol) on elderly male patients with coronary heart disease.] *Chung Hua. Nei. Ko Tsa. Chih.* 1993; 32 (4): 235–238.

181. Wu, S.Z., and X.Z Weng. Therapeutic effects of androgenic preparation on myocardial ischemia and cardiac function in 62 elderly male coronary heart disease patients. *Chin. Med. J. (Engl.)* 1993; 106 (6): 415–418.

182. Rabijewski, M., M. Adamkiewicz, and S. Zgliczynksi. [The influence of testosterone replacement therapy on well-being, bone mineral density and lipids in elderly men.] *Pol. Arch. Med. Wewn.* 1998; 100 (3): 212–221.

183. English, K.M., R.P. Steeds, T.H. Jones, et al. Low-dose transdermal testosterone therapy improves angina threshold in men with chronic stable angina: A

randomized, double-blind, placebo-controlled study. *Circulation* 2000; 102 (16: 1906–1911.

184. Webb, C.M., J.G. McNeill, C.S. Hayward, et al. Effects of testosterone on coronary artery vasomotor regulation in men with coronary heart disease. *Circulation* 1999; 100 (16): 1690–1696.

185. Kimura, N., A. Mizokami, T. Oonuma, et al. Immunocytochemical localization of androgen receptor with polyclonal antibody in paraffin-embedded human tissues. *J. Histochem. Cytochem.* 1993; 41 (5): 671–678.

186. Deslypere, J.P., and A. Vermeulen. Aging and tissue androgens. *J. Clin. Endocrinol. Metab.* 1981; 53: 430–463.

187. Deslypere, J.P., A. Sayad, L. Verdonc, et al. Androgen concentrations in sexual and non-sexual skins as well as in striated muscle in man. *J. Steroid Biochem.* 1980; 13: 1455–1460.

188. Kimura, N., A. Mizokami, T. Oonuma, et al. Immunocytochemical localization of androgen receptor with polyclonal antibody in paraffin-embedded human tissues. *J. Histochem. Cytochem.* 1993; 41 (5): 671–678.

189. Marsh, J.D., M.H. Lehmann, R.H. Ritchie, et al. Androgen receptors mediate hypertrophy in cardiac myocytes. *Circulation* 1998; 98 (3): 256–261.

190. Deslypere, J.P., and A. Vermeulen. Influence of age on steroid concentrations in skin and striated muscle in women and cardiac muscle and lung tissue in men. *J. Clin. Endocrinol. Metab.* 1985; 61: 648–653.

191. Schumacher, M., P. Robel, E.E. Baulieu, et al. Development and regeneration of the nervous system: role for neurosteroids. *Dev. Neurosci.* 1996; 18 (1–2): 6–21.

192. Jordan, C.L. Glia as mediators of steroid hormone action on the nervous system: an overview. *J. Neurobiol.* 1999; 40 (4): 434–445.

193. Schumacher, M., F. Robert, and E.E. Baulieu. [Neurosteroids: trophic effects in the nervous system.] *J. Soc. Biol.* 1999; 193 (3): 285–292.

194. Zwain, I.H., and S.S. Yen. Dehydroepiandrosterone: biosynthesis and function. *Endocrinology* 1999; 140 (2): 880–887.

195. Baulieu, E.E., and R. Robel. Neurosteroids: a new brain function? *J. Steroid Biochem. Mol. Biol.* 1990; 37 (3): 395–403.

196. Baulieu, E.E., and R. Robel. Neurosteroids: biosynthesis and function. *Crit. Rev. Neurobiol.* 1995; 9 (4): 383–394.

197. Celotti, F., P. Negri-Cesi, and A. Poletti. Steroid metabolism in the mammalian brain: 5alpha-reduction and aromatization. *Brain Bull.* 1997; 44 (4): 365–375.

198. Tsutsui, K., K. Ukena, M. Usui, et al. Novel brain function: biosynthesis and actions of neurosteroids in neurons. *Neurosci. Res.* 2000; 36 (4): 261–273.

199. Su, T.P., M. Pagliaro, P.J. Schmidt, et al. Neuropsychiatric effects of anabolic steroids in male normal volunteers. *JAMA* 1993; 269 (21): 2760–2764.

200. Janne, O.A., J.J. Palvimo, P. Kallio, et al. Androgen receptor and mechanism of androgen action. *Ann. Med.* 1993; 25 (1): 83–89.

201. Rubinow, D.R., and P.J. Schmidt. Androgens, brain, and behavior. *Am. J. Psychiatry* 1996; 153 (8): 974–984.

202. Frye, C.A., K.R. Van Keuren, P.N. Rao, et al. Analgesic effects of the neurosteroid 3 alpha-androstanediol. *Brain Res.* 1996; 709 (1): 1–9.

203. Lambert, J.J., D. Belelli, C. Hill-Venning, et al. Neurosteroid modulation of native and recombinant GABA (A) receptors. *Cell. Mol. Neurobiol.* 1996; 16 (2): 155–174.

204. Spindler, K.D. Interactions between steroid hormones and the nervous system. *Neurotoxicology* 1997; 18 (3): 745–754.

205. Baulieu, E.E. Neurosteroids: of the nervous system, by the nervous system, for the nervous system. *Recent Prog. Horm. Res.* 1997; 52: 1–32.

206. Wolf, O.T., O. Neumann, D.H. Hellhammer, et al. Effects of a two-week physiological dehydroepiandrosterone substitution on cognitive performance and well-being in healthy elderly women and men. *J. Clin. Endocrinol. Metab.* 1997; 82 (7): 2363–2367.

207. Wolkowitz, O.M., V.I. Reus, E. Roberts, et al. Dehydroepiandrosterone (DHEA) treatment of depression. *Boil. Psychiatry* 1997; 41 (3): 311–318.

208. Gasior, M., R.B. Carter, and J.M. Witkin. Neuroactive steroids: potential therapeutic use in neurological and psychiatric disorders. *Trends Pharmacol. Sci.* 1999; 22 (9): 107–112.

209. Zinder, O., and D.E. Dar. Neuroactive steroids: their mechanism of action and their function in the stress response. *Acta Physiol. Scand.* 1999; 167 (3): 181–188.

210. Park-Chung, M., A. Malyev, R.H. Purdy, et al. Sulfated and unsulfated steroids modulate gama-aminobutyric acid A receptor function through distinct sites. *Brain Res.* 1999; 830 (1): 72–87.

211. Maurice, T., V.L. Phan, A. Urani, et al. Neuroactive neurosteroids as endogenous effectors for the sigma 1 (sigma 1) receptor: pharmacological evidence and therapeutic opportunities. *JPn. J. Pharmacol.* 1999; 81 (2): 125–155.

212. Van Honk, J., A. Tuiten, R. Veraten, et al. Correlations among salivary testosterone, mood, and selective attention to threat in humans. *Horm. Behav.* 1999; 36 (1): 17–24.

213. Rupprecht, R., and F. Holsboer. Neuroactive steroids: mechanisms of action and neuropsychopharmacological perspectives. *Trends Neurosci.* 1999; 22 (9): 410–416.

214. Stomati, M., S. Rubino, A. Spinetti, et al. Endocrine, neuroendocrine and behavioral effects of oral dehydroepiandrosterone sulfate supplementation in postmenopausal women. *Gynecol. Endocrinol.* 1999; 13 (1): 15–25.

215. Green, A.R., A.H. Hainsworth, and D.M. Jackson. GABA potentiation: a logical pharmacological approach for the treatment of acute ischemic stroke. *Neuropharmacology* 2000; 39 (9): 1483–1494.

216. Morrison, M.F., E. Redei, T. TenHave, et al. Dehydroepiandrosterone sulfate and psychiatric measures in a frail, elderly residential care population. *Biol. Psychiatry* 2000; 47 (2): 144–150.

217. Barbaccia, M.L., S. Lello, T. Sidiropoulou, et al. Plasma 5alpha-androstane-3alpha, 17betadiol, and endogenous steroid that positively modulates GABA (A) receptor function and anxiety: a study in menopausal women. *Psychoneuroendocrinology* 2000; 25 (7): 659–675.

218. Johansson, P., A. Lindqvist, F. Nyberg, et al. Anabolic androgenic steroids affects alcohol intake, defensive behaviors and brain opioid peptides in the rat. *Pharmacol. Biochem. Behav.* 2000; 67 (2): 271–279.

219. Hillen, T., A. Lun, F.M. Reishies, et al. DHEA-S plasma levels and incidence of Alzheimer's disease. *Biol. Psychiatry* 2000; 47 (2): 161–163.

220. Drake, E.B., V.W. Henderson, F.Z. Stanczyk, et al. Associations between circulating sex steroid hormones and cognition in normal elderly women. *Neurology* 2000; 54 (3): 599–603.

221. Magri, F., F. Terenzi, T. Ricarciardi, et al. Associations between changes in adrenal secretion and cerebral morphometric correlates in normal aging and senile dementia. *Dement. Geriatr. Cogn. Discord.* 2000; 11 (2): 90–99.

222. Harlan, R.E., H.E. Brown, C.S. Lynch, et al. Androgenic-anabolic steroids blunt morphine-induced c-fos expression in the rat striatum: possible role in beta-endorphin. *Brain Res.* 2000; 853 (1): 99–104.

223. Lapchak, P.A., D.F. Chapman, S.Y. Nunez, et al. Dehydroepiandrosterone sulfate is neuroprotective in a reversible spinal cord ischemia model: a possible involvement of GABA (A) receptors. *Stroke* 2001; 31 (8): 1953–1957.

224. Semkova, I., and J. Krieglestein. Neuroprotection mediated via neurotrophic factors and induction of neurotrophic factors. *Brain Res. Brain Res. Rev.* 1999; 30 (2): 176–188.

225. Cardounel, A., W. Regelson, and M. Kalimi. Dehydroepiandrosterone protects hippocampal neurons against neurotoxin-induced cell death: mechanism of action. *Proc. Soc. Biol. Med.* 1999; 222 (2): 145–149.

226. Fox, H.S. Sex steroids and the immune system. *Ciba Found. Symp.* 1995; 191: 203–211.

227. Loria, R.M., D.A. Padgett, and P.N. Huynh. Regulation of the immune system by dehydroepiandrosterone and its metabolites. *J. Endocrinol.* 1996; 150 (Suppl.): S209–220.

228. Bebo, B.F., J.C. Schuster, A.A. Vanderbark, et al. Androgens alter the cytokine profile and reduce encephalogenicity in myelin-reactive T-cells. *J. Immunol.* 1999; 162 (1): 35–40.

229. Verthelyi, D., and D.M. Klinman. Sex hormone levels correlate with the activity of cytokine-secreting cells in vivo. *Immunology* 2000; 100 (3): 384–390.

230. Lye, M.D., and A.E. Ritch. A double-blind trial of an anabolic steroid (stanozolol) in the disabled elderly. *Rheumatol. Rehabil.* 1977; 16 (1): 62–69.

231. Bashski, V., M. Elliot, A. Gentili, et al. Testosterone improves rehabilitation outcomes of ill older men. *J. Am. Geriatr. Soc.* 2000; 48 (5): 550–553.

232. Tenover, J.S. Effects of testosterone supplementation in the aging male. *J. Clin. Endocrinol. Metab.* 1992; 75 (4): 1092–1098.

233. Bross, R., R. Casaburi, T.W. Storer, et al. Androgen effects on body composition and muscle function: implication for the use of androgens as anabolic agents in sarcopenic states. *Baillieres Clin. Endocrinol. Metab.* 1998; 12 (3): 365–378.

234. Katznelson, L. Therapeutic role of androgens in the treatment of osteoporosis in men. *Baillieres Clin. Endocrinol. Metab.* 1998; 12 (3): 453–470.

235. Bross, R., T. Storer, and S. Bhasin. Aging and muscle loss. *Trends Endocrinol. Metab.* 1999; 19 (5): 194–198.

236. Tenover, J.S. Androgen replacement therapy to reverse and/or prevent age-related sarcopenia in men. *Baillieres Clin. Endocrinol. Metab.* 1998; 12 (3): 419–425.

237. Creutzberg, E.C., and A.M. Schols. Anabolic steroids. *Curr. Opin. Clin. Nutr. Metab. Care* 1999; 2 (3): 243–253.

238. Nieschlag, E., D. Buchter, S. Von Eckardstein, et al. Repeated intramuscular injections of testosterone undecanoate for substitution therapy in hypogonadal men. *Clin. Endocrinol. (Oxf.)* 1999; 51 (6): 757–763.

239. Basaria, S., and A.S. Dobs. Risks versus benefits of testosterone therapy in elderly men. *Drugs Aging* 1999; 15 (2): 131–142.

240. Snyder, P.J., H. Peachey, J.A. Berlin, et al. Effects of testosterone replacement in hypogonadal men. *J. Clin. Endocrinol. Metab.* 2000; 85 (8): 2670–2677.

241. Adami, S., and M. Rossini. Anabolic steroids in corticosteroid-induced osteoporosis. *Wein. Med. Wochenschr.* 1993; 143 (15–16): 395–397.

242. Adachi, J.D., W.G. Bensen, and A.B. Hodsman. Corticosteroid-induced osteoporosis. *Semin. Arthritis Rhem.* 1993; 22 (6): 375–384.

243. Reid, I., D.J. Wattie, M.C. Evans, et al. Testosterone therapy in glucocorticoid-treated men. *Arch. Intern. Med.* 1996; 156 (11): 1173–1177.

244. Fitzgerald, R.C., S.J. Skingle, and A.J. Crisp. Testosterone concentrations in men on chronic glucocorticoid therapy. *J. R. Coll. Physicians Lond.* 1997; 31 (2): 168–170.

245. Kemink, S.A., A.R. Hermus, L.M. Swinkels, et al. Osteopenia in insulin-dependent diabetes mellitus; prevalence and aspects of pathophysiology. *J. Endocrinol. Invest.* 2000; 23 (5): 295–303.

246. Sheffield-Moore, M. Androgens and the control of skeletal muscle protein synthesis. *Ann. Med.* 2000; 32 (3): 181–186.

247. Wilmore, D.H. Deterrents to the successful clinical use of growth factors that enhance protein anabolism. *Curr. Opin. Clin. Nutr. Metab. Care* 1999; 2 (1): 15–21.

248. Wilmore, D.H. Impediments to the successful use of anabolic agents in clinical care. *J. Parenter. Enteral. Nutr.* 1999; 23 (Suppl.): S210–213.

249. Pollock, A.S., L. Legg, P. Langhorne, et al. Barriers to achieving evidence-based stroke rehabilitation. *Clin. Rehabil.* 2000; 14 (6): 611–617.

250. Garcia De Leorenzo, A., and J.M. Culebras. [Hormones, growth factors, and drugs in metabolism and nutrition.] *Nutr. Hosp.* 1995; 10 (5): 297–305.

251. Roubenoff, R. Sarcopenia: a major modifiable cause of frailty in the elderly. *J. Nutr. Health Aging* 2000; 4 (3): 140–143.

252. Dutta, C., and E.C. Hadley. The significance of sarcopenia in old age. *J. Gerontol. A. Biol. Sci. Med. Sci.* 1995; 50 (Spec. No.): 1–4.

253. Basaria, S. and A.S. Dobs. Risks versus benefits of testosterone therapy in elderly men. *Drugs Aging* 1999; 15 (2): 131–142.

254. Vermeulen, A. [Senile hypogonadism in man and hormone replacement therapy.] *Acta Med. Austriaca* 2000; 27 (1): 11–17.

255. Conway, A.J., D.J. Handelsman, D.W. Lording, et al. Use, misuse and abuse of androgens. The Endocrine Society of Australia consensus guidelines for androgen prescribing. *Med. J. Aust.* 2000; 172 (5): 220–224.

256. Lund, B.C., K.A. Bever-Stille, and P.J. Perry. Testosterone and andropause: the feasibility of testosterone replacement therapy in elderly men. *Pharmacotherapy* 1999; 19 (8): 951–956.

257. Vermeulen, A. Andropause. *Maturitas* 2000; 34 (1): 5–15.

258. Prehn, R.T. On the prevention and therapy of prostate cancer by androgen administration. *Cancer Res.* 1999; 59 (17): 4161–4164.

Part 3

*Anabolic Therapy for
Autoimmune Diseases*

7

Rationale for Anabolic Therapy in Autoimmune Diseases

Introduction: Abnormal Sex Steroid Profiles?

Autoimmune diseases represent an array of conditions that are primarily a failure of control in the immune system.[1] This failure of control in the immune system results in a loss of crucial functions that leads to the inability to distinguish and tolerate "self" from "nonself." In this manner, the immune system turns the body's mechanisms of removing nonself on itself. This results in catabolic, destructive, and degenerative alterations in specific tissues or target organs. The ability to distinguish self from nonself is not fully inherent in the immune system, but rather is acquired and continuously maintained. Unfortunately, the mechanisms that maintain the balance between self-tolerance and self-destruction are not perfect, and at times break down. In these instances, an autoimmune disease or condition may result.[2]

Initiation of autoimmune disease involves complex interactions between the neuroendocrine system and the innate and specific immune systems.[3] Under normal conditions T lymphocytes initiate normal immune responses, but it is now clear that T lymphocytes can also *initiate* pathologic immune responses and autoimmune diseases.

Differentiated T lymphocytes produce a restricted set of cells allowing for their subdivision into two major subsets: Th1 (T helper 1) and Th2 (T helper 2) cells. Evidence has accumulated suggesting that polarized Th1 and Th2 cells secrete defined cytokine profiles that have major roles in autoimmunity.[4] In recent years, it has become clear that Th1 and Th2 cells play different roles not only in protection against exogenous offending agents, but also in immunopathology. The cytokines that these T cells

119

secrete (and the balance of these cytokines) play both a crucial role in the development of immune responses towards infectious agents and a major role in the pathogenesis and modulation of autoimmune responses.[5]

A strict compartmentalization of T cells into Th1 and Th2 is clearly an oversimplification owing to the fact that regulatory and effector mechanisms in the immune system encompass much more than Th1 and Th2 cells. However, this oversimplification is useful to the investigational evaluation of autoimmune diseases. In general, it has been shown that Th1 cells contribute to the pathogenesis of several organ-specific autoimmune diseases, whereas Th2 cells may inhibit disease development. It follows that the rational manipulation of the balance of these T cells (and the cytokines that they secrete) may ultimately lead to an effective control of Th1 and Th2 cells and potentially alter the natural course of autoimmune diseases.[6]

Many autoimmune diseases are caused by or are associated with an imbalance between Th1 and Th2 cells. In some diseases an increased ratio of Th1 to Th2 cells results in the Th1 cells becoming overly aggressive and secreting cytokines that attack specific tissues within the body. Examples of Th1 dominant autoimmune diseases include multiple sclerosis (MS), insulin dependent diabetes mellitus (IDDM), and inflammatory bowel disease (IBD). In other diseases, a decreased ratio of Th1 to Th2 cells results in the Th2 cells becoming overly aggressive and secreting cytokines that attack the body. Examples of Th2 dominant autoimmune diseases include systemic lupus erythematosus (SLE), rheumatoid arthritis (RA), and Sjogren's syndrome (SS).[7] Because Th1 and Th2 cells cross-regulate each other, it is likely that therapeutic interventions designed to reinitiate normal Th1-Th2 balance may provide a strategy to prevent or modulate autoimmune diseases.[8, 9] Such therapeutic strategies have included the use of cytotoxic drugs to reduce the dominant Th cell quantity and function and the use of immunomodulating agents, such as androgens, to boost the quantity and function of the opposing Th cells.

Gender Dimorphism in Autoimmune Diseases

Autoimmune diseases are much more common in women than men. The actual prevalence ranges from ten to 15 women for each man for systemic lupus erythematosus (SLE), to four women for every man with rheumatoid arthritis (RA). Sex steroids are believed to be responsible for much of this disparity in gender prevalence. Sex steroids have been shown to exert a substantial influence on the control mechanisms of T lymphocytes, specifically the balance between Th1 and Th2 cells. Androgens have also been shown to play a major role in the inactivation of self-reactive T lymphocytes resulting in a suppressive effect that *reduces* destructive autoimmune responses.[10] In comparison, therapy involving other sex steroids, such as estrogenic steroids used with postmenopausal women, has been shown to *increase* the risk for developing SLE.[11]

Many lines of evidence suggest that autoimmune diseases are the result of *chronic immune activation* of self-reactive T lymphocytes in genetically susceptible individuals following specific environmental exposures. Much of the progress in treating these conditions has been inhibited by the relative rarity and heterogeneity of autoimmune diseases and the lack of understanding of the exact pathogenetic mechanisms. However, continued information is being gathered from genetic encoding of histocompatibility molecules, immunoglobulins, complement components, peptide transporter proteins, T-cell receptors, sex hormones, cytokines, and metabolic enzymes important for drug and toxin elimination, to identify risk factors for one or more autoimmune diseases.[12]

Defects in the immune regulatory processes, which are fundamental to immune disorders, may lie in the immune system itself, or the neuroendocrine system, or both. Defects in the hypothalamus-pituitary-thymus-adrenal-gonadal axis have been observed in autoimmune and rheumatic diseases, neuromuscular diseases, chronic inflammatory diseases, chronic fatigue syndrome, and fibromyalgia. These defects may either result from or cause decreased levels of sex hormones. It is likely that a better understanding of neuroimmunoregulation holds the promise of new approaches to the treatment of immune and inflammatory diseases with the use of sex hormones alone, or in combination with neurotransmitters, neuropeptides, and other drugs that modulate these newly recognized immune regulators.[13]

Reciprocal communication exists between the neuroendocrine and immune systems, and this communication is critical to the regulation of host homeostatic defense mechanisms. This reciprocal communication involves the production of common ligands, peptides, hormones, growth factors, cytokines, and the interaction of these molecules with receptors by cells of both the immune and neuroendocrine systems. This molecular communication constitutes a biochemical information circuit between and within the immune and neuroendocrine systems.[14]

Sex hormones influence the onset and severity of immune-mediated pathologic conditions by modulating T lymphocytes by mechanisms that are not fully understood.

However, using sex hormones for the modulation of immune responses for the treatment of autoimmune disorders continues to be a promising area for further clinical use and investigation.[15] Sex steroids play a substantial role in many autoimmune diseases, and in fact, many of these diseases are associated with the elaboration of autoantibodies or the production of self-reactive T lymphocytes that may have high levels of immune complexes and defects in T cell-mediated immunity. Some of these diseases tend to blend together and coexist such that these conditions can present with a kaleidoscope of common autoimmunity pathophysiology that is linked to sex steroids in a broad sense.[16]

In this chapter, the role of sex hormones, specifically androgens and other anabolic hormones and agents, as they relate to autoimmune diseases will be reviewed in both general and specific terms. Following these reviews, the use of these anabolic molecules as therapy for specific autoimmune diseases and conditions will be presented. Due to the rapid growth of scientific knowledge in this area, the information presented will consist of both information gathered from recognized experimental animal models for autoimmune diseases and studies conducted on human patients. The inherent complexities that relate to autoimmune diseases cross many traditional medical disciplines that correspond to the diversity of medical publications that will be utilized in these discussions.

Androgens Are Immunomodulating Agents

Autoimmune diseases afflict women at a much higher rate than they do men. This fact led to the theory that androgen deficiency may be a factor in the pathogenesis and that androgen (testosterone or anabolic steroid) treatment may be used in autoimmune diseases. Several studies, that utilized androgen therapy on an empirical basis to treat autoimmune diseases, showed promising results decades ago.[17, 18, 19, 20]

In recent times, a substantial body of evidence has accumulated that supports gonadal (testes or ovaries) or adrenal roles in the regulation of the immune system. Much of this evidence, prior to 1990, was based on the following astute observations. It was known that[21, 22, 23, 24]

(1) there was the existence of an *androgen-dependent gender dimorphism* in the immune response.

(2) there was the existence of an *androgen-dependent gender dimorphism* in the occurrence and prevalence of autoimmune diseases.

(3) there were alterations noted in the immune system responses to gonadectomy.

(4) there were alterations noted in the immune system responses to sex steroid therapies.

(5) there were alterations noted in the immune system responses to pregnancy and concomitant remissions or exacerbations of autoimmune diseases in women.

(6) there were findings that sex steroid receptors exist in the thymus tissue that affect T cell function via thymic hormones produced within the gland;

(7) there were suggestions of an identification of a functional axis, the so-called "hypothalamic-pituitary-gonadal-thymic" axis that exerts important regulatory actions on the immune system.

(8) there were findings that sex steroids could influence the immune system by acting on target sites in nonthymic lymphoid organs, the central nervous system, the macrophage-macrocyte system, and the skeletal system.

More recent studies with experimental animal models of human autoimmune diseases have clearly shown that sex hormones regulate the expression, severity, and the progression of these diseases. Many of the modulation effects of sex steroids on the immune system were unequivocal, but the exact mechanisms of action for these modulation effects remain uncertain. To further define these mechanisms, the burgeoning advances in cellular immunology, endocrinology, and molecular biology have provided a better understanding of[25, 26, 27]

(1) the interactions of sex steroids and hormones with the immune system.

(2) the activation of specific genes by sex steroids.

(3) the exact methods that sex steroids influence intracellular communications within the immune system.

(4) the clinical use of nonvirilizing androgenic therapy for immunomodulatory effects.

Recent findings have expanded our knowledge of the androgen-dependent gender dimorphism of the immune system as it relates to autoimmune diseases.[28] These findings include:

(1) that this dimorphism extends to both the humoral (B lymphocytes) and cell mediated (T lymphocytes) and appears to be mechanistically based on the concentrations of sex steroids in males versus females.[29, 30, 31, 32]

(2) that this dimorphism extends to the manner in which cytokines

and lymphokines are influenced by sex hormones during inflammation.[33, 34, 35, 36, 37, 38, 39, 40, 41]

(3) that, in gonadectomized animals, androgen treatment protects against autoimmune disease responses in both genders, especially during the acute phase of autoimmune inflammatory processes.[42, 43, 44]

(4) that this dimorphism extends, in general, to indicate that androgens are protective against autoimmune disease, while estrogens suppress antigen-specific T-cell dependent immune reactions and enhance B-cell activities.[45, 46, 47, 48]

(5) that this dimorphism extends to the genes regulated by sex steroids that affect the immune system and autoimmune responses.[49, 50, 51, 52]

(6) that men, women, and children with a variety of autoimmune diseases and immunity disorders tend to have lower plasma androgen levels than normal age-matched people.[53, 54, 55, 56, 57, 58, 59, 60, 61, 62, 63, 64, 65, 66, 67, 68, 69, 70, 71, 72]

(7) that this dimorphism extends to a gender-related difference in insulin-like growth factor-1 (IGF-1) and serum androgen levels.[73] In general, low androgen levels in men and women are correlated with low levels of IGF-1.[74] Androgen therapy elevates IGF-1 levels independently and via a synergistic effect with growth hormone stimulation.[75] Androgen therapy also has been shown to decrease the levels of IFG-1 binding proteins (IGFBP) and increase the bioavailability of IGF-1.[76] In midadulthood, men have higher IGF-1 levels than women, likely due to the direct simulation by androgens of IGF-1 levels.[77] Insulin-like growth factors have anabolic influences on cell growth and tissue repair.[78] These growth factors promote anabolic and growth actions through binding to IGF-1 receptors found throughout the body.[79] Elevated IFG-1 levels and IGF-1 therapy have been found to have beneficial effects in animal models of human autoimmune diseases and in patients with a variety of autoimmune diseases.[80, 81, 82, 83, 84, 85, 86, 87, 88, 89]

(8) that this dimorphism extends to the manner in which women respond to acute illness by significantly increasing serum estrogen levels and reducing serum androgen levels (causing a significant cytokine imbalance) that may make them more prone to autoimmune diseases than men.[90]

(9) that this dimorphism extends to provide a strong rationale for ongoing clinical trials and clinical use of exogenous androgens in therapy in autoimmune diseases.[91, 92, 93]

(10) that relative androgen deficiency may play a pathogenic role in autoimmune diseases and androgen replacement may represent a valuable concomitant or adjuvant treatment when used with other disease-modifying therapies. [94, 95, 96]

It is clear that androgens play a substantial regulatory or modulating role within the neuroendocrine and neuroimmune systems. Androgen deficiency has become recognized as a risk factor for developing a variety of autoimmune diseases in genetically susceptible individuals. Treatment of autoimmune diseases with androgens has shown promising results, but continues to be a largely overlooked form of therapy in these conditions. It is likely that future studies will indicate that androgen therapy is a disease-modifying form of treatment in a variety of autoimmune diseases due to the multifaceted influences that they exert on the immune, neuromuscular, and endocrine systems within the body.

Androgen therapy in autoimmune diseases *is not* an alternative treatment. However, many patients with autoimmune diseases resort to the use of various alternative treatments due primarily to the lack of success with current standard therapies. One study reports that 42 percent of patients with multiple sclerosis had used alternative therapies.[97] Adequate training of physicians and changes in our present approach in caring for patients may be the greatest obstacles to overcome for the full application of anabolic agents and growth factor therapy in catabolic diseases.[98]

Androgens Are Neuroprotective and Neuroregenerative Agents

There is a growing body of evidence that supports the concept that androgens exhibit neuroprotective and neuroregenerative properties. Besides the general anabolic influences, androgens have been shown to directly:

(1) exert a protective effect in animal models of human autoimmune disease by suppressing myelin basic protein (MBP)-specific T lymphocytes that attack myelin.

Specifically, androgens have been shown to exert a protective effect in experimental autoimmune encephalomyelitis (EAE)—an animal model of multiple sclerosis—by enhanced production of IL-10 by autoantigen-specific T lymphocytes and by inducing a T helper 2 cell bias.[99]

(2) exert a protective effect in EAE to a significant degree during the acute-phase of demyelination associated with the disease.[100]

(3) exert an anabolic effect on motoneurons by elevating the levels of specific mRNAs throughout the spinal cord suggesting that motoneuronal characteristics are modulated by circulating androgen levels.[101]

(4) exert a protective effect by a mechanism that blocks the toxin-

induced production of pathophysiological levels of the destructive influences of endogenous molecules such as tumor necrosis factor-alpha (TFN-alpha) and interleukin-1.[102, 103]

(5) exert a balancing effect brought about by the dissociation between androgens and corticogenic steroids often exhibited by autoimmune disease, inflammatory processes, and aging.[104, 105, 106, 107, 108]

(6) exert a direct effect on the balance of cytokines during the induction of the immune response that can alter the development of effector T cells and reduce the severity of an autoimmune insult by myelin-reactive T cells.[109, 110, 111]

(7) exert a direct effect on the macrophage activator enzymes within macrophages that play an important role for local immunomodulation at a tissue level.[112]

(8) exert a direct neuroprotective effect, via GABA(A) receptors in the CNS, in relation to a variety of insults, including ischemia, to the spinal cord, and excitotoxicity.[113]

(9) exert a direct neuroprotective effect by exhibiting an antiglucocorticoid action in the brain.[114, 115]

Androgens have also been shown to directly and significantly elevate IGF-1 levels and decrease IGFBP levels, thus further increasing the bioavailability of circulating IGF-1. This anabolic effect reverses the catabolic changes seen in many autoimmune and wasting disease conditions that are marked by depressed IGF-1 levels, increased IGFBP levels, and reduced bioavailability of circulating IFG-1.[116] These anabolic and stimulatory effects have been shown in normal men,[117] aging men and women,[118, 119, 120, 121] and in both genders afflicted by autoimmune diseases and wasting conditions.[122, 123] Specifically, androgen therapy results in:

(1) elevating IGF-1 levels that, in turn, reduces clinical deficits, decreases lesion severity and upregulates synthesis of myelin proteins including mRNA levels of MPB, proteolipid (PLP) and 2',3' cyclic nucleotide 3'-phosphodiesterase (CNP) that promote myelin regeneration in EAE.[124, 125]

(2) elevating IGF-1 levels that, in turn, assists in the maintenance of the integrity and homeostasis of the nervous system. The widespread distribution of IGF-1 receptors allows IGF-1 to affect the survival of numerous populations of neurons and glial cells in the central and peripheral nervous systems and provide a general means of reducing or slowing down neuronal losses following various brain and nerve insults.[126, 127, 128]

(3) elevating IGF-1 which, that, in turn, promotes preoligodendrocytes to divide or migrate or both in response to signals present in demyelinating lesions and thus facilitates remyelination.[129]

(4) elevating IGF-1 levels which, in turn, reduces the clinical deficits during the first attack and during subsequent relapses of inflammatory and demyelinating lesions in animal models for human autoimmune diseases.[130]

In summary, androgen therapy has been shown to have neuroprotective, regenerative, and anabolic influences on both the CNS and PNS, either directly, or indirectly via IGF-1 stimulation. Androgen therapy produces these effects in a very-cost effective manner (less than $1,000 annually) compared to the annual cost of recombinant IGF-1 costs of over $43,000.[131] Androgen therapy also has many other beneficial anabolic and neuroactive influences in patients with autoimmune diseases. In nonvirilizing doses, it should be considered in all patients with autoimmune neurological conditions. Research is ongoing with androgen therapy for these conditions.

Androgens Are Potent Neurosteroids

Patients with autoimmune diseases often suffer from deficits in cognition, disturbances in mood and sense of well-being, and loss of libido or sexual dysfunction. These conditions can be caused by the autoimmune disease itself or from prescribed medications to treat the disease.

In animals, the effects of androgens on the brain structure are well established and profound, with behavioral implications extending far beyond reproduction. Androgens play a prominent role in the organization and programming of brain circuits that are activated by sex steroids.[132] Androgens exert these behavioral influences via direct binding to a variety of receptors throughout the brain and by modulating the effects and levels of other neurotransmitters.[133, 134, 135, 136, 137, 138, 139, 140, 141, 142, 143, 144, 145, 146]

Thus, animal studies have shown that androgens:

(1) have a major role in the organization and programming of brain circuits.

(2) are direct neurotransmitters that bind to numerous neuroreceptors throughout the brain.

(3) modulate the actions and levels of a variety of other neurotransmitters throughout the brain.

(4) can induce changes in number and concentration of various neuroreceptors in brain tissues.

(5) are required in levels to activate and maintain the function of the brain's neurotransmitter circuit network.

It is likely that much of this information regarding the role of androgens in animal brain tissues will correlate with that of human studies. Even though animals and humans have very different behaviors, the biochemical neurotransmission via receptors is likely to be very similar.

In humans, roles for androgens have been described in the regulation of sexuality, aggression, cognition, emotion, well-being, and personality.[147] Androgens are potent neurosteroids that have been shown to be in reduced levels in the presence of several autoimmune diseases. Androgens have receptors throughout the human brain and consequently have manifest effects on behavior.[148] When androgen levels are reduced, subjects have been shown to exhibit:

    (1) increased risk for senile dementia.[149, 150]

    (2) reduced cognitive performance.[151, 152, 153, 154]

    (3) increase risk factor for Alzheimer's disease.[155, 156, 157, 158]

    (4) increased risk for mental depression.[159, 160]

    (5) reduced libido, self-esteem, energy levels, and sense of well-being.[161, 162, 163, 164]

Low-dose androgen therapy has been shown to:

    (1) play a role in the psychological and physical well-being of post-menopausal women acting via a restoration of neuroendocrine control of anteropituitary beta-endorphin secretion.[165, 166]

    (2) provide for characteristics of a positive mood in normal, young subjects, including euphoria, increased energy level, and increased libido.[167]

    (3) enhance libido, enhance orgasmic responses, and reduce erectile dysfunction in patients with reduced serum androgen levels.[168, 169, 170, 171, 172, 173, 174, 175, 176, 177, 178, 179, 180, 181, 182]

    (4) increase energy levels, self-esteem, sense of well-being, and quality of life.[183, 184, 185, 186 187, 188, 189, 190]

    (5) reduce mental depression, fatigue, and anxiety.[191, 192, 193, 194, 195, 196, 197, 198, 199]

    (6) improve cognitive function in healthy elderly women and men.[200, 201, 202, 203]

    (7) improve cognitive function in patients with autoimmune diseases and idiopathic causes of secondary hypogonadism.[204, 205]

Androgens Are Anabolic Agents

Loss of muscle mass, neuromuscular strength, fatigue, and osteo-porosis are common sequelae of many autoimmune diseases. These conditions occur both from the autoimmune disease, acquired secondary hypogonadism, age-related decreased androgen production, age-related adrenal androgen production, and from the heavy use of catabolic corticogenic steroids and cytotoxic drug therapies commonly prescribed to treat the disease. Androgen and other anabolic therapies should be used to counteract and reverse these catabolic influences and conditions.

Participants in competitive sports have demonstrated that the use of androgens, growth hormone, growth factors, and other anabolic agents enhance muscle mass, neuromuscular strength, and human performance, yet physicians have been slow to adopt this approach in patients who have disease-related decrease in muscle mass, strength, and activity.[206] Anabolic modification of the neuroendocrine systems may both decrease the loss of body proteins and promote and accelerate recovery, thus shortening the hospital stay, and reducing convalescence time.[207] The sarcopenia associated with disabling diseases, such as autoimmune diseases and aging, represents a major threat of epidemic of frailty which can be overcome by developing public health interventions that deliver an anabolic stimulus to the muscles of afflicted adults on a mass scale.[208]

Androgen therapy has been shown to improve rehabilitation outcomes of both men and women by improving neuromuscular strength and functional activities of daily living.[209, 210, 211] Androgen therapy has also been shown to reverse many of the catabolic effects on muscle and bone tissues caused by prolonged or repetitive corticogenic steroid therapy or from age-related alterations in adrenocortical function[212, 213, 214, 215, 216, 217] Androgen levels have also been positively correlated with the physical fitness and activity levels of independent community-dwelling older men and women.[218]

Androgens exert major anabolic influences on muscle and bone tissues and are paramount in maintaining lean body mass, neuromuscular strength, bone density and bone strength. Many of the mechanisms by which androgens affect these tissues are known and include the following:

(1) directly stimulating androgen receptors resulting in activation of mRNA and RNA-polymerase in skeletal muscle cell nuclei.[219, 220, 221, 222]

(2) directly stimulating the fractional synthetic rate by 44 percent above normal levels of skeletal muscle protein by increasing the total concentration of mRNA and the intracellular reutilization of amino acids.[223]

(3) directly stimulating the fractional synthetic rate by 94 percent of skeletal muscle protein above normal levels when combined with a continuous infusion of a commercial amino acid mixture (10 percent Travasol)[224] indicating that both anabolic stimulus and availability of an amino acid pool are important to the net muscle protein synthesis.[225]

(4) directly elevating serum levels of IGF-1 above normal levels.[226]

(5) directly enhancing GH secretion above normal via increased GHRH pulse amplitude.[227]

(6) directly increasing skeletal muscle mass and strength.[228, 229, 230, 231, 232, 233, 234, 235, 236, 237, 238]

Androgens Are Osteoblast Stimulators

Although the relative contributions of androgens and estrogens to bone metabolism are still being defined, androgens have been found to be direct osteoblast stimulators. Over the past decades, investigation into androgen effects on bone has been overshadowed by interest (by most investigators) in estrogen effects.[239]

Androgen therapy (or self-use) combined with progressive strength-training protocols have been shown to:

(1) increase skeletal muscle size and strength by muscle hypertrophy and hyperplasia mechanisms (statistically significant). The activation of satellite cells has been shown to be a key process that is enhanced by androgens, which results in the formation of new muscle fibers.[240]

(2) increase the androgen receptor concentration of skeletal muscle cells over and above the effects of strength training alone (statistically significant).[241]

(3) increase muscle mass and strength over and above resistance training alone in athletes (statistically significant).[242, 243, 244, 245, 246, 247, 248]

(4) increase muscle mass and strength over and above resistance training alone in patients with hypogonadism and compromised immune systems.[249, 250, 251]

Summary

In this chapter it has been shown that androgens play an important role in the pathogenesis, course, and sequelae of autoimmune diseases. The available scientific evidence has been utilized to show that androgens are:

(1) immunomodulating agents.
(2) neuroprotective agents.
(3) neuroregenerative agents.
(4) neurosteroid agents.
(5) anabolic agents.
(6) osteoblast stimulating agents.

These powerful and multifaceted beneficial characteristics make androgen therapy powerful and multifaceted beneficial characteristics make an appropriate therapeutic modality in the treatment of autoimmune diseases. No other class of drugs offers such a wide array of beneficial effects for therapy in autoimmune diseases.

Notes

1. Jones, D.E., and A.G. Diamond. The basis of autoimmunity: an overview. *Baillieres Clin. Endocrinol. Metab.* 1995; 9 (1): 1–24.

2. Richardson, B.C. T cell receptor usage in rheumatic disease. *Clin. Exp. Rheumatol.* 1992; 10 (3): 271–283.

3. Goverman, J., T. Brabb, A. Paez, et al. Initiation and regulation of CNS autoimmunity. *Crit. Rev. Immunol.* 1997; 17 (5–6): 469–480.

4. De Carli, M., M.M. D'Elios, G. Zancuoghi, et al. Human Th1 and Th2 cells: functional properties, regulation of development and role in autoimmunity. *Autoimmunity* 1994; 18 (4): 301–308.

5. Berger, S., H. Ballo, and H.J. Stutte. Distinct antigen-induced cytokine pattern upon stimulation with antibody-complexed antigen consistent with a Th1--> Th2-shift. *Res. Virol.* 1996; 147 (2–3): 103–108.

6. Adorini, L., J.C. Guery, and S. Trembleau. Manipulation of the Th1/Th2 cell balance: an approach to treat human autoimmune diseases? *Autoimmunity* 1996; 23 (1): 53–68.

7. Ishida, H., H. Ota, H. Yanagida, et al. [An imbalance between Th1 and Th2–like cytokines in patients with autoimmune diseases— differential diagnosis between Th1 dominant autoimmune diseases and Th2 dominant autoimmune diseases.] *Nippon Rinsho* 1997; 55 (6): 1438–1443.

8. Nicholson, L.B. and V.K. Kuchroo. Manipulation of the Th1/Th2 balance in autoimmune disease. *Curr. Opin. Immunol.* 1996; 8 (6): 837–842.

9. Kroemer, G., F. Hirsch, A. Gonzalez-Garcia, et al. Differential involvement of Th1 and Th2 cytokines in autoimmune diseases. *Autoimmunity* 1996; 24 (1): 25–33.

10. Lahita, R.G. The connective tissue diseases and the overall influence of gender. *Int. J. Fertil. Menopausal Stud.* 1996; 41 (2): 156–165.

11. Sanchez-Guerrero, J., M.H. Liang, E.W. Karlson, et al. Postmenopausal estrogen therapy and the risk for developing systemic lupus erythematosus. *Ann. Intern. Med.* 1995; 122 (6): 430–433.

12. Miller, F.W. Genetics of autoimmune diseases. *Exp. Clin. Immunogenet.* 1995; 12 (3): 182–190.

13. Anisman, H., M.G. Baines, I. Berczi, et al. Neuroimmune mechanisms in health and disease: 2. Disease. *CMAJ* 1996; 155 (8): 1075–1082.

14. Weigent, D.A. Immunoregulatory properties of growth hormone and pro-lactin. *Pharmacol. Ther.* 1996; 69 (3): 237–257.

15. Ahmed, S.A., W.J. Penhale, and N. Talal. Sex hormones, immune responses, and autoimmune diseases. Mechanisms of sex hormone action. *Am. J. Pathol.* 1985; 121 (3): 531–551.

16. Lorber, M., M.E. Gershwin, and Y. Shoenfeld. The coexistence of systemic lupus erythematosus with other autoimmune diseases: the kaleidoscope of autoimmunity. *Semin. Arthritis Rheum.* 1994; 24 (2): 105–113.

17. Szabo, S., R.C. Wagner, E.G. Malatinszky, T. Becus, et al. [The effect of anabolic steroids on blood proteins and autoantibodies in multiple sclerosis.] *Stud. Cercet. Neurol.* 1967; 12 (6): 457–461.

18. Mall, G., A. Heibrunn, H.F. Paarmann, et al. [The treatment of multiple sclerosis with anabolic steroids.] *Med. Klin.* 1968; 63 (51): 2075–2077.

19. Husemann, F., J. Kugler, and I. Frank. [Relaxation-promoting effect of vitamin B with anabolics.] *Arzneimittelforschung* 1970; 20 (4): 557–60.

20. Cendrowski, W., and W. Kuran. [Results of combined administration of anabolic steroids in patients with multiple sclerosis.] *Neurol. Neurochir. Pol.* 1972; 6 (4): 573–576.

21. Seiki, K., K., Sakabe, I. Kawashima, et al. Hormone and immune response, with special reference to steroid hormone 1. A short review. *Tokai J. Exp. Clin. Med.* 1990; 15 (2–3): 191–199.

22. Dorner, G., R. Eckert, and G. Hinz. Androgen-dependent sexual dimorphism in the immune system. *Endokrinologie* 1980; 76 (1): 112–114.

23. Ahmed S. A., W.J. Penhale, and N. Talal. Sex hormones, immune responses, and autoimmune diseases. Mechanisms of sex hormone action. *Am. J. Pathol.* 1985; 121 (3): 531–551.

24. Steinberg, A.D., K.A. Melez, E.S. Ravenche, et al. Approach to the study of the role of sex hormones in autoimmunity. *Arthritis Rheum.* 1979; 22 (11): 1170–1176.

25. Schuurs, A.H., and H.A. Verheul. Effects of gender and sex steroids on the immune response. *J. Steroid Biochem.* 1990; 35 (2): 157–172.

26. Ahmed, S.A., and N. Talal. Sex hormones and the immune system "Part 2. Animal data. *Baillieres Clin. Rheumatol.* 1990; 4 (1): 13–31.

27. Ahmed, S.A., W.J. Penhale, and N. Talal. Sex hormones, immune responses, and autoimmune diseases. Mechanisms of sex hormone action. *Am. J. Pathol.* 1985; 121 (3): 531–551.

28. Paavonen, T. Hormonal regulation of immune responses. *Ann. Med.* 1994; 26 (4): 255–258.

29. Weinstein, Y., and S. Berkovich. Testosterone effect on bone marrow, thymus, and suppressor T cells in the (NZB X NZW)F mice: its relevance to autoimmunity. *J. Immunol.* 1981; 126 (3): 998–1002.

30. Grossman, C.J., G.A. Roselle, and C.L. Mendenhall. Sex steroid regulation of autoimmunity. *J. Steroid Biochem. Mol. Biol.* 1991; 40 (4–6): 649–659.

31. Bebo, B.F., K. Adlard, J.C. Schuster, et al. Gender differences in protection from EAE induced by oral tolerance with a peptide analogue of MBP-Acl–11. *J. Neurosci. Res.* 1999; 55 (4): 432–440.

32. Culp, M., and R.L. Wilder. Different roles for androgens and estrogens in the susceptibility to autoimmune rheumatic diseases. *Rheum. Dis. Clin. North Am.* 2000; 26 (4): 825–839.

33. Angioni, S., F. Petraglia, and A.R. Genezzani. Immune-neuroendocrine correlations: a new aspect of human physiology. *Acta Eur. Fertil.* 1991; 22 (3): 167–170.

34. Compston, A. Future prospects for the management of multiple sclerosis. *Ann. Neurol.* 1994; 36 (Suppl.): S146–150.

35. Bebo, B.F., A.A. Vanderbark, and H. Offner. Male SJL mice do not relapse after induction of EAE with PLP 139–151. *J. Neurosci. Res.* 1996; 45 (6): 680–689.

36. Elenkov, I.J., J. Hoffman, and R.L. Wilder. Does differential neuroendocrine control of cytokine production govern the expression of autoimmune diseases in pregnancy and the postpartum period? *Mol. Med. Today* 1997; 3 (9): 379–383.

37. Bebo, B.F. J.C. Schuster, A.A. Vandenbark, et al. Androgens alter the cytokine profile and reduce encephalitogenicity of myelin-reactive T cells. *J. Immunol.* 1999; 162 (1): 35–40.

38. Wilcoxen, S.C., E. Kirkman, K.C. Dowdell, et al. Gender-dependent IL-12 secretion by APC is regulated by IL-10. *J. Immunol..* 2000; 164 (12): 6237–6243.

39. Verthelyi, D., and D.M. Klinman. Sex hormone levels correlate with the activity of cytokine-secreting cells in vivo. *Immunology* 2000; 100 (3): 384–390.

40. Papdopoulos, A.D., and S.L. Wardlaw. Testosterone suppresses the response of the hypothalamic-pituitary-adrenal axis to interleukin-6. *Neuroimmunomodulation* 2000; 8 (1): 39–44.

41. Giron-Gonzalez, J.A., F.J. Moral, J. Elvira, et al. Consistent production of a higher TH1: TH2 cytokine ratio stimulated T cells in men compared with women. *Eur. J. Endocrinol.* 2000; 143 (1): 31–36.

42. Spinedi, E., M.O. Suescun, R. Hadid, et al. Effects of gonadectomy and sex hormone therapy on the endotoxin-stimulated hypothalamo-pituitary-adrenal axis: evidence for a neuroendocrine-immunological sexual dimorphism. *Endocrinology* 1992; 131 (5): 2430–2436.

43. Gaillard, R.C., and E. Spinedi. Sex- and stress-steroids interactions and the immune system: evidence for a neuroendocrine-immunological sexual dimorphism. *Domest. Anim. Endocrinol.* 1998; 15 (5): 345–352.

44. Bebo, B.F., J.C. Schuster, A.A. Vandebark, et al. Gender differences in experimental autoimmune encephalomyelitis develop during the induction of the immune response to encephalitogenic peptides. *J. Neurosci. Res.* 1998; 52 (4): 420–426.

45. Schuurs, A.H., and H.A. Verheul. Sex hormones and autoimmune disease. *Br. J. Rheumatol.* 1989; 28 (Suppl. 1): 59–61.

46. Cuchacovich, M., H. Gatica, and A.N. Tchernichin. [Role of sex hormones in autoimmune diseases.] *Rev. Med. Chil.* 1993; 121 (9): 1045–1052.

47. Beeson, P.B. Age and sex associations in 40 autoimmune diseases. *Am. J. Med.* 1994; 96 (5): 457–462.

48. Dalal, M., S. Kim, and R.R. Voskuhl. Testosterone therapy ameliorates experimental autoimmune encephalomyelitis and induces a T helper 2 bias in the autoantigen-specific T lymphocyte response. *J. Immunol.* 1997; 159 (1): 3–6.

49. Fox, H.S. Sex steroids and the immune system. *Ciba Found. Symp.* 1995; 191: 203–211.

50. Holmdahl, R. Female preponderance for development of arthritis in rats is influenced by both sex chromosomes and sex steroids. *Scand. J. Immunol.* 1995; 42 (1): 104–109.

51. Voskuhl, R.R., H. Pitchekian-Halabi, A. MacKenzie-Graham, et al. Gender differences in autoimmune demyelination in the mouse: implications for multiple sclerosis. *Ann. Neurol.* 1996; 39 (6): 724–733.

52. Bebo, B.F., E. Zelinka-Vincent, G. Adamus, et al. Gonadal hormones influence the immune response to PLP 139–151 and the clinical course of relapsing experimental autoimmune encephalomyelitis. *J. Neuroimmunol.* 1998; 84 (2): 122–130.

53. Dougados, M., N. Nahoul, L.O. Benhamou, et al. [Study of plasma androgens in women with autoimmune diseases.] *Rev. Rhum. Mal. Osteoartic.* 1984; 51 (3): 145–149.

54. Klapps, P., S. Seyfert, T. Fischer, et al. Endocrine function in multiple sclerosis. *Acta Neurol. Scand.* 1992; 85 (5): 353–357.

55. Lahita, R.G. The effects of sex hormones on the immune system in pregnancy. *Am. J. Reprod. Immunol.* 1992; 28 (3–4): 136–137.

56. Valentino, R., S. Savastano, A.P. Tommaselli, et al. Hormonal pattern in women affected by rheumatoid arthritis. *J. Endocrinol. Invest.* 1993; 16 (8): 619–624.

57. Athreya, B.H., J. H. Rafferty, G.S. Sehgal, et al. Adenohypophyseal and sex hormones in pediatric rheumatic diseases. *J. Rheumatol.* 1993; 20 (4): 725–730.

58. Munoz, J.A., A. Gil, J.M. Lopez-Dupla, et al. Sex hormones in chronic systemic lupus erythematosus. Correlation with clinical and biological parameters. *Ann. Med. Interne. (Paris)* 1994; 145 (7): 459–463.

59. van Vollenhoven, R.F., and J. L. McGuire. Estrogen, progesterone, and testosterone: can they be used to treat autoimmune diseases? *Cleve. Clin. J. Med.* 1994; 61 (4): 276–284.

60. Nilsson, E., B. de la Torre, M. Hedman, et al. Blood dehydroepiandrosterone sulphate (DHEAS) levels in polymyalgia rheumatica/giant cell arthritis and primary fibromyalgia. *Clin. Exp. Rheumatol.* 1994; 12 (4): 415–417.

61. Masi, A.T., S.L. Feigenbaum, and R.T. Chatterton. Hormonal and pregnancy relationships to rheumatoid arthritis: convergent effects with immunologic and microvascular systems. *Semin. Arthritis Rheum.* 1995; 25 (1): 1–27.

62. Lahita, R.G. The connective tissue diseases and the overall influence of gender. *Int. J. Fertil. Menopausal Stud.* 1996; 41 (2): 156–165.

63. Wilder, R.L. Adrenal and gonadal steroid hormone deficiency in the pathogenesis of rheumatoid arthritis. *J. Rheumatol. Suppl.* 1996; 44: 10–12.

64. Davies, J.S., N.P. Hinds, and M.F. Scanlon. Growth hormone deficiency and hypogonadism in a patient with multiple sclerosis. *Clin. Endocrinol. (Oxf.)* 1996; 44 (1): 117–119.

65. Wei, T., and S.L. Lightman. The neuroendocrine axis in patients with multiple sclerosis. *Brain* 1997; 120 (6): 1067–1076.

66. Kumpfel, T., F. Then Bergh, E. Friess, et al. Dehydroepiandrosterone response to the adrenocorticotropin test and the combined dexamethasone and corticotrophin-releasing hormone test in patients with multiple sclerosis. *Neuroendocrinology* 1999; 70 (6): 431–438.

67. Tsuki, K., D. Furutama, M. Tagami, et al. Specific binding and effects of dehydroepiandrosterone sulfate (DHEA-S) on skeletal muscle cells: possible implication for DHEA-S replacement therapy in patients with myotonic dystrophy. *Life Sci.* 1999; 65 (1): 17–26.

68. Gebre-Medhin, G., E.S. Husebye, H. Mallmin, et al. Oral dehydroepiandrosterone (DHEA) replacement therapy in women with Addison's disease. *Clin. Endocrinol. (Oxf.)* 2000; 52 (6): 775–780.

69. James, W.H. Androgen levels of patients with ankylosing spondylitis. *J. Rheumatol.* 1999; 26 (8): 1850–1851.

70. Straub, R.H., T. Gluck, M. Cutolo, et al. The adrenal steroid status in relation to inflammatory cytokines (interleukin-6 and tumor necrosis factor) in polymyalgia rheumatica. *Rheumatology (Oxf.)* 2000; 39 (6): 624–631.

71. Johansson, A., K. Carstrom, B. Ahren, et al. Abnormal cytokine and adrenocortical hormone regulation in myotonic dystrophy. *J. Clin. Endocrinol. Metab.* 2000; 85 (9): 3169–3176.

72. James, W.H. Androgen levels of patients with ankylosing spondylitis. *J. Rheumatol.* 2000; 27 (2): 556–557.

73. Kostka, T., L.M. Arsac, M. C. Patricot, et al. Leg extensor power and dehydroepiandrosterone sulfate, insulin-like growth factor-I and testosterone in healthy active elderly people. *Eur. J. Appl. Physiol.* 2000; 82 (1–2): 83–90.

74. Proctor, D.N., P. Balagopal, and K.S. Nair. Age-related sarcopenia in humans is associated with reduced synthetic rates of specific muscle proteins. *J. Nutr.* 1998; 128 (2 Suppl.): 351S–355S.

75. Eakman, G.D., J.S. Dallas, S.W. Ponder, et al. The effects of testosterone and dihydrotestosterone on hypothalamic regulation of growth hormone secretion. *J. Clin. Endocrinol. Metab.* 1996; 81 (3): 1217–1223.

76. Hobbs, C. J., S.R. Plymate, C.J. Rosen, et al. Testosterone administration increases insulin-like growth factor-1 levels in normal men. *J. Clin. Endocrinol. Metab.* 1993; 77 (3): 776–779.

77. Jorgensen, J. O., N. Vahl, T.B. Hansen, et al. Determinants of serum insulin-like growth factor I in growth hormone deficient adults as compared to healthy adults. *Clin. Endocrinol. (Oxf.)* 1998; 48 (4): 479–486.

78. Zapt, J., M.Y. Donath, and C. Schmid. [Spectrum of effectiveness of insulin-like growth factors.] *Schweiz. Med. Wochenschr.* 2000; 130 (6): 190–195.

79. Hall, K., P. Bang, and K. Brismar. [Insulin-like growth factors. Future treatment in catabolism?] *Lakartidningen* 1995; 92 (26–27): 2888–2891.

80. Festoff, B.W., S.X. Yang, J. Vaught, et al. The insulin-like growth factor signaling system and ALS neurotrophic factor treatment strategies. *J. Neurol. Sci.* 1995; 129 (Suppl.): 114–121.

81. Yao, D.L., X. Liu, L.D. Hudson, et al. Insulin-like growth factor 1 treatment reduces demyelination and up-regulates gene expression of myelin-related proteins in experimental autoimmune encephalomyelitis. *Proc. Natl. Acas. Sci. U.S.A.* 1995; 92 (13): 6190–6194.

82. Liu, X., D.L. Yao, and H. Webster. Insulin-like growth factor 1 treatment reduces clinical deficits and lesion severity in acute demyelinating experimental autoimmune encephalomyelitis. *Mult. Scler.* 1995; 1 (1): 2–9.

83. Yao, D.L., X. Liu, L.D. Hudson, et al. Insulin-like growth factor-1 given subcutaneously reduces clinical deficits, decreases lesion severity and upregulates synthesis of myelin proteins in experimental autoimmune encephalomyelitis. *Life Sci.* 1996; 58 (16): 1301–1306.

84. Lai, E.C., K.J. Felice, B.W. Festoff, et al. Effect of recombinant human insulin-like growth factor-I on progression of ALS. A placebo-controlled study. The North America ALS/IGF-I Study Group. *Neurology* 1997; 49 (6): 1621–1630.

85. Liu, X., C. Linnington, H.D. Webster, et al. Insulin-like growth factor-1 treatment reduces immune cell responses in acute non-demyelinative experimental autoimmune encephalomyelitis. *J. Neurosci. Res.* 1997; 47 (5): 531–538.

86. Webster, H.D. Growth factors and myelin regeneration in multiple sclerosis. *Mult. Scler.* 1997; 3 (2): 113–120.

87. Li, W., L. Quigley, D.L. Yao, et al. Chronic relapsing experimental auto-immune encephalomyelitis: effects of insulin-like growth factor-1 treatment on clinical deficits, lesion severity, glial responses, and blood brain barrier defects. *J. Neuropathol. Exp. Neurol.* 1998; 57 (5): 426–438.

88. Corse, A.M., M.M. Bilak, S.R. Bilak, et al. Preclinical testing of neuroprotective neurotrophic factors in a model of chronic motor neuron degeneration. *Neurobiol. Dis.* 1999; 6 (5): 335–346.

89. Dubois-Dalcq, M., and K. Murry. Why are growth factors important in oligodendrocyte physiology? *Pathol. Biol. (Paris)* 2000; 48 (1): 80–86.

90. Spratt, D.I., C. Longcope, P.M. Cox, et al. Differential changes in serum

concentrations of androgens and estrogens (in relation with cortisol) in post-menopausal women with acute illness. *J. Clin. Endocrinol. Metab.* 1993; 76 (6): 1542–1547.

91. Merrill, J.T., A.R. Dinu, and R.G. Lahita. Autoimmunity: The female connection. *Medscape Womens Health* 1996; 1 (11): 5.

92. Shahar, E., R. Bergman, and S. Pollack. Autoimmune progesterone dermatitis: effective prophylactic treatment with danazol. *Int. J. Dermatol.* 1997; 36 (9): 708–711.

93. Bijlsma, J.W. Can we use steroid hormones to immunomodulate rheumatic diseases? Rheumatoid arthritis as an example. *Ann. N.Y. Acad. Sci.* 1999; 876: 366–376.

94. James, W.H. Rheumatoid arthritis, the contraceptive pill, and androgens. *Ann. Rheum. Dis.* 1993; 52 (6): 470–474.

95. Masi, A.T. Sex hormones and rheumatoid arthritis: cause or effect relationships in a complex pathophysiology? *Clin. Exp. Rheumatol.* 1995; 13 (2): 227–240.

96. Cutolo, M. Sex hormone adjuvant therapy in rheumatoid arthritis. *Rheum. Dis. Clin. North. Am.* 2000; 26 (4): 881–895.

97. Van der Ploeg, H.M., M.J. Molenaar, and C.W. van Tiggelen. [Use of alternative treatments by patients with multiple sclerosis.] *Ned. Tijdschr. Geneeskd.* 1994; 138 (6): 296–299.

98. Wilmore, D.W. Impediments to the successful use of anabolic agents in clinical care. *J. Parenter. Enteral Nutr.* 1999; 23 (6): S210–213.

99. Dalal, M., S. Kim, and R.R. Voskuhl. Testosterone therapy ameliorates experimental autoimmune encephalomyelitis and induces T helper 2 bias in the autoantigen-specific T lymphocyte response. *J. Immunol.* 1997; 159 (1): 3–6.

100. Voskuhl, R.R., H. Pitchekian-Halabi, A. Mackenzie-Graham, et al. Gender differences in autoimmune demyelination in the mouse: implications for multiple sclerosis. *Ann. Neurol.* 1996; 39 (6): 724–733.

101. Blanco, C.E., P. Popper, and P. Micevych. Anabolic-androgenic steroid induced alterations in choline acetyltransferase messenger RNA levels of spinal cord motoneurons in the male rat. *Neuroscience* 1997; 78 (3): 873–882.

102. Loria, R.M., D.A. Padgett, and P.N. Huynh. Regulation of the immune system by dehydroepiandrosterone and its metabolites. *J. Endocrinol.* 1996; 150 (Suppl.): S209–220.

103. Ben-Nathan, D., D.A. Padgett, and R.M. Loria. Androstenediol and dehydroepiandrosterone protect mice against lethal bacterial infections and lipopolysaccharide toxicity. *J. Med. Microbiol.* 1999; 48 (5): 425–431.

104. Zeitz, B., R. Reber, M. Oertel, et al. Altered function of the hypothalamic stress axes in patients with moderately active systemic lupus erythematosus. II. Dissociation between androstenedione, cortisol, or dehydroepiandrosterone and interleukin 6 or tumor necrosis factor. *J. Rheumatol.* 2000; 27 (4): 911–918.

105. Fiter, J., J.M. Nolla, M.A. Navarro, et al. Weak androgens, glucocorticoid therapy, and bone mineral density in postmenopausal women with rheumatoid arthritis. *Joint Bone Spine* 2000; 67 (3): 199–203.

106. Padgett, D.A., and J.F. Sheridan. Androstenediol (AED) prevents neuroendocrine-mediated suppression of the immune system response to an influenza viral infection. *J. Neuroimmunol.* 1999; 98 (2): 121–129.

107. Harper, A.J., J.E. Bruster, and P.R. Casson. Changes in adrenocortical function with aging and therapeutic implications. *Semin. Reprod. Endocrinol.* 1999; 17 (4): 327–338.

108. van Vollenhoven, R.F., J.L. Park, M.C. Genovese, et al. A double-blind, placebo-controlled, clinical trial of dehydroepiandrosterone in severe systemic lupus erythematosus. *Lupus* 1999; 8 (3): 181–187,

109. Bebo, B.F., J.C. Schuster, A.A. Vandenbark, et al. Androgens alter the cytokine profile and reduce encephaliogenicity of myelin-reactive T cells. *J. Immunol.* 1999; 162 (1): 35–40.

110. Wilcoxen, S.C., E. Kirkman, K.C. Dowdell, et al. Gender-dependent IL-2 secretion by APC is regulated by IL-10. *J. Immunol.* 2000; 164 (12): 6237–6243.

111. Schifitto, G., M.P. McDermott, T. Evans, et al. Autonomic performance and dehydroepiandrosterone sulfate levels in HIV-1 infected individuals: relationship to TH1 and TH2 cytokine profile. *Arch. Neurol.* 2000; 57 (7): 1027–1032.

112. Schmidt, M., M. Kruetz, G. Loffler, et al. Conversion of dehydroepiandrosterone to downstream steroid hormones in macrophages. *J. Endocrinol.* 2000; 164 (2): 161–169.

113. Lapchak, P.A., D.F. Chapman, S.Y. Nunez, et al. Dehydroepiandrosterone sulfate is neuroprotective in a reversible spinal cord ischemia model: a possible involvement of GABA (A) receptors. *Stroke* 2000; 31 (8): 1953–1957.

114. Ledlhuber, F., C. Neubauer, M. Peichl, et al. Age and sex differences of dehydroepiandrosterone sulfate (DHEAS) and cortisol (CRT) plasma levels in normal controls and Alzheimer's disease (AD). *Psychopharmacology (Berl.)* 1993; 111 (1): 23–26.

115. Cardounel, A., W. Regelson, and M. Kalimi. Dehydroepiandrosterone protects hippocampal neurons against neurotoxin-induced cell death: mechanism of action. *Proc. Soc. Exp. Biol. Med.* 1999; 222 (2): 145–149.

116. Gelato, M.C., and R.A. Frost. IGFBP-3. Functional and structural implications in aging and wasting syndromes. *Endocrine* 1997; 7 (1): 81–85.

117. Hobbs, C.J., S.R. Plymate, C.J. Rosen, et al. Testosterone administration increases insulin-like growth factor-1 levels in normal men. *J. Clin. Endocrinol. Metab.* 1993; 77 (3): 776–779.

118. Morales, A.J., J.J. Nolan, J.C. Nelson, et al. Effects of replacement dose of dehydroepiandrosterone in men and women of advancing age. *J. Clin. Endocrinol. Metab.* 1994; 78 (6): 1360–1367.

119. Morales, A.J., R.H. Haubrich, J.Y. Hwang, et al. The effect of six months treatment with a 100mg daily dose of dehydroepiandrosterone (DHEA) on circulating sex steroids, body composition and muscle strength in age-advanced men and women. *Clin. Endocrinol. (Oxf.)* 1998; 49 (4): 421–432.

120. Casson, P.R., N. Santoro, K. Elkind-Hirsch, et al. Postmenopausal dehydroepiandrosterone administration increases free insulin-like growth factor-1 and decreases high density lipoprotein: a six month trial. *Fertil. Steril.* 1998; 70 (1): 107–110.

121. Arfvat, E., F. Broglio, and E. Ghigo. Insulin-like growth factor-1: implications in aging. *Drugs Aging* 2000; 16 (1): 29–40.

122. Gebre-Medhin, G., E.S. Husebye, H. Mallmin, et al. Oral dehydroepiandrosterone (DHEA) replacement therapy in women with Addison's disease. *Clin. Endocrinol. (Oxf.)* 2000; 52 (6): 775–780.

123. van Vollenhoven, R.F. Dehydroepiandrosterone in systemic lupus erythematosus. *Rheum. Dis. Clin. North Am.* 2000; 26 (2): 349–362.

124. Yao, D.L., X. Liu, L.D. Hudson, et al. Insulin-like growth factor-1 given subcutaneously reduces clinical deficits, decreases lesion severity and upregulates synthesis of myelin proteins in experimental autoimmune encephalomyelitis. *Life Sci.* 1996; 58 (16): 1301–1306.

125. Webster, H.D. Growth factors and myelin regeneration in multiple sclerosis. *Mult. Scler.* 1997; 3 (2): 113–120.

126. Lewis, M.E., N.T. Neft, P.C. Contreras, et al. Insulin-like growth factor-1: potential for treatment of motor neuronal disorders. *Exp. Neurol.* 1993; 124 (1): 73–88.

127. Vaught, J.L., P.C. Contreras, M.A. Glicksman, et al. Potential utility of rhIGF-1

in neuromuscular and/or degenerative disease. *Ciba Found. Symp.* 1996; 196: 18–27.

128. Dore, S., S. Kar, and R. Quirion. Rediscovering an old friend, IGF-1: potential use in the treatment of neurodegenerative diseases. *Trends Neurosci.* 1997; 20 (8): 326–331.

129. Armstrong, R.C., H.H. Dorn, C.V. Kufta, et al. Pre-oligodendrocytes from adult human CNS. *J. Neurosci.* 1992; 12 (4): 1538–1547.

130. Li, W., L. Quigley, D.L. Yao, et al. Chronic relapsing experimental autoimmune encephalomyelitis: effects of insulin-like growth factor-1 treatment on clinical deficits, lesion severity, glial responses, and blood brain barrier defects. *J. Neuropathol. Exp. Neurol.* 1998; 57 (5): 426–438.

131. Ackerman, S.J., E.M. Sullivan, K.M. Beusterien, et al. Cost effectiveness of recombinant human insulin-like growth factor-1 therapy in patients with ALS. *Pharmacoeconomics* 1999; 15 (2): 179–195.

132. Rubinow, D.W. and P.J. Schmidt. Androgens, brain, and behavior. *Am. J. Psychiatry* 1996; 153 (8): 974–984.

133. Masonis, A.E., and M.P. McCarthy. Direct effects of the anabolic/androgenic steroids, stanozolol and 17 alpha-methyltesosterone, on benzodiazepine binding to the gamma-aminobutyric acid (a) receptor. *Neurosci. Lett.* 1995; 189 (1): 35–38.

134. Frye, C.A., J.E. Duncan, M. Brasham, et al. Behavioral effects of 3 alpha-androstanediol. II. Hypothalamic and preoptic area actions via a GABAergic mechanism. *Behav. Brain Res.* 1996; 79 (1–2): 119–130.

135. Masoinis, A.E., and M. P. McCarthy. Effects of the androgenic/anabolic steroid stanolzolol on GABA (A) receptor function: GABA-stimulated 36Cl–influx and [35S] TBPS binding. *J. Pharmacol. Exp. Ther.* 1996; 279 (1): 186–193.

136. Masonis, A.E., and M.P. McCarthy. Direct interactions of androgenic/anabolic steroids with the peripheral benzodiazepine receptor in rat brain: implications for the psychological and physical manifestations of androgenic/anabolic steroid abuse. *J. Steroid Biochem. Mol. Biol.* 1996; 58 (5–6): 551–555.

137. Bitran, D., R.J. Hilvers, C.A. Frye, et al. Chronic anabolic-androgenic steroid treatment affects brain GABA (A) receptor-gated chloride ion transport. *Life Sci.* 1996; 58 (7): 573–583.

138. Tirassa, P., I. Thiblin, G. Agren, et al. High-dose anabolic androgenic steroids modulate concentrations of nerve growth factor and expression of its low affinity receptor (p75–NGFr) in male rat brain. *J. Neurosci. Res.* 1997; 47 (2): 198–207.

139. Le Greves, P., W Huang, P. Johansson, et al. Effects of an anabolic-androgenic steroid on the regulation of the NMDA receptor NR1, NR2A and NR2B subunit mRNAs in brain regions of the male rat. *Neurosci. Lett.* 1997; 226 (1): 61–64.

140. Frye, C.A., and T.A. Reed. Androgenic neurosteroids: anti-seizure effects in an animal model of epilepsy. *Psychoneuroendocrinology* 1998; 23 (4): 385–399.

141. Thiblin, I., A. Finn, S.B. Ross, et al. Increased dopaminergic and 5–hytryptaminergic activities in male rat brain following long-term treatment with anabolic androgenic steroids. *Br. J. Pharmacol.* 1999; 126 (6): 1301–1306.

142. Thiblin, I., A. Finn, S.B. Ross, et al. Increased dopaminergic and 5–hytryptaminergic activities in the male rat brain following long-term treatment with anabolic androgenic steroids. *Br. J. Pharmacol.* 1999; 126 (6): 1301–1306.

143. Jorge-Rivera, J.C., K.L. McIntyre, and L.P. Henderson. Anabolic steroids induce region- and subunit-specific rapid modulation of GABA (A) receptor-mediated currents in the rat forebrain. *J. Neurophysiol.* 2000; 83 (6): 3299–3309.

144. Hallberg, M., P. Johansson, A.M. Kindlundh, et al. Anabolic-androgenic

steroids affect the content of substance P and substance P (1–7) in the rat brain. *Peptides* 2000; 21 (6): 845–852.

145. Pasquariello, A., R. Di Toro, F. Nyberg, et al. Down-regulation of delta opioid receptor mRNA by an anabolic steroid in neuronal hybrid cells. *Neuroreport* 2000; 11 (4): 863–867.

146. Frye, C.A., and C.M. McCormick. The neurosteroid, 3alpha-androstanediol, prevents inhibitory avoidance deficits and pyknotic cells in the granule layer of the dentate gyrus induced by adrenalectomy in rats. *Brain Res.* 2000; 855 (1): 166–170.

147. Rubinow, D.R., and P.J. Schmidt. Androgens, brain, and behavior. *Am. J. Psychiatry* 1996; 153 (8): 974–984.

148. Isacsson, G. and U. Bergman. [Can anabolic steroids cause personality changes?] *Nord. Med.* 1993; 108 (6–7): 180–181.

149. Magri, F., F. Terenzi, T. Ricciardi, et al. Associations between changes in adrenal secretion and cerebral morphometric correlates in normal aging and senile dementia. *Dement. Geriatr. Cogn. Disord.* 2000; 11 (2): 90–99.

150. Baulieu, E.E. 'New' active steroids and an unforeseen mechanism of action. *C.R. Acad. Sci. III.* 2000; 323 (6): 513–518.

151. Hier, D.B., and W.F. Crowley. Spatial ability in androgen-deficient men. *New Engl. J. Med.* 1982; 306 (20): 1202–1205.

152. Tan, R.S., and P. Phillip. Attitudes of older males toward the andropause. *Am. Geriatr. Soc.* 1998; 46 (9): S74.

153. Drake, E.B., V.W. Henderson, F.Z. Stanczyk, et al. Associations between circulating sex steroid hormones and cognition in normal elderly women. *Neurology* 2000; 54 (3): 599–603.

154. Morrison, M.F., E. Redei, T. TenHave, et al. Dehydroepiandrosterone sulfate and psychiatric measures in a frail, elderly residential care population. *Bio. Psychiatry* 2000; 47 (2): 144–150.

155. Leblhuber, F., C. Neubauer, M. Peichl, et al. Age and sex differences of dehydroepiandrosterone sulfate (DHEAS) and cortisol (CRT) plasma levels in normal controls and Alzheimer's disease (AD). *Psychopharmacology (Berl.)* 1993; 111 (1): 23–26.

156. Attal-Khemis, S., V. Dalmeyda, J.L. Michot, et al. Increase total 7 alpha-hydroxy-dehydroepiandrosterone in serum of patients with Alzheimer's disease. *J. Gerontol. A. Biol. Med. Sci.* 1998; 53 (2): B125–B132.

157. Hillen, T., A. Lun, F.M. Reischies, et al. DHEA-S plasma levels and incidence of Alzheimer's disease. *Biol. Psychiatry* 2000; 47 (2): 161–163.

158. Murialdo, G., A. Barreca, F. Nobili, et al. Dexamethasone effects on cortisol secretion in Alzheimer's disease: some clinical and hormonal features in suppressor and nonsuppressor patients. *J. Endocrinol. Invest.* 2000; 23 (3): 178–186.

159. Barhal, H.S. Testosterone in male involutional melancholia. *Psychiatric Quarterly* 1938; 12: 743–749.

160. Kurzrok, L., C.H. Birnberg, and S. Livingston. The treatment of the female menopause with male sex hormone. *Endocrinol.* 1939; 24: 347–350.

161. Hallstrom, T. Sexuality in the climacteric. *Clin. Obstet. Gynecol.* 1977; 4: 227–239.

162. Longcope, C., C. Franz, C. Morello, et al. Steroid and gonadotrophin levels in women during the peri-menopausal years. *Maturitas* 1986; 8: 189–196.

163. Frock, J., and J. Money. Sexuality and the menopause. *Psycholther. Psychosom.* 1992; 57: 29–32.

164. Zumoff, B., G.W. Strain, L.K. Miller, et al. Twenty-four hour mean plasma testosterone concentration declines with age in normal premenopausal women. *J. Clin. Endocrinol. Metab.* 1995; 80: 3537–3545.

165. Rubino, S. M., Stomati, C. Bersi, et al. Neuroendocrine effect of a short-term treatment with DHEA in postmenopausal women. *Maturitas* 1998; 28 (3): 251–257.

166. Stomati, M., S. Rubino, A. Spinetti, et al. Endocrine, neuroendocrine and behavioral effects of oral dehydroepiandrosterone sulfate supplementation in post-menopausal women. *Gynecol. Endocrinol.* 1999; 13 (1): 15–25.

167. Su, T.P., M. Pagliar, P.J. Schmidt, et al. Neuropsychiatric effects of anabolic steroids in male normal volunteers. *JAMA* 1993; 269 (21): 2760–2764.

168. Turner, H.H. The clinical use of synthetic male sex hormone. *Endocrinol.* 1939; 24 (6): 763–773.

169. Greenblatt, R.B. Androgenic therapy in women. *J. Clin. Endocrinol. Metab.* 1942; 2: 65–66.

170. Salmon, U.J., and S.H. Geist. Effect of androgens upon libido in women. *J. Clin. Endocrinol. Metab.* 1943; 3: 235–238.

171. Bancroft, J., D. Sanders, D. Davidson, et al. Mood, sexuality, hormones, and the menstrual cycle. III. Sexuality and the role of androgens. *Psychosom. Med.* 1983; 45 (6): 509–516.

172. Nankin, H.R., T.U. Lin, and J. Osterman. Chronic testosterone cypionate therapy in men with secondary impotence. *Fertil. Steril.* 1986; 46 (2): 300–307.

173. Sherwin, B.B., and M.M. Gelfand. The role of androgen in the maintenance of sexual functioning in oophorectomized women. *Psychosom. Med.* 1987; 49: 137–142.

174. Greenblatt, R.B. The use of androgens in the menopause and other gyneic disorders. *Obstet. Gynecol. N. Am.* 1987; 14 (1): 251.

175. Taylor, W.N., and C. Alanis. Triple sex steroid replacement therapy for osteoporosis after surgical menopause. *J. Neurol. Orthop. Med. Surg.* 1992; 13: 16–19.

176. Warnick, J.K., J.C. Bundren, and D.W. Morris. Female hypoactive sexual desire disorder due to androgen deficiency: clinical and psychometric issues. *Psychopharmacol. Bull.* 1997; 33 (4): 761–766.

177. Reiter, W.J., A. Pycha, G. Schatzl, et al. Dehydroepiandrosterone in the treatment of erectile dysfunction: a prospective, double-blind, randomized, placebo-controlled study. *Urology* 1999; 53 (3): 590–594.

178. Reiter, W.J., and A. Pycha. [Placebo-controlled dehydroepiandrosterone substitution in elderly men.] *Gynakol. Geburtshilfiche Rundsch.* 1999; 39 (4): 208–209.

179. Anderson, R.A., C.W. Martin, A.W. Kung, et al. 7Alpha-methyl-19–nor-testosterone maintains sexual behavior and mood in hypogonadal men. *J. Clin. Endocrinol. Metab.* 1999; 84 (10): 3556–3562.

180. Warnock, J.K., J.C. Bundren, and D.W. Morris. Female hypoactive sexual disorder: case studies of physiologic androgen replacement. *J. Sex. Marital. Ther.* 1999; 25 (3): 175–182.

181. Baulieu, E.E., G. Thomas, S. Legrain, et al. Dehydroepiandrosterone (DHEA), DHEA sulfate, and aging: contribution of the DHEAge Study to a sociobiomedical issue. *Proc. Natl. Acad. Sci. U.S.A.* 2000; 97 (8): 4279–4284.

182. Vandekerckhove, P., R. Lilford, A. Vail, et al. Androgens versus placebo or no treatment for idiopathic oligo/asthenospermia. *Cochrane Database Syst. Rev.* 2000; (2): CD000150.

183. Sherwin, B.B., and M.M. Gelfand. Differential symptom response to parenteral estrogen and/or androgen administration in the surgical menopause. *Am. H. Obstet. Gynecol.* 1985; 151: 153–159.

184. Foster, G.V., H.A. Zacur, and J.A. Rock. Hot flashes in postmenopausal women ameliorated by danazol. *Fertil. Steril.* 1985; 43 (3): 401–404.

185. Morales, A.J., J.J. Nolan, J.C. Nelson, et al. Effects of replacement dose of

dehydroepiandrosterone in men and women of advancing age. *J. Clin. Endocrinol. Metab.* 1994; 78 (6): 1360–1367.

186. Carter, W.J. Effect of anabolic hormones and insulin-like growth factor-1 on muscle mass and strength in elderly persons. *Clin. Geriatr. Med.* 1995; 11 (4): 735–748.

187. Wolf, O.T., O. Neumann, D.H. Hellhammer, et al. Effects of a two-week physiological dehydroepiandrosterone substitution on cognitive performance and well-being in healthy elderly women and men. *J. Clin. Endocrinol. Metab.* 1997; 82 (7): 2363–2367.

188. Sarrel, P., B. Dobay, and B. Wiita. Estrogen and estrogen-androgen replacement in postmenopausal women dissatisfied with estrogen-only therapy. Sexual behavior and neuroendocrine responses. *J. Reprod. Med.* 1998; 43 (10): 847–856.

189. Shifren, J.L., G. D. Braunstein, J.A. Simon, et al. Transdermal testosterone treatment in women with impaired sexual function after oophorectomy. *N. Engl. J. Med.* 2000; 343: 682–688.

190. English, K. M., et al. Low-dose transdermal testosterone therapy improves angina threshold in men with chronic stable angina: A randomized, double-blind placebo-controlled study. *Circulation* 2000; 102: 1906–1911.

191. Thomas, H.B., and R.T. Hill. Testosterone propionate and the male climacteric. *Endocrinol.* 1941; 26: 953–954.

192. Davidoff, E., and G.L. Goodstone. Use of testosterone propionate in treatment of involutional psychosis in the male. *Arch. Neuro. Psych.* 1942; 11 (5): 181–183.

193. Werner, A.A. The male climacteric: additional observations of thirty-seven patients. *J. Urol.* 1943; 49: 872–882.

194. Freed, S.C. Therapeutic use of testosterone in aqueous suspension. *J. Clin. Endocrinol. Metab.* 1946 (6): 571–572.

195. Szarvas, F. [The male climacteric from the practical viewpoint.] *Wien. Med. Wochenschr.* 1992; 142 (5–6): 100–103.

196. Arlt, W., F. Callies, J.C. van Vlijmen, et al. Dehydroepiandrosterone replacement in women with adrenal insufficiency. *N. Engl. J. Med.* 1999; 341 (14): 1013–1020.

197. Barbaccia, M.L., S. Lello, T. Sidiropoulou, et al. Plasma 5alpha-androstane-3alpha, 17betadiol, an endogenous steroid that positively modulates GABA (A) receptor function and anxiety: a study in menopausal women. *Psycholneuroendocrinology* 2000; 25 (7): 659–675.

198. Rabkin, J.G., S.J. Ferrando, G.J. Wagner, et al. DHEA treatment for HIV+ patients: effects on mood, androgenic and anabolic parameters. *Psychoneuroendocrinology* 2000; 25 (1): 53–68.

199. Rabkin, J.G., S.J. Ferrando, G.J. Wagner, et al. DHEA treatment for HIV+ patients: effects on mood, androgenic and anabolic parameters. *Psychomeuroendocrinology* 2000; 25 (1): 53–68.

200. Lamar, C.P. Clinical endocrinology of the male with special reference to the male climacteric. *J. Florida Med. Assoc.* 1940; 26 (8): 398–404.

201. Simonson, E., W.E. Kearns, and N. Enzer. Effect of methyl testosterone on the muscular performance and central nervous system of older men. *J. Clin. Endocrinol.* 1944; 4: 528–534.

202. Wolf, O.T., O. Neumann, D.H. Hellhammer, et al. Effects of a two-week physiological dehydroepiandrosterone substitution on cognitive performance and well-being in healthy elderly women and men. *J. Clin. Endocrinol. Metab.* 1997; 82 (7): 2363–2367.

203. Wolkowitz, O.M., V.I. Reus, E. Roberts, et al. Dehydroepiandrosterone (DHEA) treatment of depression. *Biol. Psychiatry* 1997; 41 (3): 311–318.

204. Hier, D.B., and W.F. Crowley. Spatial ability in androgen-deficient men. *N. Engl. J. Med.* 1982; 306 (20): 1202–1205.

205. van Vollenhoven, R.F. Dehydroepiandrosterone in systemic lupus erythematosus. *Rheum. Dis. Clin. North Am.* 2000; 26 (2): 349–362.

206. Wilmore, D.W. Deterrents to the successful clinical use of growth factors that enhance protein anabolism. *Curr. Opin. Clin. Nutr. Metab. Care* 1999; 2 (1): 15–21.

207. Garcia de Lorenzo, A., and J.M. Culebras. [Hormones, growth factors, and drugs in metabolism and nutrition.] *Nutr. Hosp.* 1995; 10 (5): 297–305.

208. Roubenoff, R. Sarcopenia: A major modifiable cause of frailty in the elderly. *J. Nutr. Health Aging* 2000; 4 (3): 140–142.

209. Lye, M.D., and A.E. Ritch. A double-blind trial of an anabolic steroid (stanozolol) in the disabled elderly. *Rheumatol. Rehabil.* 1977; 16 (1): 62–69.

210. Drosos, A.A., E. van Vliet-Dascalopoulou, A.P. Andonopoulos, et al. Nandrolone decanoate (deca-durabolin) in primary Sjogren's syndrome: a double blind pilot study. *Clin. Exp. Rheumatol.* 1988; 6 (1): 53–57.

211. Bakhshi, V., M. Elliott, A. Gentili, et al. Testosterone improves rehabilitation outcomes in ill older men. *J. Am. Geriatr. Soc.* 2000; 48 (5): 550–553.

212. Brochner-Mortensen, K., G. Steffen, and J.H. Thaysen. The metabolic effect of new anabolic 19–nor-steroids. Metabolic studies on patients with chronic rheumatoid arthritis during combined therapy with Prednisone and anabolic steroid. *Acta Med. Scand.* 1959; 165 (3): 197–205.

213. Morley, K.D., A. Parke, and G.R.V. Hughes. Systemic lupus erythematosus: two patients treated with danazol. *Br. Med. J.* 1982; 284: 1431–1432.

214. Nilsson, B., R. Sodergard, M. Damber, et al. Free testosterone levels during danazol therapy. *Fertil. Steril.* 1983; 39 (4): 505–509.

215. Reid, I.R., D.J. Wattie, M.C. Evans, et al. Testosterone therapy in glucocorticoid-treated men. *Arch. Intern. Med.* 1996; 156 (11): 1173–1177.

216. Harper, A.J., J.E. Buster, and P.R. Casson. Changes in adrenocortical function with aging and therapeutic implications. *Semin. Reprod. Endocrinol.* 1999; 17 (4): 327–338.

217. Fiter, J., J.M. Nolla, M. A. Navarro, et al. Weak androgen levels, glucocorticoid therapy, and bone mineral density in postmenopausal women with rheumatoid arthritis. *Joint Bone Spine* 2000; 67 (3): 199–203.

218. Abbasi, A., E.H. Duthie, L. Sheldahl, et al. Association of dehydroepiandrosterone sulfate, body composition, and physical fitness in independent community-dwelling older men and women. *J. Am. Geriatr. Soc.* 1998; 46 (3): 263–273.

219. Bullock, G., A.M. White, and J. Worthington. The effects of catabolic and anabolic steroids on amino acid incorporation by skeletal-muscle ribosomes. *Biochem. J.* 1968; 108 (3): 417–425.

220. Rogozkin, V. Metabolic effects of anabolic steroid on skeletal muscle. *Med. Sci. Sports* 1979; 11 (2): 160–163.

221. Janne, O.A., J.J. Palvimo, P. Kallio, et al. Androgen receptor and mechanism of androgen action. *Ann. Med.* 1993; 25 (1): 83–89.

222. Wu, F.C. Endocrine aspects of anabolic steroids. *Clin. Chem.* 1997; 43 (7): 1289–1292.

223. Sheffield-Moore, M., R.J. Urban, S.E. Wolf et al. Short-term oxandrolone administration stimulates net muscle protein synthesis in young men. *J. Clin. Endocrinol. Metab.* 1999; 84 (8): 2705–2711.

224. Sheffield-Moore, M., R.R. Wolfe, D.C. Gore, et al. Combined effects of hyperaminoacidemia and oxandrolone on skeletal muscle protein synthesis. *Am. J. Physiol. Endocrinol. Metab.* 2000; 278 (2): E273–279.

225. Wolfe, R., A. Ferrando, M. Sheffield-Moore, et al. Testosterone and muscle protein metabolism. *Mayo Clinc. Proc.* 2000; 75 (Suppl.): S55–59.

226. Hobbs, C.J., S.R. Plymate, C.J. Rosen, et al. Testosterone administration increases insulin-like growth factor-1 levels in normal men. *J. Clin. Endocrinol. Metab.* 1993; 77 (3): 776–779.

227. Eakman, G.D., J.S. Dallas, S.W. Ponder, et al. The effects of testosterone and dihydrotestosterone on hypothalamic regulation of growth hormone secretion. *J. Clin. Endocrinol. Metab.* 1996; 81 (3): 1217–1223.

228. Simonson, E., W.E. Kearns, and N. Enzer. Effect of methyltestosterone on the muscular performance and central nervous system of older men. *J. Clin. Endocrinol.* 1944; 4: 528–534.

229. Lye, M.D., and A.E. Ritch. A double-blind trial of an anabolic steroid (stanozolol) in the disabled elderly. *Rheumatol. Rehabil.* 1977; 16 (1): 62–69.

230. Tenover, S. Effects of testosterone supplementation in the aging male. *J. Clin. Endocrinol. Metab.* 1992; 75 (4): 1092–1098.

231. Reid, I.R., D.J. Wattie, M.C. Evans, et al. Testosterone therapy in glucocorticoid-treated men. *Arch. Intern. Med.* 1996; 156 (11): 1173–1177.

232. Morales, A.J., R.H. Haubrich, J.Y. Hwang, et al. Effects of six months' treatment with 100mg daily dose of dehydroepiandrosterone (DHEA) on circulating sex steroids, body composition and muscle strength in age-advanced men and women. *Clin. Endocrinol. (Oxf.)* 1998; 49 (4): 421–432.

233. Tenover, J.S. Androgen replacement therapy to reverse and/or prevent age-related sarcopenia in men. *Baillieres Clin. Endocrinol. Metab.* 1998; 12 (3): 419–425.

234. Bross, R., R. Casaburi, T.W. Storer, et al. Androgen effects on body composition and muscle function: implications for the use of androgens as anabolic agents in sarcopenic states. *Baillieres Clin. Endocrinol. Metab.* 1998; 12 (3): 365–378.

235. Synder, P.J., H. Peachey, P. Hannoush, et al. Effect of testosterone treatment on body composition and muscle strength in men over 65 years of age. *J. Clin. Endocrinol. Metab.* 1999; 84 (8): 2646–2653.

236. Strawford, A., T. Barbieri, R. Neese, et al. Effects of nandrolone decanoate therapy in borderline hypogonadal men with HIV-associated weight loss. *J. Acquir. Immune Defic. Syndr. Human Retrovirol.* 1999; 20 (2): 137–146.

237. Bakhski, V., M. Elliott, A. Gentili, et al. Testosterone improves rehabilitation outcomes in ill older men. *J. Am. Geriatr. Soc.* 2000; 48 (5): 550–553.

238. Sheffield-Moore, M. Androgens and the control of skeletal muscle protein synthesis. *Ann. Med.* 2000; 32 (3): 181–186.

239. Khosla, S. The effects of androgens on osteoblast function in vitro. *Mayo Clin. Proc.* 2000; 75 (Suppl): S51–S54.

240. Kadi, F., A. Eriksson, S. Holmner, et al. Effects of anabolic steroids on the muscle cells of strength-trained athletes. *Med. Sci. Sports. Exerc.* 1999; 31 (11): 1528–1534.

241. Kadi, F., P. Bonnerud, A. Eriksson, et al. The expression of androgen receptors in human neck and limb muscles: effects of training and self-administration of androgenic-anabolic steroids. *Histochem. Cell Biol.* 2000; 113 (1): 25–29.

242. O'Shea, J.P., and W. Winkler. Biochemical and physical effects of an anabolic steroid in competitive swimmers and weight lifters. *Nutr. Rpts. Intern.* 1970; 2; 351–365.

243. O'Shea, J.P. The effects of an anabolic steroid on dynamic strength levels of weight lifters. *Nutr. Rpts. Intern.* 1971; 4: 363–370.

244. Bowers, R.W., and J. P. Reardon. Effects of methandrostenolone (Dianabol) on strength development and aerobic capacity. *Med. Sci. Sports* 1972; 4: 54.

245. Ward, P. The effect of an anabolic steroid on strength and lean body mass. *Med. Sci. Sports* 1973; 5: 277–282.

246. Stanford, B.A., and R. Moffatt. Anabolic steroid: Effectiveness as an ergogenic aid to experienced weight trainers. *J. Sports Med. Phys. Fitness* 1974; 14: 191–197.

247. O'Shea, P. Biochemical evaluation of effects of stanozolol on adrenal, liver and muscle function in man. *Nutr. Rpts. Intern.* 1974; 10: 381–388.

248. Freed, D.L.J., and A.J. Banks. A double-blind crossover trial of methandieonone (Dianabol, Ciba) in moderate doses on highly trained experienced athletes. *Br. J. Sports Med.* 1975; 9: 78–81.

249. Romeyn, M., and N. Gunn. Resistance exercise and oxandrolone for men with HIV-related weight loss. *JAMA* 2000; 284 (2): 176.

250. Bhasin, S., T.W. Storer, M. Javanbakht, et al. Testosterone replacement and resistance exercise in HIV-infected men with weight loss and low testosterone levels. *JAMA* 2000; 283 (6): 763–770.

251. Sattler, F.R., S.V. Jaque, E.T. Schroeder, et al. Effects of pharmacological doses of nandrolone decanoate and progressive resistance training in immunodeficient patients infected with human immunodeficiency virus. *J. Clin. Endocrinol. Metab.* 1999; 84 (4): 1268–1276.

8

Rationale for Anabolic Therapy in Amyotrophic Lateral Sclerosis

Introduction: Anabolic and Neurotrophin Factor Deficiency?

Amyotrophic lateral sclerosis (ALS) is a progressive, adult-onset, neurodegenerative disease that results in the degeneration of lower and upper motor neurons in the brain and spinal cord. The exact cause of ALS remains unknown. Among the possible causes are deficiency of anabolic and nerve growth factors, deficient glutamate reuptake, autoimmunity, mutation of superoxide dimutase 1 gene, and history of previous trauma with axonal injury.[1, 2, 3]

ALS, also referred to as motor neuron disease in the United Kingdom, Australia and other Commonwealth countries, Lou Gehrig's disease in the United States, and maladie de Charcot in France, is a fatal disease that is characterized clinically by progressive muscle weakness, muscle atrophy, spasticity, and eventual paralysis.[4, 5] Traditionally thought to affect solely the lower motor neurons and corticospinal tracts, recent studies have shown that the pathogenic process of ALS is more extensive, involving dysfunction of cortical gray and white matter with clinical correlates of impairment in cognition and language.[6] The mean age at onset of ALS is 55 years and the mean duration of the disease is approximately 4 years. In the United States, it has been estimated that there are 20,000 to 30,000 cases of ALS. The incidence of new cases of ALS is about 1 per 100,000 population, with about 10 percent of these cases inheriting the disease as a dominant trait of the autosome.[7] Death usually occurs from paralysis and respiratory failure.[8]

ALS is more common in men than in women (male to female ratio of approximately 2:1), suggesting a role for a gender-linked factor in the disease. It has been suggested that polymorphisms of the androgen receptor gene may reduce androgen-binding capacities, which reduces anabolic and trophic functions and increases the susceptibility to ALS.[9]

Current data on the neurotrophic effects of steroid hormones suggest that, in brain and spinal cord regions containing receptor systems, steroids act at the level of RNA and protein synthesis to effect metabolic changes associated with nerve-cell survival, elaboration and maintenance of dendritic and axonal processes, synaptogenesis, and neurotransmission. Both androgens and estrogens appear to exert these growthlike effects on neurons through receptor-mediated genomic activation. The brain and spinal cord, injured by either disease or by experimentally induced trauma, is responsive in an anabolic and reparative manner to exogenous and endogenous sex steroids.[10]

It has been hypothesized that ALS may be related to sex steroid hormone/receptor deficiencies or defects and that sex steroid therapy could be candidates for treating this disease.[11, 12] This has been suggested by the male-to-female ratio of the disease, the age of onset, and the sparing of neurons of cranial nerves III, IV, and VI that coincidentally lack androgen receptors. Reduced or altered androgen receptors may result in an inability to respond in anabolic fashions to a variety of insults including axonal damage.[13] It has been shown that patients with ALS have hyperestrogenemia and lower androgen-to-estrogen ratios, presumably from increased peripheral androgen-to-estrogen conversion.[14] Serum androgens have been shown to be reduced in some patients with ALS.[15] The status of the patient's sex hormonal status and androgen levels should be taken into account in ALS.[16, 17]

Besides androgens, many neurotrophic factors have been shown to enhance survival of embryonic motor neurons and influence their response to injury. These anabolic and protective effects of neurotrophic factors on mature motor neurons have been suggested as a rationale for pharmacologic therapy for neurodegenerative diseases.[18, 19] Recently, considerable research has focused on anabolic and neurotrophic therapies for ALS, primarily with growth hormone (GH) and insulin-like growth factor-1 (IGF-1) administration.[20, 21, 22, 23, 24] An early study reported that serum concentrations of IGF-1 and IGF-1 receptor binding capacity in patients with ALS were not been found to be reduced compared to controls.[25] More recent studies have indicated that serum IGF-1 levels tend to be reduced.[26] However, a general upregulation of the IGF-1 receptors throughout the spinal cord of ALS patients has been reported with significant increases observed in the cervical and sacral segments compared to controls.[27, 28, 29]

The widespread distribution of its receptor allows IGF-1 to affect the survival of numerous populations of neurons and glial cells in both the central and peripheral nervous systems. Recent evidence has supported the significance of IGF-1 in the maintenance of the integrity and homeostasis of the nervous systems.[30]

Anabolic Therapy for ALS

Recent investigational studies have evaluated recombinant GH and IGF-1 in ALS patients. Overall, the results of these studies have been mixed and less promising than had been hoped.

With GH therapy, 75 ALS patients were treated for up to 18 months and survival analysis did not reveal a difference between the treatment and placebo groups.[31] Two large studies with IGF-1 therapy in ALS patients have been published. In one study (the North America ALS/IGF-1 Study Group) recombinant IGF-1 therapy was shown to slow the progression of functional impairment and the decline in health-related quality of life in patients with ALS with no medically important adverse effects.[32] In another large study (European ALS/IGF-1 Study Group) recombinant IGF-1 therapy resulted in no significant difference in the change of disease progression compared to placebo.[33] The overall cost per quality-adjusted life-year (QALY) gained for ALS patients treated with IGF-1 therapy has been estimated to be over $67,000.[34]

Summary

Although there is still no truly effective disease-specific therapy for any of the motor neuron diseases, rapid progress in our understanding of the pathophysiology of some of these diseases is being made.[35] No scientific studies have been published about androgen therapy alone or in combination with other anabolic hormones and factors. Investigational studies utilizing anabolic and neurotrophic factor therapy (GH and IGF-1) have revealed mixed results in ALS patients. Further studies with androgen therapy in combination with other anabolic and neurotrophic factors are warranted.

Notes

1. Drachman, D.B., P.S. Fishman, J.D. Rothstein, et al. Amyotrophic lateral sclerosis. An autoimmune disease? *Adv. Neurol.* 1995; 68: 59–65.

2. Riggs, J.E. Trauma, axonal injury, and amyotrophic lateral sclerosis: a clinical correlate of a neuropharmacologic model. *Clin. Neuropharmacol.* 1995; 18 (3): 273–276.

3. Milonas, I. Amyotrophic lateral sclerosis: an introduction. *J. Neurol.* 1998; 245 (Suppl. 2): S1–S3.

4. Festoff, B.W. Amyotrophic lateral sclerosis: current and future treatment strategies. *Drugs* 1996; 51 (1): 28–44.

5. Martin, L.J., A.C. Price, A. Kaiser, et al. Mechanisms for neuronal degeneration in amyotrophic lateral sclerosis and in models of motor neuron death. *Int. J. Mol. Med.* 2000; 5 (1): 3–13.

6. Strong, M.J., G.M. Grace, J.B. Orange, et al. Cognition, language, and speech in amyotrophic lateral sclerosis: a review. *J. Clin. Exp. Neuropsychol.* 1996; 18 (2): 291–303.

7. Brown, R.H. Amyotrophic lateral sclerosis. Insights from genetics. *Arch. Neurol.* 1997; 54 (10): 1246–1250.

8. Bromberg, M.B. Pathogenesis of amyotrophic lateral sclerosis: a critical review. *Curr. Opin. Neurol.* 1999; 12 (5): 581–588.

9. Garafalo, O., D.A. Figlewicz, P.N. Leigh, et al. Androgen receptor gene polymorphism in amyotrophic lateral sclerosis. *Neuromuscul. Disord.* 1993; 3 (3): 195–199.

10. Jones, K.J. Steroid hormones and neurotrophism: relationship to nerve injury. *Metab. Brain Dis.* 1988; 3 (1): 1–18.

11. Jones, K.J. Steroid hormones and neurotrophism: relationship to nerve injury. *Metab. Brain Dis.* 1988; 3 (1): 1–18.

12. Ogata, A., T. Matsuura, K. Tashiro, et al. Expression of androgen receptor in X-linked spinal and bulbar muscular atrophy and amyotrophic lateral sclerosis. *J. Neurol. Neurosurg. Psychiatry* 1994; 57 (10): 1274–1275.

13. Weiner, L.P. Possible role of androgen receptors in amyotrophic lateral sclerosis. A hypothesis. *Arch. Neurol.* 1980; 37 (3): 129–131.

14. Usuki, F., O. Nakazato, M. Osame, et al. Hyperestrogenemia in neuromuscular diseases. *J. Neurol. Sci.* 1989; 89 (2–3): 189–197.

15. Eisen, A., J. Pearmain, and H. Stewart. Dehydroepiandrosterone sulfate (DHEAS) concentrations and amyotrophic lateral sclerosis. *Muscle Nerve* 1995; 18 (12): 1481–1483.

16. Jones, T.M., R. Yu, and J.P. Antel. Response of patients with amyotrophic lateral sclerosis to testosterone therapy: endocrine evaluation. *Arch. Neurol.* 1982; 39 (11): 721–722.

17. Miller, S.C., and J.E. Warnick. Protirelin (thyrotropin-releasing hormone) in amyotrophic lateral sclerosis. The role of androgens. *Arch. Neurol.* 1989; 46 (3): 330–335.

18. Yuen, E.C., and W.C. Mobley. Therapeutic applications of neurotrophic factors in disorders of motor neurons and peripheral nerves. *Mol. Med. Today* 1995; 1 (6): 278–286.

19. Corse, A.M., M.M. Bilak, S.R. Bilak, et al. Preclinical testing of neuroprotective neurotrophic factors in a model of chronic motor neuron degeneration. *Neurobiol. Dis.* 1999; 6 (5): 335–346.

20. Smith, R.A., S. Melmed, B. Sherman, et al. Recombinant growth hormone treatment of amyotrophic lateral sclerosis. *Muscle Nerve* 1993; 16 (6): 624–633.

21. Lewis, M.E., N.T. Neff, P.C. Contreras, et al. Insulin-like growth factor-1: potential for treatment of motor neuronal disorders. *Exp. Neurol.* 1993; 124 (1): 73–88.

22. Festoff, B.W., S.X. Yang, J. Vaught, et al. The insulin-like growth factor signaling system and ALS neurotrophic factor treatment strategies. *J. Neurol. Sci.* 1995; 129 (Suppl.): 114–121.

23. Vaught, J.L., P.C. Contreras, M.A. Glickman, et al. Potential utility of rhIGF-1 in neuromuscular and/or degenerative disease. *Ciba Found. Symp.* 1996; 196: 18–27.

24. Rothstein, J.D. Therapeutic horizons for amyotrophic lateral sclerosis. *Curr. Opin. Neurobiol.* 1996; 6 (5): 679–687.

25. Braunstein, G.D., and A.L. Reviczky. Serum insulin-like growth factor-1 levels in amyotrophic lateral sclerosis. *J. Neurol. Neurosurg. Psychiatry* 1987; 50 (6): 792–794.

26. Torres-Aleman, I., V. Barrios, and J. Bericano. The peripheral insulin-like growth factor system in amyotrophic lateral sclerosis and in multiple sclerosis. *Neurology* 1998; 59 (3): 772–776.

27. Adem, A., J. Ekblom, P.G. Gillberg, et al. Insulin-like growth factor-1 receptors in human spinal cord: changes in amyotrophic lateral sclerosis. *J. Neural Transm. Gen. Sect.* 1994; 97 (1): 73–84.

28. Adem, A., J. Ekblom, and P.G. Gillberg. Growth factor receptors in amyotrophic lateral sclerosis. *Mol. Neurobiol.* 1994; 9 (1–3): 225–231.

29. Dore, S., C. Kriegr, S. Kar, et al. Distribution and levels of insulin-like growth factor (IGF-I and IGF-II) and insulin receptor binding sites in the spinal cords of amyotrophic lateral sclerosis (ALS) patients. *Brain. Res. Mol. Brain Res.* 1996; 41 (1–2): 128–133.

30. Dore, S., S. Kar, and R. Quirion. Rediscovering an old friend, IGF-1: potential use in the treatment of neurodegenerative diseases. *Trends Neurosci.* 1997; 29 (8): 326–331.

31. Smith, R.A., S. Melmed, B. Sherman, et al. Recombinant growth hormone treatment of amyotrophic lateral sclerosis. *Muscle Nerve* 1993; 16 (6): 624–633.

32. Lai, E.C., K.J. Felice, B.W. Festoff, et al. Effect of recombinant human insulin-like growth factor-1 on progression of ALS. A placebo-controlled study. The North America ALS/IGF-1 Study Group. *Neurology* 1997; 49 (6): 1621–1630.

33. Borasio, G.D., W. Robberecht, P.N. Leigh, et al. A placebo-controlled trial of insulin-like growth factor-1 in amyotrophic lateral sclerosis. European ALS/IGF-1 Study Group. *Neurology* 1998; 51 (2): 583–586.

34. Ackerman, S.J., E.M. Sullivan, K.M. Beusterien, et al. Cost effectiveness of recombinant human insulin-like growth factor 1 therapy in patients with ALS. *Pharmacoeconomics* 1999; 15 (2): 179–195.

35. Miller, R.G. Carrell-Krusen Symposium invited lecture. Clinical trials in motor neuron diseases. *J. Child. Neurol.* 1999; 14 (3): 173–179.

9

Rationale for Anabolic Therapy in Chronic Fatigue Syndrome

Introduction: Chronic Fatigue Syndrome: A Neurosteroid Deficiency?

Chronic fatigue syndrome, CFS, is an illness that results in debilitating fatigue as well as rheumatological, infectious, and neuropsychiatric symptoms.[1] The exact etiology of CFS remains an enigma,[2] although there is substantial evidence that its onset may be linked to viral or toxic agents.[3, 4, 5, 6] CFS has remained an ill-defined clinical problem that is perceived as a complex of multiple symptomatologies with unexplained persistent fatigue. The major symptoms include fatigue lasting for more than six months, fatigue after minor exertion, low-grade fever, moderate lymphadenopathy, muscle and joint pain, various psychological presentations, and idiosyncrasies in short-term memory and cognitive processing, often occurring in cycles.[7, 8, 9, 10] Often, the symptomatology of patients with CFS overlaps the symptomatologies of those with other autoimmune diseases and conditions such as major depression, fibromyalgia, and Gulf War Syndrome.[11, 12, 13, 14, 15, 16, 17, 18, 19, 20, 21, 22,]

Hypoandrogenemia and CFS

There is a growing body of scientific evidence to indicate that CFS is a disease of deficient neuroendocrine-immune communication. This results in an immune dysregulation that ushers in neuropsychological, neuroendocrine, and neurobiological abnormalities in most patients with CFS.[23] Recent studies have shown that these alterations may give rise to the profound fatigue and array of diffuse somatic symptoms.

Abnormalities in neuroendocrine-immune communication have

recently been demonstrated in patients with CFS by utilizing specific laboratory tests. In response to provocative, activating chemical stimuli, patients with CFS have been shown to have a relative resistance of the immune system to regulation by the neuroendocrine system as demonstrated by:

(1) impaired activation of the hypothalamic-pituitary-adrenal (HPA) axis that may be the essential neuroendocrine abnormality.[24, 25, 26, 27, 28, 29, 30]

(2) significantly reduced T-cell proliferation, decreased natural killer (NK) cell activity, imbalanced cytokine (tumor necrosis factor-alpha and interleukin-10) production by monocytes, and abnormal release of cytokines within the CNS.[31, 32, 33, 34, 35, 36]

(3) significantly lower adrenal androgen levels (DHEA and DHEA-S) that may provide a role for androgens, both therapeutically and as a diagnostic tool.[37, 38, 39, 40, 41, 42] Lower adrenal androgen production in response to provocative stimuli in CFS has been identified as resembling that seen in several autoimmune diseases. This androgen deficiency condition may result in a deficiency of neurosteroids, leading to the psychophysiological phenomena of memory less, increased perceived stress, anxiety, insomnia, and depression. Patients with CFS have been shown to have significant (over 50 percent smaller adrenal glands than controls) adrenal atrophy by CT studies.[43]

(4) significant imbalance in the DHEA/cortisol ratio that represents a divergence in the synthetic pathways of androgen production within the adrenal cortex in response to provocative stimuli and stressors.[44]

Studies with Anabolic Therapy in CFS

To date, there have been no published studies on the use of androgen therapy in patients with CSF. However, patients with CSF who have or develop hypoandrogenemia should be candidates for androgen therapy.

Summary

In this chapter the rationale for anabolic therapy in CFS has been presented. It is likely that future studies will show that androgen therapy:

(1) can reduce fatigue and depression and improve cognitive functions.

(2) can elevate hemoglobin concentrations that improve aerobic capacity.

(3) can prevent or reverse sarcopenia and osteoporosis.

(4) can provide for improved outcomes for patients undergoing traditional rehabilitative modalities.

(5) can modulate pathogenic cytokine profiles.

(6) correct hypoandrogenemia and prevent the mental and physical sequelae of hypoandrogenemia.

For these reasons, androgen therapy should be included in research efforts and therapeutic trials in the area of CFS.

Notes

1. Deluca, J., S.K. Johnson, and B.H. Natelson. Neuropsychiatric status of patients with chronic fatigue syndrome: an overview. *Toxicol. Ind. Health* 1994; 10 (4–5): 513–522.

2. van der Steen, W.J. Chronic fatigue syndrome: a matter of enzyme deficiencies? *Med. Hypotheses* 2000; 54 (5): 853–854.

3. Buchwald, D., J. Umali, T. Pearlman, et al. Postinfectious chronic fatigue: a distinct syndrome? *Clin. Infect. Dis.* 1996; 23 (2): 385–387.

4. Johnson, S.K., J. Deluca, and B.H. Natelson. Chronic fatigue syndrome: reviewing the research findings. *Ann. Behav. Med.* 1999; (21 (3): 258–271.

5. Glaser, R., and J.K. Kiecolt-Glaser. Stress-associated immune modulation: relevance to viral infections and chronic fatigue syndrome. *Am. J. Med.* 1998; 105 (3A): 35S–42S.

6. Zhang, Q.W., B.H. Natelson, J.E. Ottenweller, et al. Chronic fatigue syndrome beginning suddenly occurs seasonally over the years. *Chronobiol. Int.* 2000; 17 (1): 95–99.

7. Kanayama, Y. [Chronic fatigue syndromeùsymptoms, signs, laboratory tests, and prognosis.] *Nippon Rinsho* 1992; 50 (11): 2586–2590.

8. Lanham, R.J. Chronic fatigue syndrome: a diagnostic challenge for the laboratory. *Clin. Lab. Sci.* 1994; 7 (5): 279–282.

9. Fry, A.M., and M. Martin. Fatigue in the chronic fatigue syndrome: a cognitive phenomenon? *J. Psychosom. Res.* 1996; 41 (5): 415–426.

10. Dipino, R.K. and R.L. Kane. Neurocognitive functioning in chronic fatigue syndrome. *Neurospsychol. Rev.* 1996; 6 (1): 47–60.

11. Abbey, S.E., and P.E. Garfinkel. Chronic fatigue syndrome and depression: cause, effect, or covariate. *Rev. Infect. Dis.* 1991; 13 (Suppl. 1): S73–S83.

12. Pepper, C.M., L.B. Krupp, F. Friedberg, et al. A comparison of neuropsychiatric characteristics in chronic fatigue syndrome, multiple sclerosis, and major depression. *J. Neuropsychiatry Clin. Neurosci.* 1993; 5 (2): 200–205.

13. Buchwald, D. Fibromyalgia and chronic fatigue syndrome: similarities and differences. *Rheum. Dis. Clin. North Am.* 1996; 22 (2): 219–243.

14. Haley, R.W., T.L. Kurt, and J. Hom. Is there a Gulf War Syndrome? Searching for syndromes by factor analysis of symptoms. *JAMA* 1997; 277 (3): 215–222.

15. Rook, G.A., and A. Zumla. Is the Gulf War syndrome an immunologically mediated phenomenon? *Hosp. Med.* 1998; 59 (1): 10–11.

16. Rook, G.A., and A. Zumla. Gulf War syndrome: is it due to a systemic shift in cytokine balance towards a Th2 profile? *Lancet* 1997; 349 (9086): 1831–1833.

17. Crofford, L.J. The hypothalamic-pituitary-adrenal stress axis in fibromyalgia and chronic fatigue syndrome. *Z. Rheumatol.* 1998; 57 (Suppl 2): 67–71.

18. Demitrack, M.A., and L.J. Crofford. Evidence for and pathophysiologic implications of hypothalamic-pituitary-adrenal axis dysregulation in fibromyalgia and chronic fatigue syndrome. *Ann. N.Y. Acad. Sci.* 1998; 840: 684–697.

19. Zhang, Q, X.D. Zhou, T. Denny, et al. Changes in immune parameters seen in Gulf War veterans but not in civilians with chronic fatigue syndrome. *Clin. Diagn. Lab. Immunol.* 1999; 6 (1): 6–13.

20. Everson, M.P., K. Kotler, and W.D. Blackburn. Stress and immune dysfunction in Gulf War veterans. *Ann. N.Y. Acad. Sci.* 1999; 876: 413–418.

21. Frost, S.D. Gulf War syndrome: proposed causes. *Cleve. Clin. Med.* 2000; 67 (1): 17–20.

22. Asa, P.B., Y. Cao, and R.F. Garry. Antibodies to squalene in Gulf War syndrome. *Exp. Mol. Pathol.* 2000; 68 (1): 55–64.

23. Gonzales, M.B., J.C. Cousins, and P.M. Doraiswamy. Neurobiology of chronic fatigue syndrome. *Prog. Neuropsychopharmacol. Biol. Psychiatry* 1996; 20 (5): 749–759.

24. Bearn, J., T. Allain, P. Coskeran, et al. Neuroendocrine responses to d-fenfluramine and insulin-induced hypoglycemia in chronic fatigue syndrome. *Biol. Psychiatry* 1995; 37 (4): 245–252.

25. Sterzl, I., and V. Zamrazil. [Endocrinopathy in the differential diagnosis of chronic fatigue syndrome.] *Vnitr. Lek.* 1996; 42 (9): 624–626.

26. Dinan, T.G., T. Majeed, E. Lavelle, et al. Blunted serotonin-mediated activation of the hypothalamic-pituitary-adrenal axis in chronic fatigue syndrome. *Psychoneuroendocrinology* 1997; 22 (4): 261–267.

27. Demitrack, M.A., and L.J. Crofford. Evidence for and pathopysiologic implications of hypothalamic-pituitary-adrenal axis dysregulation in fibromyalgia and chronic fatigue syndrome. *Ann. N.Y. Acad. Sci.* 1998; 840: 684–697.

28. Komaroff, A.L., and D.S. Buchwald. Chronic fatigue syndrome: an update. *Annu. Rev. Med.* 1998; 49: 1–13.

29. Crofford, L.J. The hypothalamic-pituitary-adrenal stress axis in fibromyalgia and chronic fatigue syndrome. *Z. Rheumatol.* 1998; 57 (Suppl 2): 67–71.

30. Scott, L.V., and T. G. Dinan. Urinary free cortisol excretion in chronic fatigue syndrome, major depression and in healthy volunteers. *J. Affect. Disord.* 1998; 47 (1–3): 49–54.

31. Uschida, A. [Therapy of chronic fatigue syndrome.] *Nippon Rinsho* 1992; 50 (11): 2679–2683.

32. Lloyd, A., I. Hickie, C. Hickie, et al. Cell-mediated immunity in patients with chronic fatigue syndrome, healthy control subjects and patients with major depression. *Clin. Exp. Immunol.* 1992; 87 (1): 76–79.

33. Whiteside, T.L., and D. Friberg. Natural killer cells and natural killer cell activity in chronic fatigue syndrome. *Am. J. Med.* 1998; 105 (3A): 27S–34S.

34. Glaser, R., and J.K. Kieclot-Glasser. Stress-associated immune modulation: relevance to viral infections and chronic fatigue syndrome. *Am. J. Med.* 1998; 105 (3A): 35S–42S.

35. Vollmer-Conna, U., A. Lloyd, A Hickie, et al. Chronic fatigue syndrome: an immunological perspective. *Aust. N. Z. J. Psychiatry* 1998; 32 (4): 523–527.

36. Kavelaars, A., W. Kuis, L. Knook, et al. Disturbed neuroendocrine-immune interactions in chronic fatigue syndrome. *J. Clin. Endocrinol. Metab.* 2000; 85 (2): 692–696.

37. Kodama, M., T Kodama, and M. Murakami. The value of dehydroepiandrosterone-annexed vitamin C infusion treatment in the clinical control of chronic fatigue

syndrome (CFS). A pilot study of the new vitamin C infusion treatment with a volunteer CFS patient. *In Vivo* 1996; 10 (6): 575–584.

38. Kuratsune, H., K. Yamasguti, M. Sawada, et al. Dehydroepiandrosterone sulfate deficiency in chronic fatigue syndrome. *Int. J. Mol. Med.* 1998; 1 (1): 143–146.

39. Scott, L.V., S. Medbak, and T.G. Dinan. The low dose ACTH test in chronic fatigue syndrome and in health. *Clin. Endocrinol. (Oxf.)* 1998; 48 (6): 733–737.

40. Scott, L.V., F. Salahuddin, J. Cooney, et al. Differences in adrenal steroid profile in chronic fatigue syndrome, in depression, and in health. *J. Affect. Disord.* 1999; 54 (1–2): 129–137.

41. Adachi, M., and H. Nawata. [Dehydroepiandrosterone (DHEA), dehydroepiandrosterone sulfate (DHEA-S).] *Nippon Rinsho* 1999; 57 (Suppl): 157–161.

42. De Becker, P., K. De Meileir, J. Joos, et al. Dehydroepiandrosterone (DHEA) response to i.v. ACTH in patients with chronic fatigue syndrome. *Horm. Metab. Res.* 1999; 31 (1): 18–21.

43. Scott, L.V., J. The, R. Reznek, et al. Small adrenal glands in chronic fatigue syndrome: a preliminary computer tomography study. *Pschoneuroendocrinology* 1999; 24 (7): 759–768.

44. Scott, L.V., F. Svec, and T. Dinan. A preliminary study of dehydroepiandrosterone response to low-dose ACTH in chronic fatigue syndrome and in healthy subjects. *Psychiatry Res.* 2000; 97 (1): 21–28.

10

Rationale for Anabolic Therapy in Multiple Sclerosis

Introduction: A Major Loss of Anabolic Potentials to Counteract Severe Catabolism

Multiple sclerosis (MS) is a chronic autoimmune inflammatory demyelinating disease of the central nervous system that can be characterized clinically by a remitting-relapsing or a chronic progressive course.[1] One of the earliest pathologic changes seen with MS involves the inflammatory activation of vascular endothelial cells and a loss of control of the neuroimmune response to this activation.[2, 3] However, the exact cause of MS remains uncertain.

It has long been suspected that sex hormones contribute directly and indirectly to the etiology and pathogenesis of MS.[4, 5] Basic and clinical research suggests that disturbed neuroendocrine function may be involved in the pathogenesis and clinical course of MS.[6, 7, 8] It has also been demonstrated by both basic and clinical research that there is a gender dimorphism with MS, in that females have a higher incidence of MS (experimental autoimmune encephalomyelitis, EAE, in animal models) compared to males.[9, 10, 11, 12, 13]

The susceptibility of women to MS has been related to sex steroid influences when onset occurs at an early age or a delayed age. Pregnancy has been shown to have a short-term favorable effect on the course of MS, but there is an increased rate of relapse during the postpartum period. In addition, women often report premenstrual exacerbation of their MS symptoms, with subsequent remission during menses.[14]

155

Hypoandrogenemia and Hyposomatomedinemia in MS

The fact that aging curves for sex steroids show a striking similarity to the MS incidence curves has further implicated these steroids in the pathogenesis of the disease.[15] Androgens have been shown to have an important beneficial impact on the immune response to MS and animal models of MS.[16, 17, 18, 19] A number of studies have shown that patients with MS have hypoandrogenemia.[20, 21, 22] Alterations in the hypothalamic-pituitary-adrenal (HPA) and hypothalamic-pituitary-gonadal axes have been implicated in the hypoandrogenemia associated with MS.[23, 24]

Hypoandrogenemia has been associated with altered and often pathologic cytokine imbalances. Considerable scientific investigation has been focused on the cytokine imbalances associated with MS.[25, 26] Most MS prognostic indicators seem to act through the neuroendocrine-immune network, modulating the immune response in the context of the Th1/Th2 cytokine paradigm.[27] These pathologic cytokine profiles, seen with MS, have been associated with other diseases, such as other autoimmune diseases, stroke, Alzheimer's disease, and traumatic brain injury, that are associated with hypoandrogenemia.[28, 29, 30] However, very little investigation has been given to the "upstream" immunomodulation by androgens to the "downstream" cytokine imbalance abnormalities in MS. It is well known that androgens play a beneficial role in correcting and modulating autoimmune cytokine profiles. This connection of hypoandrogenemia and altered and pathologic cytokine profiles in MS seems obvious, and androgen therapy to correct both hypoandrogenemia and pathologic cytokine profiles should be considered as a disease-modifying treatment even while further scientific studies are conducted.

Besides hypoandrogenemia, other research groups have shown that MS is associated with other defects in anabolic hormone deficiency mechanisms that give rise to hyposomatomedinemia.[31] These deficits have included growth hormone (GH) and insulin-like growth factor-1 (IGF-1).[32, 33, 34] Considerable research has been conducted into the hyposomatomedinemia of and IGF-1 therapy for MS via animal models of the disease.[35, 36, 37, 38, 39, 40, 41, 42] Other basic research studies have focused on the use of alternative anabolic therapies, including gene therapy, myelin basic protein-derived peptide, and GHRH-GH-IGF-IGFBP axis stimulatory analogues.[43, 44, 45, 46, 47, 48, 49] However, because of the perceived failures of the current standard of care, many MS patients have resorted to using alternative treatments to treat themselves and some of these regimes include anabolic therapies.[50]

Anabolic Therapy for MS Patients in Rehabilitation

Unlike other areas of rehabilitation, which typically follow a single incident such as trauma or stroke and are followed by improvement (or at least an expectation of stable impairment), MS presents the problem of progressive impairment and disability.[51] Therefore, a comprehensive strategy for the management of MS should involve modalities that limit the inflammatory processes *and* repair the catabolic damages and sequelae.[52] Many of these damages and sequelae are associated with hypoandrogenemia and hyposomatomedinemia and can be treated. These include:

(1) sexual dysfunction, reduced orgasmic response, and erectile dysfunction.[53]

(2) reduced fibrinolytic activity, microvascular disease, and thromboembolic complications.[54, 55, 56, 57]

(3) clinical depression and deficits in cognition.[58, 59, 60, 61, 62, 63, 64, 65]

(4) osteoporosis.[66, 67, 68]

(5) sarcopenia and reduced exercise tolerance.[69, 70, 71]

(6) myocardial dysfunction.[72]

(7) Raynaud's phenomenon.[73, 74]

Although many of the conditions associated with MS can be diagnosed and treated, a recent study has indicated that they are not. For example, in the diagnosis and treatment of osteoporosis in women patients with MS, the evidence shows:[75]

(1) that despite multiple risk factors, 85 percent of women MS patients have never had a bone density test, even with past, heavy corticosteroid therapy.

(2) that 81 percent of postmenopausal women have never had a bone density test, 50 percent have not been prescribed calcium supplementation, and 70 percent have not been prescribed any type of hormone-replacement therapy.

(3) that even though osteoporosis screening, prevention, and treatment protocols must be a part of the medical plan for all women with MS, inexcusable deficits are widespread in this area among physicians.

This recent report exemplifies the huge gap that exists between the scientific evidence-based information and the current treatment with MS patients. This gap can be narrowed by understanding the mechanisms of hypoandrogenemia and hyposomatomedinemia and how they relate to the entire disease mechanisms of patients with MS.

In a large 16-year study, it has been shown that less than half of the causes of mortality in MS patients are directly attributed to the complications of MS. Other causes of death in MS patients include:

(1) 28 percent from suicide (7.5 times that for age-matched individuals).

(2) 32 percent from thromboembolic events such as acute myocardial infarction and stroke (similar for age-matched individuals).

(3) 30 percent from malignancy (similar for age-matched individuals).

(4) 10 percent from miscellaneous causes.

This evidence suggests that diagnosing and treating dysthymia in MS should be a major consideration. The potential roles of neuroendocrine and molecular mechanisms in dysthymia in MS patients have been identified.[76] In addition, it has been shown that subjective well-being plays an important role in rehabilitation outcomes in patients with MS.[77]

Summary

There have been no recent studies published with regards to androgen therapy for patients with MS. A few studies have been published in the late 1960s and early 1970s indicated that androgen therapy had some beneficial effects in MS.[78, 79, 80, 81]

An appropriate rationale for androgen therapy in MS patients should include a therapeutic modality that:

(1) provides for an overall anabolic effect to combat or reverse sarcopenia.

(2) provides for stimulation of osteoblasts to prevent or reverse osteoporosis.

(3) provides for an overall anabolic effect to prevent or reverse the catabolic actions of corticosteroid or cytotoxic drug therapies.

(4) reduces corticosteroid therapy requirements.

(5) provides for correction or improvement of pathologic cytokine imbalances.

(6) provides for enhanced myelin synthesis and regeneration, for neuroprotection, and for enhanced nerve growth factor activities.

(7) provides for mood enhancement via mechanisms such as direct and indirect neurosteroid neurotransmitter activities.

(8) provides for an enhanced fibrinolytic effect.

(9) corrects hypoandrogenemia and hyposomatomedinemia and prevents or reverses the associated sequelae.

(10) corrects hypoandrogenemia secondary to estrogen monotherapy.

(11) improves overall well-being.

(12) improves fatigue, aerobic capacity, and corrects anemic states, including autoimmune anemic conditions.

(13) prevents or improves deficits in cognition.

(14) improves libido and sexual function.

(15) corrects or improves dyslipidemias.

(16) improves rehabilitation outcomes and hastens traditional rehabilitation modalities.

There is little doubt that androgen therapy will be shown, via future research efforts, to have disease-modifying effects for patients with MS. No other class of drugs has such a plethora of proven beneficial effects that can be offered to MS patients.

Notes

1. Whitacre, C.C, I.E. Gienapp, A. Meyer, et al. Treatment of autoimmune disease by oral tolerance to autoantigens. *Clin. Immunol. Immunopathol.* 1996; 80 (3 Pt. 2): S31–S39.

2. Tintore, M., A.L. Fernandez, A. Rovira, et al. Antibodies against endothelial cells in patients with multiple sclerosis. *Acta Neurol. Scand.* 1996; 93 (6): 416–420.

3. Onodera, H., I. Nakashima, K. Fujihara, et al. Elevated plasma level of plasminogen activator inhibitor-1 (PAI-1) in patients with relapsing-remitting multiple sclerosis. *Toholu J. Exp. Med.* 1999; 198 (4): 259–265.

4. Sandyk, R. Estrogen's impact on cognitive functions in multiple sclerosis. *Int. J. Neurosci.* 1996; 86 (1–2): 23–31.

5. D'Agostino, P., S. Milano, C. Barbera, et al. Sex hormones modulate inflammatory mediators produced by macrophages. *Ann. N.Y. Acad. Sci.* 1999; 876: 426–429.

6. Anisman, H., M.G. Baines, I. Berczi, et al. Neuroimmune mechanisms in health and disease: 2. Disease. *Canad. Med. Assoc. J.* 1996; 155 (8): 1075–1082.

7. Whitacre, C.C., K. Dowdell, and A.C. Griffin. Neuroendocrine influences on experimental autoimmune encephalomyelitis. *Ann. N.Y. Acad. Sci.* 1998; 840: 705–716.

8. Kumpfel, T., F. Then Bergh, E. Friess, et al. Dehydroepiandrosterone response to the adrenocorticotropin test and the combined dexamethasone and corticotropin-releasing hormone test in patients with multiple sclerosis. *Neuroendocrinology* 1999; 70 (6): 431–438.

9. Voskuhl, R.R., H. Pitchenkian-Halabi, A. MacKenzie-Graham, et al. Gender differences in autoimmune demyelination in the mouse: implications for multiple sclerosis. *Ann. Neuro.* 1996; 39 (6): 724–733.

10. Bebo, B.F., A.A. Vandenbark, H. Offner. Male SJL mice do not relapse after induction of EAE with PLP 139–151. *J. Neurosci. Res.* 1996; 45 (6): 680–689.

11. Ding, M., J.L. Wong, N.E. Rogers, et al. Gender differences of inducible nitric oxide production in SJL/J mice with experimental autoimmune encephalomyelitis. *J. Neuroimmunol.* 1997; 77 (1): 99–106.

12. Bebo, B.F., E. Zelinka-Vincent, G. Adamus, et al. Gonadal hormones influence the immune response to PLP 139–151 and the clinical course of relapsing experimental autoimmune encephalomyelitis. *J. Neuroimmunol.* 1998; 84 (2): 122–130.

13. Bebo, B.F., J.C. Schuster, A.A. Vandenbark, et al. Gender differences in experimental autoimmune encephalomyelitis develop during the induction of the immune response to encephalitogenic peptides. *J. Neurosci. Res.* 1998; 52 (4): 420–426.

14. Sandyk, R. Estrogen's impact on cognitive functions in multiple sclerosis. *Int. J. Neurosci.* 1996; 86 (1–2): 23–31.

15. Fischman, H.R. Multiple sclerosis: a two-stage process? *Am. J. Epidemiol.* 1981; 114 (2): 244–252.

16. Dalal, M., S. Kim, and R.R. Voskuhl. Testosterone therapy ameliorates experimental autoimmune encephalomyelitis and induces a T helper 2 bias in the autoantigen-specific T lymphocyte response. *J. Immunol.* 1997; 159 (1): 3–6.

17. Bebo, B.F., E. Zelinka-Vincent, G. Adamus, et al. Gonadal hormones influence the immune response to PLP 139–151 and the clinical course of relapsing experimental autoimmune encephalomyelitis. *J. Neuroimmunol.* 1998; 84 (2): 122–130.

18. Bebo, B.F., J.C. Schuster, A.A. Vandenbark, et al. Androgens alter the cytokine profile and reduce encephalitogenicity of myelin-reactive T cells. *J. Immunol.* 1999; 162 (1): 35–40.

19. Bebo, B.F., K. Adlard, J.C. Schuster, et al. Gender differences in protection from EAE induced by oral tolerance with a peptide analogue of MBP-Acl–11. *J. Neurosci. Res.* 1999; 55 (4): 432–440.

20. Klapps, P., S. Seyfert, T. Fischer, et al. Endocrine function in multiple sclerosis. *Acta Neurol. Scand.* 1992; 85 (5): 353–357.

21. Davies, J.S., N.P. Hinds, and M.F. Scanlon. Growth hormone deficiency and hypogonadism in a patient with multiple sclerosis. *Clin. Endocrinol. (Oxf.)* 1996; 44 (1): 117–119.

22. Kumpfel, T., F. Then Bergh, E. Friess, et al. Dehydroepiandrosterone response to the adrenocorticotropin test and the combined dexamethasone and corticotrophin-releasing hormone test in patients with multiple sclerosis. *Neuroendocrinoloy* 1999; 70 (6): 431–438.

23. Wei, T., and S.L. Lightman. The neuroendocrine axis in patients with multiple sclerosis. *Brain* 1997; 120 (6): 1067–1076.

24. Martinelli, V. Trauma, stress and multiple sclerosis. *Neurol. Sci.* 2000; 21 (4 Suppl. 2): S849–S852.

25. Navikas, V., and H. Link. Review: cytokines and the pathogenesis of multiple sclerosis. *J. Neurosci. Res.* 1996; 45 (4): 322–333.

26. Ledeen, R.W., and G. Chakraborty. Cytokines, signal transduction, and inflammatory demyelination: review and hypothesis. *Neurochem. Res.* 1998; 23 (3): 277–289.

27. Zaffaroni, M., and A. Ghezzi. The prognostic value of age, gender, pregnancy and endocrine factors in multiple sclerosis. *Neurol. Sci.* 2000; 21 (4 Suppl. 2): S857–S860.

28. Miller, F.W. Genetics of autoimmune diseases. *Exp. Clin. Immunogenet.* 1995; 13 (3): 182–190.

29. Hays, S.J. Therapeutic approaches to the treatment of neuroinflammatory diseases. *Curr. Pharm. Des.* 1998; 4 (4): 335–348.

30. Elkarim, R.A., M. Mustafa, P. Kivisakk, et al. Cytokine autoantibodies in

multiple sclerosis, aseptic meningitis and stroke. *Eur. J. Clin. Invest.* 1998; 28 (4): 295–299.

31. Armstrong, R.C., H.H. Dorn, C.V. Kufta, et al. Pre-oligodendrocytes from adult human CNS. *J. Neurosci.* 1992; 12 (4): 1538–1547.

32. Nowak, S., D. Kowalski, K. Kowalska, et al. [Growth hormone levels in the blood serum and cerebrospinal fluid of patients with multiple sclerosis.] *Neurol. Neurochir. Pol.* 1987; 21 (4–5): 315–318.

33. Fisher, K. Multiple sclerosis and the evolution of growth hormone mechanisms in man. *Med. Hypotheses* 1988; 27 (2): 99–106.

34. Weigent, D.A. Immunoregulatory properties of growth hormone and prolactin. *Pharmacol. Ther.* 1996; 69 (3): 237–257.

35. Yao, D.L., X. Liu, L.D. Hudson, et al. Insulin-like growth factor-1 treatment reduces demyelination and up-regulates gene expression of myelin-related proteins in experimental autoimmune encephalomyelitis. *Proc. Natl. Acad. Sci. U.S.A.* 1995; 92 (13): 6190–6194.

36. Liu, X., D.L. Yao, and H. Webster. Insulin-like growth factor-1 treatment reduces clinical deficits and lesion severity in acute demyelinating experimental autoimmune encephalomyelitis. *Mult. Scler.* 1995; 1 (1): 2–9.

37. Yao, D.L., X. Liu, L.D. Hudson, et al. Insulin-like growth factor-1 given subcutaneously reduces clinical deficits, decreases lesion severity and upregulates synthesis of myelin proteins in experimental autoimmune encephalomyelitis. *Life Sci.* 1996; 58 (16): 1301–1306.

38. Liu, X., C. Linnington, H.D. Webster, et al. Insulin-like growth factor-1 treatment reduces immune cell responses in acute non-demyelinative experimental autoimmune enchpalomyelitis. *J. Neurosci. Res.* 1997; 47 (5): 531–538.

39. Webster, H.D. Growth factors and myelin regeneration in multiple sclerosis. *Mult. Scler.* 1997; 3 (2): 113–120.

40. Li, W., L Quigley, D.L. Yao, et al. Chronic relapsing experimental autoimmune encephalomyelitis: effects of insulin-like growth factor-1 treatment on clinical deficits, lesion severity, glial responses, and blood brain barrier defects. *J. Neuropathol. Exp. Neurol.* 1998; 57 (5): 426–438.

41. Ye, P., and A.J. D'Erole. Insulin-like growth factor 1 protects oligodendrocytes from tumor necrosis factor-alpha-induced injury. *Endocrinology* 1999; 140 (7): 3063–3072.

42. DuboiS–Dalcq, M., and K. Murray. Why are growth factors important in oligodendrocyte physiology? *Pathol. Biol. (Paris)* 2000; 48 (1): 80–86.

43. Bitar, D.M., and C.C. Whitacre. Suppression of experimental autoimmune encephalomyelitis by the oral administration of myelin basic protein. *Cell Immunol.* 1988; 112 (2): 364–370.

44. Chen, Y., V.K. Kuchroo, J. Inobe, et al. Regulatory T cell clones induced by oral tolerance: suppression of autoimmune encephalomyelitis. *Science* 1994; 265 (5176): 1237–1240.

45. Marusic, S. and S. Tonegawa. Tolerance induction and autoimmune encephalomyelitis amelioration after administration of myelin basic protein-derived peptide. *J. Exp. Med.* 1997; 186 (4): 507–515.

46. Liu, J.Q., X.F. Bai, F.D. Shi, et al. Inhibition of experimental autoimmune enchpalomyelitis in Lewis rats by nasal admistration of encephalitogenic MBP peptides: synergistic effects of MBP 68–86 and 87–99. *Int. Immunol.* 1998; 10 (8): 1139–1148.

47. Jewell, S.D., I.E. Gienapp, K.L. Cox, et al. Oral tolerance as therapy for experimental autoimmune encephalomyelitis and multiple sclerosis: demonstration of T cell anergy. *Immunol. Cell Biol.* 1998; 76 (1): 74–82.

48. Chen, L.Z., G.M. Hochwald, C. Huang, et al. Gene therapy in allergic encephalomyelitis using myelin basic protein-specific T cells engineered to express latent transforming growth factor-beta 1. *Proce. Natl. Acad. Sci. U.S.A.* 1998; 95 (13): 12516–12521.

49. Benson, J.M., S.S. Stuckman, K.L. Cox, et al. Oral administration of myelin basic protein is superior to myelin in suppressing established relapsing experimental autoimmune encephalomyelitis. *J. Immunol.* 1999; 162 (10): 6247–6254.

50. Van der Ploeg, H.M., M.J. Molenaar, and C.W. van Tiggelen. [Use of alternative treatments by patients with multiple sclerosis.] *Ned. Tijdchr. Geneeskd.* 1994; 138 (6): 296–299.

51. C. Ko Ko. Effectiveness of rehabilitation for multiple sclerosis. *Clin. Rehabil.* 1999; 13 (Suppl. 1): 33–41.

52. Compston, A. Future prospects for the management of multiple sclerosis. *Ann. Neurol.* 1994; 36 (Suppl.): S146–S150.

53. Stenager, E., E.N. Stenager, K. Jensen, et al. Sexual function in multiple sclerosis. A 5-year follow-up study. *Ital. J. Neurol. Sci.* 1996; 17 (1): 67–69.

54. Menon, I.S., H.A. Dewar, and D.J. Newell. Fibrinolytic activity of venous blood of patients with multiple sclerosis. *Neurology* 1969; 19 (1): 101–104.

55. Brunetti, A., G.L. Ricchieri, G.M. Patrassi, et al. Rheological and fibrinolytic findings in multiple sclerosis. *J. Neurol. Neurosurg. Psychiatry* 1981; 44 (4): 340–343.

56. Paterson, P.Y., C.S. Koh, and H.C. Kwaan. Role of the clotting system in the pathogenesis of neuroimmunologic disease. *Fed. Proc.* 1987; 46 (1): 91–96.

57. LaBan, M.M., T. Martin, J. Pechur, et al. Physical and occupational therapy in the treatment of patients with multiple sclerosis. *Phys. Med. Rehabil. Clin. N. Am.* 1998; 9 (3): 603–614.

58. Holsboer, F., A. Grasser, E. Friess, et al. Steroid effects on central neurons and implications for psychiatric and neurological disorders. *Ann. N.Y. Acad. Sci.* 1994; 746: 345–359.

59. Fuhrer, M.J. Subjective well-being: implications for medical rehabilitation outcomes and models of disablement. *Am. J. Phys. Med. Rehabil.* 1994; 73 (5): 358–364.

60. Rao, S. White matter disease and dementia. *Brain Cogn.* 1996; 31 (2): 250–268.

61. Akiskal, H.S., C.L. Bolis, C. Cazzullo, et al. Dysthymia in neurological disorders. *Mol. Psychiatry* 1996; 1 (6): 478–491.

62. Andrade, V.M., O.F. Bueno, M.G. Oliveira, et al. Cognitive profile of patients with relapsing remitting multiple sclerosis. *Arq. Neuropsiquiatr.* 1999; 57 (3B): 775–783.

63. Fisher, E., R.A. Rudick, G. Cutter, et al. Relationship between brain atrophy and disability: an 8-year follow-up study of multiple sclerosis patients. *Mult. Scler.* 2000; 6 (6): 373–377.

64. Benedict, R.H., R.L. Priore, C. Miller, et al. Personality disorder in multiple sclerosis correlates with cognitive impairment. *J. Neuropsychiatry Clin. Neurosci.* 2001; 13 (1): 70–76.

65. Polliack, M., Y. Barak, and A. Achiron. Late-onset multiple sclerosis. *J. Am. Geriatr. Soc.* 2001; 49 (2): 168–171.

66. Stenager, E., and K. Jensen. Fractures in multiple sclerosis. *Acta Neurol. Belg.* 1991; 91 (5): 296–302.

67. Formica, C.A., F. Cosman, J. Nieves, et al. Reduced bone mass and fat-free mass in women with multiple sclerosis: effects of ambulatory status and glucocorticoid use. *Calcif. Tissue Int.* 1997; 61 (2): 129–133.

68. Cosman, F., J. Nieves, L. Komar, et al. Fracture history and bone loss in patients with MS. *Neurology* 1998; 51 (4): 1161–1165.

69. Petajan, J.H., E. Gappmaier, A.T. White, et al. Impact of aerobic training

on fitness and quality of life in multiple sclerosis. *Ann. Neurol.* 1996; 39 (4): 432–441.

70. Kent-Braun, J.A., A.V. Ng, M. Castro, et al. Strength, skeletal muscle composition, and enzyme activity in multiple sclerosis. *J. Appl. Physiol.* 1997; 83 (6): 1998–2004.

71. Ng., A.V., H.T. Dao, R.G. Miller, et al. Blunted pressor and intramuscular metabolic responses to voluntary isometric exercise in multiple sclerosis. *J. Appl. Physiol.* 2000; 88 (3): 871–880.

72. Ziaber, J., H. Chmielewski, T. Dryjanski, et al. Evaluation of myocardial muscle functional parameters in patients with multiple sclerosis. *Acta Neurol. Sand.* 1997; 95 (6): 335–337.

73. Linden, D. Severe Raynaud's phenomenon associated with interferon-beta treatment for multiple sclerosis. *Lancet* 1998; 352 (9131): 878–879.

74. Cruz, B.A., E.D. Queiroz, S.V. Nunes, et al. [Severe Raynaud's phenomenon associated with interferon-beta therapy for multiple sclerosis: case report.] *Arq. Neuropsiquiatr.* 2000; 58 (2B): 556–559.

75. Shabas, D., and H. Weinreb. Preventive healthcare in women with multiple sclerosis. *J. Womens Health Gend. Based Med.* 2000; 9 (4): 389–395.

76. Akiskal, H.S., C.L. Bolis, C. Cazzullo, et al. Dysthymia in neurological disorders. *Mol. Psychiatry* 1996; 1 (6): 478–491.

77. Fuhrer, M.J. Subjective well-being: implications for medical rehabilitation outcomes and models of disablement. *Am. J. Phys. Med. Rehabil.* 1994; 73 (5): 358–364.

78. Szabo, S., R.C. Wagner, E.G. Malatinsky, et al. [The effect of anabolic steroids on blood proteins and autoantibodies in multiple sclerosis.] *Stud. Cercet. Neurol.* 1967; 12 (6): 457–461.

79. Mall, G., A. Heibrunn, H.F. Paarmann, et al. [The treatment of multiple sclerosis with anabolic steroids.] *Med. Klin.* 1968; 63 (51): 2075–2077.

80. Husemann, F., J. Kugler, and I. Frank. [Relaxation-promoting effect of vitamin B with anabolics.] *Arzneimittelforschung* 1970; 20 (4): 557–560.

81. Cendrowski, W., and W. Kuran. [Results of combined administration of anabolic steroids in patients with multiple sclerosis.] *Neurol. Neurochir. Pol.* 1972; 6 (4): 573–576.

11

Rationale for Anabolic Therapy in Rheumatoid Arthritis

Introduction: Androgens, the Missing Hormones in RA

Rheumatoid arthritis (RA) is a heterogeneous autoimmune rheumatic disease with a diverse spectrum of manifestations and course of illness. Multiple factors are believed to contribute to its etiology; these include:[1]

(1) an increased familial or immunogenetic risks in younger-onset disease.

(2) a strong female predisposition, particularly during child-bearing years.

(3) a clinical improvement during pregnancy and worsening post-partum.

(4) an increased incidence with aging.

RA may result from a combination of several predisposing factors, including genetic factors, triggering agents, the status of the stress response system, and sex hormone status.[2] It is now documented that androgens and estrogens modulate susceptibility and progression to autoimmune rheumatic diseases. At any concentration, androgens seem primarily to suppress cellular and humoral immunity, whereas at physiologic concentrations, estrogens seem to enhance humoral immunity.[3]

Sex steroid concentrations have been evaluated in RA patients prior to therapy and have frequently been found to indicate hypoandrogenemia, especially in premenopausal women, postmenopausal women, and aging men.[4, 5, 6, 7, 8, 9] In particular, low levels of gonadal and adrenal androgens (testosterone, DHT, DHEA, and DHEAS) and reduced androgen-to-estrogen ratios have been detected in a variety of body fluids of male and female RA patients. These body fluids include blood, synovial fluid, and saliva.[10, 11] Such observations support a pathogenic role for hypoandrogenemia and the decreased levels of the immune-suppressive androgens in RA.[12, 13] Evidence has been accumulating to indicate that hypoandrogenemia is a significant cause of rheumatoid arthritis.[14]

A number of conditions and factors have been shown to alter androgen-to-estrogen ratios. These include exposure to environmental estrogens (phytoestrogens or estrogenic xenobiotics), oral contraceptive use, estrogen monotherapy for HRT, genetic polymorphisms of genes coding for hormone metabolic enzymes or receptors, and gonadal disturbances related to stress system activation (hypothalamic-pituitary-adrenal axis) and physiologic hormonal perturbations such as those during aging, the menstrual cycle, pregnancy, the postpartum period, and menopause.[15, 16, 17, 18, 19, 20] As previously stated, estrogens tend to accelerate and androgens tend to suppress autoantibody formation. In this manner, androgen deficiency promotes the production of autoantibodies and development of RA.[21]

On a molecular basis, androgen adjuvant therapy in RA has been experimentally substantiated.[22] In animal models of RA, androgen therapy has been shown to have significant inhibitory effects on inflammation and cartilage erosion, which results in disease-modifying effects.[23, 24] In humans, androgens exert their immune-modulating effects by a number of mechanisms, including correcting abnormal cytokine imbalances and via androgen receptors in tissue and circulating immune system cells.[25, 26]

Androgen therapy has been shown to have beneficial and multifaceted effects in patients with RA.[27, 28, 29, 30, 31, 32, 33, 34] Thus, it has been suggested that androgen therapy may represent a valuable concomitant or adjuvant treatment associated with other disease-modifying antirheumatic drugs in the management of RA.[35]

Mechanisms of Hypoandrogenemia in RA

Numerous scientific reports have suggested that gonadal and adrenal sex hormones, and specifically low androgen levels accounts for the gender dimorphism in the immune response and for the greater incidence of RA in women and older men. It has been shown that hypoandrogenemia in RA may occur via several mechanisms, including:

(1) in premenopausal women, that ovarian androgen production in

RA patients is lower (statistically significant) during the menstrual cycle when compared to healthy age-matched controls.[36]

(2) in premenopausal women, evidence of a primary adrenal dysfunction exists in RA patients which results in increased production of adrenal corticosteroids and a decreased production of adrenal androgens. This imbalanced steroid ratio tends to cause imbalanced cytokine profiles in relative adrenal androgen-deficient environments which predisposes to the development or increased activity of RA.[37, 38, 39, 40] It has been shown that low adrenal androgen production in premenopausal women with RA is associated with elevated erythrocyte sedimentation rates and platelet counts, and statistically significant increased disease activity scores.[41] It is still not established whether these abnormalities are primary or secondary, although data indicating adrenal dysfunction before the development of RA or within the first year of disease activity suggest a primary abnormality.[42] These studies suggest that adrenal cortical dysfunction, manifested mainly by adrenal androgen deficiency, may either predispose to younger-onset RA or be a longer-term marker in some women.[43] A recent cross-sectional study has shown a steeper age-associated decline in adrenal androgen production in patients who go on to develop RA than in normal age-matched controls.[44]

(3) in premenopausal and postmenopausal women with RA, there is a delay in the recovery of adrenal androgen secretion after corticosteroid therapy that may be a consequence of chronic illness, aging, immune dysfunction, or a specific defect in adrenal androgen synthesis.[45]

(4) in juvenile RA, hypoandrogenemia has been shown to correlate with low androgen levels in synovial fluid and relate to the pathogenic mechanisms and severity of the disease.[46]

(5) in men with RA, a growing body of data indicates that RA develops as a consequence of a deficiency of either adrenal and gonadal androgen production, or both, which results in pathologic cytokine imbalances and higher inflammatory indices.[47, 48, 49] Hypoandrogenemia and diminished testicular androgen biosynthesis after gonadotrophin stimuli have been shown (both statistically significant) to be associated with RA in men.[50] In men with RA, prolonged hypoandrogenemia from suppression of testicular function has been associated with flares and increased disease activity.[51] It has been shown that the immunosuppressive action exerted by androgens may be mediated by androgen receptors in synovial tissue[52] and in synovial macrophages.[53] In men with RA, hypoandrogenemia has been associated with a particular HLA haplotype, and androgen receptors have been described in synovial cells in HLA-DR positive men.[54]

(6) in men and women RA patients, corticosteroid therapy may cause

or exacerbate hypoandrogenemia. In normal men and women the concomitant secretion of adrenal corticosteroids and androgens enables a balance of anabolic and catabolic effects. It has been well established that adrenal androgen secretion diminishes during aging and chronic diseases such as RA. Also, the anti-inflammatory and immunosuppressive effects of both androgens and corticosteroids have been well established. However, corticosteroid therapy inhibits ACTH secretion, involutes the adrenal cortex, and results in further adrenal androgen deficiency that can be particularly harmful in RA. Therefore, the deleterious adverse effects of chronic or cyclical corticosteroid therapy can be from both their direct catabolic activities and the further suppression of adrenal androgens. These harmful effects are biologically and clinically important in women and older men with RA.[55]

Male patients with RA who are not on corticosteroid therapy have significantly elevated levels of FSH and LH with low normal testosterone levels, suggesting a state of compensated partial gonadal failure. When these men are treated with low-dose corticosteroid therapy, both androgen and gonadotrophin levels drop, suggesting that corticosteroids may suppress the hypothalamic-pituitary-testicular axis. Since testosterone affects the immune system function as well as exerting anabolic influences on bone and muscle tissues, hypoandrogenemia in some men with RA may predispose these patients to more severe disease and to increased complications of corticosteroid therapy, such as sarcopenia and osteoporosis.[56]

Androgen Therapy in RA and for RA-Related Sequelae

Science-based evidence supports the role of hypoandrogenemia in the pathogenesis and subsequent disease activity of RA. A number of authors have recommended that androgen therapy be utilized due to its multifaceted role in the therapy of RA patients. Yet, to date, only a few studies have been published on the effect of androgen therapy in RA patients. Physicians have continued to be slow to add androgen therapy for their RA patients who are androgen deficient. However, it has recently been suggested that androgen therapy may represent a valuable concomitant or adjuvant treatment associated with other disease-modifying antirheumatic drugs in the management of RA.[57]

Published studies regarding androgen therapy for patients with RA have shown:

(1) that androgen therapy counteracts some of the catabolic effects of corticosteroid therapy.[58]

(2) that androgen therapy has a positive effect on bone mass, mood, and general well-being in men and postmenopausal women.[59, 60, 61] Osteoporosis has been shown to be a major disease associated with RA, in patients with or without previous corticosteroid treatment.[62, 63, 64, 65, 66] Hypoandrogenemia has been linked with depression in RA.[67] Depression in patients with RA has shown to be a major factor in the clinical course, inflammation markers, pathologic cytokine profiles, neuroendocrine dysfunction, increased disease activity, and disability scores.[68, 69, 70, 71] Regarding health status, the presence of depression with concomitant RA has such a negative outcome that treatment is warranted.[72] A recent review article has concluded that some depressed older men may have state-dependent hypoandrogenemia and that some depressed men may improve with androgen therapy.[73] Another recent study has shown that androgen therapy is an effective treatment for midlife onset dysthymia in women and men.[74] A growing body of evidence has supported the role of androgen therapy for patients with depressed moods and for some aspects of cognitive and functional impairments.[75, 76, 77, 78, 79, 80, 81]

(3) that androgen therapy in men with RA leads to significant reductions in IgM rheumatoid factor concentrations, joint pain, number of joints affected, and daily intake of nonsteroidal anti-inflammatory drugs.[82]

(4) that androgen therapy (stanozolol) is a fibrinolytic agent that reduces disease activity, duration of morning stiffness, pain, and erythrocyte sedimentation rate (ESR), while improving articular index scores, and enhancing fibrinolysis.[83]

(5) that androgen therapy (danazol) has been successful in the treatment of refractory thrombocytopenia, hemolytic anemia, and pure red cell aplasia in RA patients.[84, 85, 86]

Summary

In this chapter, the rationale for utilizing anabolic therapy in rheumatoid arthritis has been presented. This evidence-based rationale is supported by the scientific literature and includes:

(1) the evidence that hypoandrogenemia has a pathogenic role in the development of RA and in the clinical course of RA.

(2) the evidence that hypoandrogenemia is very common and may be caused by several mechanisms in RA patients.

(3) the evidence that hypoandrogenemia is associated with elevated

inflammatory markers, pathologic cytokine profiles, and reduced synovial androgen receptor activities, all of which correlates with increased disease activity in RA.

(4) the evidence that hypoandrogenemia is linked to many other disease afflictions in RA patients, including mental depression, osteoporosis, sarcopenia, frailty, anemia, and impairments in fibrinolysis and cognition.

(5) the available evidence that androgen therapy has disease-modifying effects and overall beneficial health impacts. Androgen replacement therapy is a safe, effective, cost-effective, and physiologically sound adjuvant therapy for patients with RA. Both subjective and clinical measures of disease activities can be improved with androgen therapy.

(6) the evidence that androgen therapy protects against the catabolic actions of corticosteroid therapy and cytotoxic drug therapy in patients with RA.

(7) the evidence that concomitant corticosteroid and nonsteroidal anti-inflammatory drug doses can be reduced with androgen therapy.

(8) the evidence that rehabilitative outcomes may be hastened and improved with androgen therapy.

In curbing illness-related and age-related human frailty, a major effort should be made to deliver an anabolic stimulus to these patients on a mass scale.[87] This effort (addressed by the National Institute on Aging) behooves physicians to create an improved dialogue between several areas of medicine and science and to utilize multidisciplinary approaches to make anabolic therapy available to patients.[88] American physicians have been slow to adopt the approach of prescribing anabolic agents in patients who have age-related or disease-related catabolic states which result in decreased musculoskeletal strength, bone mass, and activity levels.[89]

Adequate training and retraining of physicians and changes in the present approaches and attitudes in caring for patients may be the greatest obstacles to overcome if application of anabolic agents to patient care is to be realized.[90] Androgen therapy is a well tolerated but neglected area of medical practice and such therapy is underused and very much underresearched.[91] It is time to reassess androgen therapy, clear unfounded fears, and reinforce the physiological and scientific foundations for therapeutic options.[92] Providing androgen therapy as an anabolic stimulus for patients with hypoandrogenemia seems such a correct way to allow patients the ability to achieve the full benefits of rehabilitation modalities.

Notes

1. Masi, A.T., R.T. Chatterton, and J.C. Aldag. Perturbations of hypothalamic-pituitary-gonadal axis and adrenal androgen functions in rheumatoid arthritis: an odyssey of hormonal relationships to the disease. *Ann. N.Y. Acad. Sci.* 1999; 876: 53–62.

2. Larsen, B., C.A. King, M. Simms, et al. Major histocompatibility complex phenotypes influence serum testosterone concentration. *Rheumatology (Oxf.)* 2000; 39 (7): 758–763.

3. Cutolo, M., and R.L. Wilder. Different roles for androgens and estrogens in the susceptibility to autoimmune rheumatic diseases. *Rheum. Dis. Clin. North Am.* 2000; 26 (4): 825–839.

4. Cutolo, M., E. Balleari, S. Accardo, et al. Preliminary results of serum androgen level testing in men with rheumatoid arthritis. *Arthritis. Rheum.* 1984; 27 (8): 958–959.

5. Spector, T.D., L.A. Perry, G. Tubb, et al. Low free testosterone levels in rheumatoid arthritis. *Ann. Rheum. Dis.* 1988; 47 (1): 65–68.

6. Valentino, R., S. Savastano, A.P. Tommaselli, et al. Hormonal pattern in women affected by rheumatoid arthritis. *J. Endocrinol. Invest.* 1993; 16 (8): 619–624.

7. Masi, A.T. Sex hormones and rheumatoid arthritis: cause or effect relationships in a complex pathophysiology? *Clin. Exp. Rheumatol.* 1995; 13 (2): 227–240.

8. Wilder, R.L. Adrenal and gonadal steroid hormone deficiency in the pathogenesis of rheumatoid arthritis. *J. Rheumatol. Suppl.* 1996; 44: 10–12.

9. Stafford, L. Bleasel, A. Giles, et al. Androgen deficiency and bone mineral density in men with rheumatoid arthritis. *J. Rheumatol.* 2000; 27 (12): 2786–2790.

10. De la Torre, B., M. Hedman, E. Nilsson, et al. Relationship between blood and joint tissue DHEAS levels in rheumatoid arthritis and osteoarthritis. *Clin. Exp. Rheumatol.* 1993; 11 (6): 597–601.

11. Cutolo, M. Sex hormone adjuvant therapy in rheumatoid arthritis. *Rheum. Dis. Clin. North Am.* 2000; 26 (4): 881–895.

12. Brennan, P., and A. Silman. Role of androgens in the aetiology of rheumatoid arthritis. *Ann. Rheum. Dis.* 1996; 55 (6): 404.

13. James, W.H. Further evidence that low androgen values are a cause of rheumatoid arthritis: the response of rheumatoid arthritis to seriously stressful life events. *Ann. Rheum. Dis.* 1997; 56 (9): 566.

14. James, W.H. Rheumatoid arthritis, the contraceptive pill, and androgens. *Ann. Rheum. Dis.* 1993; 53 (6): 470–474.

15. Masi, A.T., S.L. Feigenbaum, and R.T. Chatterton. Hormonal and pregnancy relationships to rheumatoid arthritis: convergent effects with immunologic and microvascular systems. *Semin. Arthritis Rheum.* 1995; 25 (1): 1–27.

16. Elenkov, I.J., J. Hoffman, and R.L. Wilder. Does differential neuroendocrine control of cytokine production govern the expression of autoimmune diseases in pregnancy and the postpartum period? *Mol. Med. Today* 1997; 3 (9): 379–383.

17. Huizinga, T.W., M.W. van der Liden, V. Deneys–Laporte, et al. Interleukin-10 as an explanation for pregnancy-induced flare in systemic lupus erythematosus and remission in rheumatoid arthritis. *Rheumatology (Oxf.)* 1999; 38 (6): 496–498.

18. Ostensen, M. Sex hormones and pregnancy in rheumatoid arthritis and systemic lupus erythematosus. *Ann. N.Y. Acad. Sci.* 1999; 876: 131–143.

19. Cutolo, M., and R.L. Wilder. Different roles for androgens and estrogens in the susceptibility to autoimmune rheumatic diseases. *Rheum. Dis. Clin. North Am.* 2000; 26 (4): 825–839.

20. Kanik, K.S., and R.L. Wilder. Hormonal alterations in rheumatoid arthritis,

including the effects of pregnancy. *Rheum. Dis. Clin. North Am.* 2000; 26 (4): 805–823.

21. Feher, K.G., T. Feher, and K. Meretey. Interrelationship between the immunological and steroid hormone parameters in rheumatoid arthritis. *Exp. Clin. Endocrinol.* 1986; 87 (1): 38–42.

22. Cutolo, M. Sex hormone adjuvant therapy in rheumatoid arthritis. *Rheum. Dis. Clin. North Am.* 2000; 26 (4): 881–895.

23. Steward, A., and D.L. Bayley. Effects of androgens in models of rheumatoid arthritis. *Agents Actions* 1992; 35 (3–4): 268–272.

24. Da Silva, J.A., J.P. Larbre, T.D. Spector, et al. Protective effect of androgens against inflammation induced cartilage degradation in male rodents. *Ann. Rheum. Dis.* 1993; 52 (4): 285–291.

25. Cutolo, M., A. Sulli, B. Villaggio, et al. Relations between steroid hormones and cytokines in rheumatoid arthritis and systemic lupus erythematosus. *Ann. Rheum. Dis.* 1998; 57 (10): 573–577.

26. Bijlsma, J.W. Can we use steroid hormones to immunomodulate rheumatic diseases? Rheumatoid arthritis as an example. *Ann. N.Y. Acad. Sci.* 1999; 876: 366–376.

27. Brochner-Mortensen, K., G. Steffen, and J.H. Thaysen. The metabolic effect of new anabolic 19–nor-steroids. Metabolic studies on patients with chronic rheumatoid arthritis during combined therapy with Prednisone and anabolic steroid. *Acta Med. Scand.* 1959; 165 (3): 197–205.

28. Belch, J.J., R. Madhok, B. McArdle, et al. The effect of increasing fibrinolysis in patients with rheumatoid arthritis: a double blind study of stanozolol. *Q.J. Med.* 1986; 58 (225): 19–27.

29. Dasqupta, B., and R. Grahame. Treatment with danazol for refractory thrombocytopenia in rheumatoid arthritis. *Br. J. Rheumatol.* 1989; 28 (6): 550–552.

30. Masson, C., C. Bregeon, N. Ifrah, et al. [Evans' syndrome caused by D-penicillamine in rheumatoid arthritis. Value of the corticoids–danazol combination.] *Rev. Rhum. Mal. Osteoartic.* 1991; 58 (7): 519–522.

31. van Vollenhoven, R.F., and J.L. McGuire. Estrogen, progesterone, and testosterone: can they be used to treat autoimmune diseases? *Cleve. Clin. J. Med.* 1994; 61 (4): 276–284.

32. Masi, A.T. Sex hormones and rheumatoid arthritis: cause or effect relationships in a complex pathophysiology? *Clin. Exp. Rheumatol.* 1995; 13 (2): 227–240.

33. Tsai, C.Y., C.L. Yu, Y.Y. Tsai, et al. Pure red cell aplasia in a man with RA. *Scand. J. Rheumatol.* 1997; 26 (4): 329–331.

34. Bijlsma, J.W. Can we use steroid hormones to immunomodulate rheumatic diseases? Rheumatoid arthritis as an example. *Ann. N.Y. Acad. Sci.* 1999; 876: 366–376.

35. Cutolo, M. Sex hormone adjuvant therapy in rheumatoid arthritis. *Rheum. Dis. Clin. North Am.* 2000; 26 (4): 881–895.

36. Valentino, R., S. Savastano, A. P. Tommaselli, et al. Hormonal pattern in women affected by rheumatoid arthritis. *J. Endocrinol. Invest.* 1993; 16 (8): 619–624.

37. Feher, K.G., T. Feher, and K. Meretey. Interrelationship between the immunological and steroid hormone parameters in rheumatoid arthritis. *Exp. Clin. Endocrinol.* 1986; 87 (1): 38–42.

38. Roubenoff, R., R.A. Roubeuoft, J.G. Cannon, et al. Rheumatic cachexia: cytokine-driven hypermetabolism accompanying reduced body cell mass in chronic inflammation. *J. Clin. Invest.* 1994; 93 (6): 2379–2386.

39. Mirone, L., L. Altomonte, P. D'Agostino, et al. A study of serum androgen and cortisol levels in female patients with rheumatoid arthritis. Correlation with disease activity. *Clin. Rheumatol.* 1996; 15 (1): 15–19.

40. Cutolo, M., M. Guisti, L. Foppiani, et al. The hypothalamic-pituitary-adreno-cortical and gonadal axis function in rheumatoid arthritis. *Z. Rheumatol.* 2000; 59 (Suppl. 2): 66–69.

41. Cutolo, M., L. Foppiani, C. Prete, et al. Hypothalamic-pituitary-adrenocor-tical axis function in premenopausal women with rheumatoid arthritis not treated with glucocorticoids. *J. Rheumatol.* 1999; 26 (2): 282–288.

42. Kanik, K.S., and R.L. Wilder. Hormonal alterations in rheumatoid arthritis, including the effects of pregnancy. *Rheum. Dis. Clin. North Am.* 2000; 26 (4): 805–823.

43. Masi, A.T., R.T. Chatterton, and J.C. Aldag. Perturbations of hypothalamic-pituitary-gonadal axis and adrenal androgen functions in rheumatoid arthritis: an odyssey of hormonal relationships to the disease. *Ann. N.Y. Acad. Sci.* 1999; 876: 53–62.

44. Kanik, K.S., G.P. Chrousos, H.R. Schumacher, et al. Adrenocorticotropin, glucocorticoid, and androgen secretion in patients with new onset synovitis/rheuma-toid arthritis: relations with indices of inflammation. *J. Clin. Endocrinol. Metab.* 2000; 85 (4): 1461–1466.

45. Hall, G.M., L.A. Perry, and T.D. Spector. Depressed levels of dehy-droepiandrosterone sulphate in postmenopausal women with rheumatoid arthritis but no relation with axial bone density. *Ann. Rheum. Dis.* 1993; 52 (3): 211–214.

46. Khalkhali-Ellis, Z., T.L. Moore, and M.J. Hendrix. Reduced levels of testos-terone and dihydrotestosterone sulfate in the serum and synovial fluid of juvenile rheumatoid arthritis patients correlates with disease severity. *Clin. Exp. Rheumatol.* 1998; 16 (6): 753–756.

47. Gordon, D., G.H. Beastall, J.A. Thomson, et al. Androgenic status and sex-ual function in males with rheumatoid arthritis and ankylosing spondylitis. *Q. J. Med.* 1986; 60 (231): 671–679.

48. Wilder, R.L. Adrenal and gonadal steroid hormone deficiency in the patho-genesis of rheumatoid arthritis. *J. Rheumatol. Suppl.* 1996; 44: 10–12.

49. Kanik, K.S., G.P. Chrousos, H.R. Schumacher, et al. Adrenocorticotrophin, glucocorticoid, and androgen secretion in patients with new onset synovitis/rheuma-toid arthritis: relations with indicies of inflammation. *J. Clin. Endocrinol. Metab.* 2000; 85 (4): 1461–1466.

50. Cutolo, M., E. Balleari, M. Giusti, et al. Sex hormone status of male patients with rheumatoid arthritis: evidence of low serum concentrations of testosterone at baseline and after human chorionic gonadotrophin stimulation. *Arthritis Rheum.* 1988; 31 (10): 1314–1317.

51. Gordon, D., G.H. Beastall, J.A. Thomson, et al. Prolonged hypogonadism in male patients with rheumatoid arthritis during flares in disease activities. *Br. J. Rheumatol.* 1988; 27 (6): 440–444.

52. Cutolo, M., S. Accardo, B. Villaggio, et al. Evidence for the presence of an-drogen receptors in the synovial tissue of rheumatoid arthritis patients and healthy controls. *Arthritis Rheum.* 1992; 35 (9): 1007–1015.

53. Castagnetta, L., M. Cutolo, O.M. Granata, et al. Endocrine end-points in rheumatoid arthritis. *Ann. N.Y. Acad. Sci.* 1999; 876: 180–191.

54. Cutolo, M., and S. Accardo. Sex hormones, HLA and rheumatoid arthritis. *Clin. Exp. Rheumatol.* 1991; 9 (6): 641–646.

55. Robinzon, B., and M. Cutolo. Should dehydroepiandrosterone replacement therapy be provided with glucocorticoids? *Rheumatology (Oxf.)* 1999; 38 (6): 488–495.

56. Martens, H.F., P.K. Sheets, J.S. Tenover, et al. Decreased testosterone levels in men with rheumatoid arthritis: effect of low dose prednisone therapy. *J. Rheuma-tol.* 1994; 21 (8): 1427–1431.

57. Cutolo, M. Sex hormone adjuvant therapy in rheumatoid arthritis. *Rheum. Dis. Clin. North. Am.* 2000; 26 (4): 881–895.

58. Brochner-Mortensen, K., S. Gjorup, and J.H. Thaysen. The metabolic effect of new anabolic 19–nor-steroids. Metabolic studies on patients with chronic rheumatoid arthritis during combined therapy with prednisone and anabolic steroid. *Acta Medica. Scand.* 1959; 165 (3): 197–205.

59. Booji, A., C.M. Biewenga-Booji, O. Huber-Bruning, et al. Androgens as adjuvant treatment in postmenopausal female patients with rheumatoid arthritis.

60. Bijlsma, J.W. Can we use steroid hormones to immunomodulate rheumatic diseases? Rheumatoid arthritis as an example. *Ann. N.Y. Acad. Sci.* 1999; 876: 366–376.

61. Bijlsma, J.W., and J.W. Jacobs. Hormonal preservation of bone in rheumatoid arthritis. *Rheum. Dis. Clin. North Am.* 2000; 26 (4): 897–910.

62. Cortet, B., R.M. Flipo, P. Pigny, et al. How useful are bone turnover markers in rheumatoid arthritis? Influence of disease activity and corticosteroid therapy. *Rev. Rhum. Engl. Ed.* 1997; 64 (3): 153–159.

63. Lange, U., B. Boss, J. Teichmann, et al. Bone mineral density and biochemical markers of bone metabolism in late onset rheumatoid arthritis and polymyalgia rheumaticaùa prospective study on the influence of glucocorticoid therapy. *Z. Rheumatol.* 2000; 59 (Suppl. 2): 137–141.

64. Cortet, B., M.H. Guyot, E. Solau, et al. Factors influencing bone loss in rheumatoid arthritis: a longitudinal study. *Clin. Exp. Rheumatol.* 2000; 18 (6): 683–690.

65. Fiter, J., J.M. Nolla, M.A. Navarro, et al. Weak androgen levels, glucocorticoid therapy, and bone mineral density in postmenopausal women with rheumatoid arthritis. *Joint Bone Spine* 2000; 67 (3): 199–203.

66. Sinigaglia, L., A. Nervetti, Q. Mela, et al. A multicenter cross sectional study on bone mineral density in rheumatoid arthritis. Italian Study Group on Bone Mass in Rheumatoid Arthritis. *J. Rheumatol.* 2000; 27 (11): 2582–2589.

67. Swinden, D.C., C.M. Deighton, K. Nott, et al. Free testosterone and depression in male rheumatoid arthritis (RA).*Br. J. Rheumatol.* 1990; 29 (5): 401–402.

68. Wright, G.E., J.C. Parker, K.L. Smarr, et al. Age, depressive symptoms, and rheumatoid arthritis. *Arthritis Rheum.* 1998; 41 (2): 298–305.

69. Fifield, J. H. Tennen, S. Reisine, et al. Depression and the long-term risk of pain, fatigue, and disability in patients with rheumatoid arthritis. *Arthritis Rheum.* 1998; 41 (10): 1851–1857.

70. O'Connor, T.M., D.J. O'Halloran, and F. Shanahan. The stress response and the hypothalamic-pituitary-adrenal axis: from molecule to melancholia. *Q.J. Med.* 2000; 93 (6): 323–333.

71. Soderlin, M.K., M. Hakala, and P. Nieminen. Anxiety and depression in a community-based rheumatoid arthritis population. *Scand. J. Rheumatol.* 2000; 29 (3): 177–183.

72. Smarr, K.L., J.C. Parker, J.F. Kosciulek, et al. Implications of depression in rheumatoid arthritis: do subtypes really matter? *Arthritis Care Res.* 2000; 13 (1): 23–32.

73. Seidman, S.N., and B.T. Walsh. Testosterone and depression in aging men. *Am. J. Geriatr. Psychiatry* 1999; 7 (1): 18–33.

74. Bloch, M., P.J. Schmidt, M.A. Danaceua, et al. Dehydroepiandrosterone treatment of midlife dysthymia. *Biol. Psychiatry* 1999; 45 (12): 1533–1541.

75. Sherwin, B.B. Estrogen and/or androgen replacement therapy and cognitive functioning in surgically menopausal women. *Psychoneuroendocrinology* 1988; 13 (4): 345–357.

76. Janowsky, J.S., S.K. Oviatt, and E.S. Orwoll. Testosterone influences spatial cognition in older men. *Behav. Neurosci.* 1994; 108 (2): 325–332.

77. Sih, R., J.E. Morley, F.E. Kaiser, et al. Testosterone replacement in older

hypogonadal men: a 12–month randomized controlled trial. *J. Clin. Endocrinol. Metab.* 1997; 82 (6): 1661–1667.

78. Alexander, G.M., R.S. Swerdloff, C. Wang, et al. Androgen-behavior correlations in hypogonadal men and eugonadal men. II. Cognitive abilities. *Horm. Behav.* 1998; 33 (2): 85–94.

79. Janowsky, J.S., B. Chavez, and E. Orwoll. Sex steroids modify working memory. *J. Cogn. Neurosci.* 2000; 12 (3): 407–414.

80. Gambineri, A., and R. Pasquali. Testosterone therapy in men: clinical and pharmacological perspectives. *J. Endocrinol. Invest.* 2000; 23 (3): 196–214.

81. Bakhshi, V., M. Elliott, A. Gentili, et al. Testosterone improves rehabilitation outcomes in ill older men. *J. Am. Geriatr. Soc.* 2000; 48 (5): 550–553.

82. Cutolo, M., E. Balleari, M. Giusti, et al. Androgen replacement therapy in male patients with rheumatoid arthritis. *Arthritis Rheum.* 1991; 34 (1): 1–5.

83. Belch, J.J., R. Madhok, B. McArdle, et al. The effect of increasing fibrinolysis in patients with rheumatoid arthritis: a double blind study of stanozolol. *Q.J. Med.* 1986; 58 (225): 19–27.

84. Dasgupta, B., and R. Grahame. Treatment with danazol for refractory thrombocytopenia in rheumatoid arthritis. *Br. J. Rheumatol.* 1989; 28 (6): 550–552.

85. Masson, C., C. Bregeon, N. Ifrah, et al. [Evan's syndrome caused by D-penicillamine in rheumatoid arthritis. Value of corticoids–danazol combination.] *Rev. Rhum. Mal. Osteoartic.* 1991; 58 (7): 519–522.

86. Tsai, C.Y., C.L. Yu, Y.Y. Tsai, et al. Pure red cell aplasia in a man with RA. *Scand. J. Rheumatol.* 1997; 26 (4): 329–331.

87. Roubenoff, R. Sarcopenia: a major modifiable cause of frailty in the elderly. *J. Nutr. Health Aging* 2000; 4 (3): 140–142.

88. Dutta, C., and E.C. Hadley. The significance of sarcopenia in old age. *J. Gerontol. A. Biol. Sci. Med. Sci.* 1995; 50 (Spec. No.): 1–4.

89. Wilmore, D.W. Deterrents to the successful clinical use of growth factors that enhance protein anabolism. *Curr. Opin. Clin. Nutr. Metab. Care* 1999; 2 (1): 15–21.

90. Wilmore, D.W. Impediments to the successful use of anabolic agents in clinical care. *J. Parenter. Enteral Nutr.* 1999; 23 (6 Suppl.): S210–213.

91. Sands, R., and J. Studd. Exogenous androgens in postmenopausal women. *Am. J. Med.* 1995; 98 (1A): 76S–79S.

92. da Silva, J.A., and A. Porto. [Sex hormones and osteoporosis: a physiological perspective for prevention and therapy.] *Acta Med. Port.* 1997; 10 (10): 689–695.

12

Rationale for Anabolic Therapy in Sjogren's Syndrome

Introduction: Hypoandrogenemia Associated with Sjogren's Syndrome

Sjogren's syndrome (SS) is a chronic, complex autoimmune and inflammatory disorder that occurs almost exclusively in women and induces extensive lymphocyte accumulation in lacrimal and salivary glands, and represents one of the leading causes of dry eye and mouth in the world.[1] It was described over 100 years ago and is related to other autoimmune rheumatic diseases. Current estimates suggest that over one million people in the United States have SS.[2] Over 5 percent of Americans above the age of 60 years have primary SS.[3]

In Sjogren's syndrome, inflammatory lymphocyte proliferation can progressively destroy exocrine glands and infiltrate other, more vital organs, and may become malignant.[4] Virtually any organ can become affected by this disease process.[5, 6]

This results in the association of SS with other autoimmune diseases and sarcopenia, osteoporosis, Raynaud's phenomenon, sexual dysfunction, hyperlipidemia, hypercoagulability, reduced fibrinolysis, renal disease, and other diseases and malignancies.[7, 8, 9, 10, 11, 12, 13, 14, 15, 16] In almost one third of patients, SS involves extraglandular sites, and approximately 5 percent of patients may develop malignancies. In addition, features of Sjogren's syndrome are frequently encountered (5–20 percent) in patients with several other autoimmune rheumatic diseases.[17, 18] Neuromuscular, neurological, and neuropsychiatric conditions, especially depression, cognitive deficits, fatigue, hearing loss, and dementia, are common in patients with SS.[19, 20, 21, 22, 23, 24, 25, 26, 27]

It has been hypothesized that androgen deficiency, which reportedly occurs in primary and secondary SS (e.g., systemic lupus erythematosus, rheumatoid arthritis), is a critical etiologic factor in the pathogenesis of dry-eye and-mouth syndromes.[28] Androgen deficiency promotes the progression of SS and its associated lacrimal gland inflammation, meibomian gland dysfunction, and severe dry-eye conditions.[29] Also, androgen deficiency has been incriminated in the pathogenesis of SS and the crossover with other rheumatic diseases, where rheumatoid factor (73 percent), antinuclear antibodies (85 percent), anti–SS-A (62 percent) and anti–SS-B (46 percent) antibodies have been found.[30] It has been shown that those patients with SS who present with these and other serologic abnormalities tend to have poor outcomes.[31, 32, 33]

Androgens have been shown to regulate the ultrastructure and secretion functions of the lacrimal gland.[34, 35] It has been suggested that a critical level of androgens is necessary to maintain lacrimal gland structure and function and that hypoandrogenemia could trigger lacrimal gland apoptosis and necrosis due to a pathologic autoimmune response.[36] Recent research has demonstrated that androgen therapy dramatically curtails lymphocyte infiltration in the lacrimal glands in animal models of SS[37, 38, 39, 40, 41, 42, 43, 44, 45, 46, 47] and in patients with SS.[48, 49, 50, 51]

Pathologic Mechanisms and Hypoandrogenemia in SS

It has been shown that patients with SS have an altered hypothalamic-pituitary-adrenal (HPA) axis, lower adrenocorticotropin (ACTH) levels, and blunted pituitary and adrenal response to ovine corticotropin releasing hormone (oCRH) stimulation.[52, 53] A growing body of data has indicated that SS develops as a consequence of a deficiency of adrenal and gonadal androgens.[54, 55] In addition, it has been suggested that significant changes in the estrogen-to-androgen ratio via enhanced aromatase activities or the ratio of their receptors alters the activity of steroid-sensitive cells that adversely affect neuroimmunomodulatory functions.[56, 57] Hypoandrogenemia may lead to the pathologic cytokine profiles associated with SS as shown in animal models and human patients.[58, 59, 60, 61, 62]

Other mechanisms of hypoandrogenemia in SS occur with estrogen monotherapy,[63] previous corticosteroid therapy, response to acute illness, and aging.[64, 65, 66, 67, 68, 69, 70] Estrogen monotherapy has been shown to exacerbate or cause hypoandrogenemia.[71, 72]

Androgen receptors are located in human lacrimal gland acinar cell nuclei as in other animals. Androgen receptors have also been found in human lacrimal interacinar interstitial and inflammatory cells suggesting that androgens may play a role in modulating both the lacrimal and non-lacrimal cells within the lacrimal gland.[73]

In animal models, experimentally induced hypoandrogenemia has been shown to cause pathologic autoimmune and ultrastructural changes (atrophy, interstitial cell apoptosis, necrosis of acinar cells, and increased lymphocytic infiltration) within the lacrimal gland similar to that encountered in SS.[74] In addition, androgen therapy has been shown to increase the secretory component mRNA levels,[75] upregulate androgen receptors in lacrimal tissue,[76] and increase gland weight and tear volumes.[77]

Studies with Androgen Therapy in SS

Despite progress in the understanding of the broad clinicopathological spectrum of SS, its treatment remains largely empirical, symptomatic, and inadequate.[78] To date, the decision for systemic therapeutic intervention is primarily based on the severity of extraglandular manifestations.[79] It has been suggested that topical androgen therapy may serve as a safe and effective therapy for the treatment of dry eye in SS.[80]

Treatment of the extraglandular and systemic aspects of SS may include systemic androgen therapy. Investigational studies have shown that systemic androgen therapy induces moderate improvement in subjective xerostomia, significant decrease in erythrocyte sedimentation rate, decrease in inflammatory disease markers, clinical remission, and overall subjective and objective well-being.[81, 82]

Summary

In this chapter the rationale for anabolic therapy in SS has been presented. It has been shown that androgen therapy corrects hypoandrogenemia associated with SS and may impact the course of the disease by correcting abnormal cytokine profiles and extraglandular infiltration while treating and/or reversing osteoporosis, sarcopenia, depression and cognitive and neurological deficits. In addition, for women on estrogen monotherapy, adding an androgen component for HRT may be indicated since estrogen monotherapy may play a role in the pathogenesis of SS in some women.[83] Further studies with androgen therapy for SS are warranted due to the multifaceted actions that androgens have in this disease. These studies may prove that androgen therapy effectively treats and discourages extraglandular infiltration in patients with SS.

Notes

1. Toda, I., B.D. Sullivan, E.M. Rocha, et al. Impact of gender on exocrine gland inflammation in mouse models of Sjogren's syndrome. *Exp. Eye Res.* 1999; 69 (4): 355–366.

2. Rhodus, N.L. Sjogren's syndrome. *Quintessence Int.* 1999; 30 (10): 698–699.

3. Fleming Cole, N., E.C. Toy, and B. Baker. Sjogren's syndrome. *Prim. Care Update Ob. Gyns.* 2001; 8 (1): 48–51.

4. Talal, N. Sjogren's syndrome: historical overview and clinical spectrum of disease. *Rheum. Dis. Clin. North Am.* 1992; 18 (3): 507–515.

5. Lahita, R.G. The connective tissue diseases and the overall influence of gender. *Int. J. Fertil. Menopausal Stud.* 1996; 41 (2): 156–165.

6. Sorensen, I.M., A. Soderlund, H.J. Haga, et al. [Symptoms in women with Sjogren's syndrome.] *Tidsskr. Nor. Laageforen.* 2000; 120 (7): 794–797.

7. Drosos, A.A., E. van Vliet-Dascaolpouluo, A.P. Andonopoulos, et al. Nandrolone decanoate (deca-durabolin) in primary Sjogren's syndrome: a double blind pilot study. *Clin. Exp. Rheumatol.* 1988; 6 (1): 53–57.

8. Tanimoto, K. [Overlapping syndrome.] *Nippon Rinsho* 1992; 50 (3): 625–628.

9. Zeher, M., G. Szegedi, A. Csiki, et al. Fibrinolysis-resistant fibrin deposits in minor labial salivary glands of patients with Sjogren's syndrome. *Clin. Immunol. Immunopathol.* 1994; 71 (2): 149–155.

10. Belilos, E., and S. Carsons. Rheumatologic disorders in women. *Med. Clin. North Am.* 1998; 82 (1): 77–101.

11. Grassi, W., R. De Angelis, G. Lapadula, et al. Clinical diagnosis found in patients with Raynaud's phenomenon: a multicentre study. *Rheumatol. Int.* 1998; 18 (1): 17–20.

12. Aasarod, K., H.J. Haga, K.J. Berg, et al. Renal involvement in primary Sjogren's syndrome. *Q.J. Med.* 2000; 93 (5): 297–304.

13. Goules, A., S. Masouridi, A.G. Tzioufas, et al. Clinically significant and biopsy-documented renal involvement in primary Sjogren's syndrome. *Medicine (Baltimore)* 2000; 79 (4): 241–249.

14. Terpos, E., M.K. Angelopoulou, E. Variami, et al. Sjogren's syndrome associated with multiple myeloma. *Ann. Hematol.* 2000; 79 (8): 449–451.

15. Izumi, M., A. Hida, Y. Takagi, et al. MR imaging of the salivary glands in sicca syndrome: comparison of lipid profiles and imaging in patients with hyperlipidemia and patients with Sjogren's syndrome. *Am. J. Roetgenol.* 2000; 175 (3): 829–834.

16. Regeczy, N., I. Balogh, G. Lakos, et al. Hypercoagulability in various autoimmune diseases: no association with factor V Leiden mutation. *Haematologia* 2000; 30 (1): 35–39.

17. Manoussakis, M.N., and H. M. Moutsopoulos. Sjogren's syndrome: autoimmune epithelitis. *Baillieres Best Pract. Res. Clin. Rheumatol.* 2000; 14 (1): 73–95.

18. Fox, R.I. Sjogren's syndrome: current therapies remain inadequate for a common disease. *Expert Opin. Investig. Drugs* 2000; 9 (9): 2007–2016.

19. Caselli, R.J., B.W. Scheithauer, C.A. Bowles, et al. The treatable dementia of Sjogren's syndrome. *Ann. Neurol.* 1991; 30 (1): 98–101.

20. Kawashima, N., R. Shindo, and M. Kohno. Primary Sjogren's syndrome with subcortical dementia. *Intern. Med.* 1993; 32 (7): 561–564.

21. Mauch, E., C. Volk, G. Kratzsch, et al. Neurological and neuropsychiatric dysfunction in primary Sjogren's syndrome. *Acta Neurol. Scand.* 1994; 89 (1): 31–35.

22. Valtydottir, S.T., B. Gudbjornsson, R. Hallgren, et al. Psychological well-being in patients with primary Sjogren's syndrome. *Clin. Exp. Rheumatol.* 2000; 18 (5): 597–600.

23. Sugai, S. Sjogren's syndrome associated with liver and neurological disorders, and malignant lymphoma. *Intern. Med.* 2000; 39 (3): 193–194.

24. Manabe, Y., C. Sasaki, H. Warita, et al. Sjogren's syndrome with acute transverse myelopathy as the initial manifestation. *J. Neurol. Sci.* 2000; 176 (2): 158–161.

25. Parke, A.L. Sjogren's syndrome: a woman's health problem. *J. Rheumatol. Suppl.* 2000; 61: 4–5.

26. Ziavra, N., E.N. Politi, I. Kastanioudakis, et al. Hearing loss in Sjogren's syndrome patients. A comparative study. *Clin. Exp. Rheumatol.* 2000; 18 (6): 725–728.

27. Rosenbaum, R. Neuromuscular complications of connective tissue diseases. *Muscle Nerve* 2001; 24 (2): 154–169.

28. Sullivan, D.A., L.A. Wickham, E.M. Rocha, et al. Androgens and dry eye in Sjogren's syndrome. *Ann. N.Y. Acad. Sci.* 1999; 876: 312–324.

29. Sullivan, D.A., K.L. Krenzer, B.D. Sullivan, et al. Does androgen insufficiency cause lacrimal gland inflammation and aqueous tear deficiency? *Invest. Ophthalmol. Vis. Sci.* 1999; 40 (6): 1261–1265.

30. Anaya, J.M., G.T. Liu, E. D'Souza, et al. Primary Sjogren's syndrome in men. *Ann. Rheum. Dis.* 1995; 54 (9): 748–751.

31. Skopouli, F.N., U. Dafni, J.P. Ioannidis, et al. Clinical evolution, and morbidity and mortality of primary Sjogren's syndrome. *Semin. Arthritis Rheum.* 2000; 29 (5): 296–304.

32. Gannot, G., H.E. Lancaster, and P.C. Fox. Clinical course of primary Sjogren's syndrome: salivary, oral, and serologic aspects. *J. Rheumatol.* 2000; 27 (8): 1905–1909.

33. Al-Hashimi, I., S. Khuder, N. Haghighat, et al. Frequency and predictive value of the clinical manifestations in Sjogren's syndrome. *J. Oral Pathol. Med.* 2001; 30 (1): 1–6.

34. Sullivan, D.A., L. Block, and J.D. Pena. Influence of androgens and pituitary hormones on the structural profile and secretory activity of the lacrimal gland. *Acta Ophthalmol. Scand.* 1996; 74 (5): 421–435.

35. Azzarolo, A.M., A.K. Mircheff, R.L. Kaswan, et al. Androgen support of lacrimal gland function. *Endocrine* 1997; 6 (1): 39–45.

36. Azzarolo, A.M., R.L. Wood, A.K. Mircheff, et al. Androgen influence on lacrimal gland apoptosis, necrosis, and lymphocytic infiltration. *Invest. Opthalmol. Vis. Sci.* 1999; 40 (3): 592–602.

37. Schot, L.P., H.A. Verheul, and A.W. Schuurs. Effect of nandrolone decanoate on Sjogren's syndrome like disorders in NZB/NZW mice. *Clin. Exp. Immunol.* 1984; 57 (3): 571–574.

38. Verheul, A.A., L.P. Schot, and H.W. Schuurs. Therapeutic effects of nandrolone decanoate, tibolone, lynesternol and ethylestrenol on Sjogren's syndrome-like disorder in NZB/W mice. *Clin. Exp. Immunol.* 1986; 64 (2): 243–248.

39. Vendramini, A.C., C. Soo, and D.A. Sullivan. Testosterone-induced suppression of autoimmune disease in lacrimal tissue of a mouse model (NZB/NZW F1) of Sjogren's syndrome. *Invest. Ophthalmol. Vis. Sci.* 1991; 32 (11): 3002–3006.

40. Sato, E.H., H. Agria, and D.A. Sullivan. Impact of androgen therapy in Sjogren's syndrome: hormonal influence on lymphocyte populations and Ia expression in lacrimal glands of MRL/Mp-lpr/lpr mice. *Invest. Ophthalmol.* 1992; 33 (8): 2537–2545.

41. Sato, E.H., H. Ariga, and D.A. Sullivan. Impact of androgen therapy in Sjogren's syndrome: hormonal influence on lymphocyte populations and Ia expression in lacrimal glands of MRL/Mp-Ipr/Ipr mice. *Invest. Ophthalmol. Vis. Sci.* 1992; 33 (8): 2537–2545.

42. Rocha, F.J., E.H. Sato, B.D. Sullivan, et al. Comparative efficacy of androgen

analogues in suppressing lacrimal gland inflammation in a mouse model (MRL/lpr) of Sjogren's syndrome. *Adv. Exp. Med. Biol.* 1994; 350: 697–700.

43. Sullivan, D.A., H. Ariga, A.C. Vendramini, et al. Androgen-induced suppression of autoimmune disease in lacrimal glands of mouse models of Sjogren's syndrome. *Adv. Exp. Med. Biol.* 1994; 350: 683–690.

44. Ono, M., F.J. Rocha, and D.A. Sullivan. Immunocytochemical location and hormonal control of androgen receptors in lacrimal tissues of the female MRL/Mp-lpr/lpr mouse model of Sjogren's syndrome. *Exp. Eye Res.* 1995; 61 (6): 659–666.

45. Rocha, E.M., L.A. Wickham, Z. Huang, et al. Presence and testosterone influence on the levels of anti- and pro-inflammatory cytokines in lacrimal tissues of a mouse model of Sjogren's syndrome. *Adv. Exp. Med. Biol.* 1998; 438; 485–491.

46. Toda, I., L.A. Wickham, and D.A. Sullivan. Gender and androgen treatment influence the expression of proto-oncogenes and apoptotic factors in lacrimal and salivary tissues of MRL/lpr mice. *Clin. Immunol. Immunopathol.* 1998; 86 (1): 59–71.

47. Toda, I., B.D. Sullivan, L.A. Wickham, et al. Gender- and androgen-related influence on the expression of proto-oncogene and apoptotic factor mRNAs in lacrimal glands of autoimmune and non-autoimmune mice. *J. Steroid Biochem. Mol. Biol.* 1999; 71 (1–2): 49–61.

48. Bizzarro, A., G. Valentini, G. Di Martino, et al. Influence of testosterone therapy on clinical and immunological features of autoimmune diseases associated with Klinefelter's syndrome. *J. Clin. Endocrinol. Metab.* 1987; 64 (1): 32–36.

49. Drosos, A.A., E. van Vliet-Dascolpoulou, A.P. Andonopoulos, et al. Nandrolone decanoate (deca-durabolin) in primary Sjogren's syndrome: a double blind pilot study. *Clin. Exp. Rheumatol.* 1988; 6 (1): 53–57.

50. Sullivan, D.A., and E.H. Sato. Potential therapeutic approach for the hormonal treatment of lacrimal gland dysfunction in Sjogren's syndrome. *Clin. Immunol. Immunopathol.* 1992; 64 (1): 9–16.

51. Sullivan, D.A., L.A. Wickhan, E.M. Rocha, et al. Androgens in dry eye in Sjogren's syndrome. *Ann. N.Y. Acad. Sci.* 1999; 876: 312–324.

52. Johnson, E.O., P.G. Vlachoyiannopoulos, F.N. Skopouli, et al. Hypofunction of the stress axis in Sjogren's syndrome. *J. Rheumatol.* 1998; 25 (8): 1508–1514.

53. Mastorakos, G., and I. Ilias. Relationship between interleukin-6 (IL-6) and hypothalamic-pituitary adrenal axis hormones in rheumatoid arthritis. *Z. Rheumatol.* 2000; 59 (Suppl. 2): 75–79.

54. Sullivan, D.A., K.L. Krenzer, B.D. Sullivan, et al. Does androgen insufficiency cause lacrimal gland inflammation and aqueous tear deficiency? *Invest. Ophthalmol. Vis. Sci.* 1999; 40 (6): 1261–1265.

55. Valtysdottir, S.T., B. Gudbjornsson, R. Hallgren, et al. Psychological well-being in patients with primary Sjogren's syndrome. *Clin. Exp. Rheumatol.* 2000; 18 (5): 597–600.

56. Onodera, K., H. Sasano, R. Ichinohasama, et al. Immunolocalization of aromatase in human minor salivary glands of the lower lip with primary Sjogren's syndrome. *Pathol. Int.* 1998; 48 (10): 786–790.

57. Johnson, E.O., F.N. Skopouli, and H. M. Moutsopoulos. Neuroendocrine manifestations in Sjogren's syndrome. *Rheum. Dis. Clin. North Am.* 2000; 26 (4): 927–949.

58. Pflugfelder, S.C., D. Jones, Z. Ji, et al. Altered cytokine balance in the tear fluid and conjunctiva of patients with Sjogren's syndrome keratoconjunctivitis sicca. *Curr. Eye Res.* 1999; 19 (3): 201–211.

59. Jabs, D.A., B. Lee, J.A. Whittum-Hudson, et al. Th1 versus Th2 immune response in autoimmune lacrimal gland disease in MRL/Mp mice. *Invest. Ophthalmol. Vis. Sci.* 2000; 41 (3): 826–831.

60. Kohriyama, K., and Y. Katayama. Disproportion of helper T cell subsets in peripheral blood of patients with primary Sjogren's syndrome. *Autoimmunity* 2000; 32 (1): 67–72.

61. Fox, R.I., and P. Michelson. Approaches to the treatment of Sjogren's syndrome. *J. Rheumatol. Suppl.* 2000; 61: 15–21.

62. Saegusa, K., N. Ishimaru, K. Yanagi, et al. Autoantigen-specific CD4+CD28low T cell subset prevents autoimmune exocrinopathy in murine Sjogren's syndrome. *J. Immunol.* 2000; 165 (4): 2251–2257.

63. Nagler, R.M., and S. Pollack. Sjogren's syndrome induced by estrogen therapy. *Semin. Arthritis Rheum.* 2000; 30 (3): 209–214.

64. Spratt, D.I., C. Longscope, P.M. Cox, et al. Differential changes in serum concentrations of androgens and estrogens (in relation with cortisol) in postmenopausal women with acute illness. *J. Clin. Endocrinol. Metab.* 1993; 76 (6): 1542–1547.

65. Parker, C.R., R. Azziz, H.D. Potter, et al. Adrenal androgen production in response to adrenocorticotropin infusions in men. *Endocr. Res.* 1996; 22 (4): 717–722.

66. Phillips, G.B. Relationship between serum dehydroepiandrosterone sulfate, androstenedione, and sex hormones in men and women. *Eur. J. Endocrinol.* 1996; 134 (2): 201–216.

67. Yen, S.S., and G.A. Laughlin. Aging and the adrenal cortex. *Exp. Gerontol.* 1998; 33 (7–8): 897–910.

68. Harper, A.J., J.E. Buster, and P.R. Casson. Changes in adrenocortical function with aging and therapeutic implications. *Semin. Reprod. Endocrinol.* 1999; 17 (4): 327–338.

69. Arlt, W., F. Callies, J.C. van Vlijmen, et al. Dehydroepiandrosterone replacement in women with adrenal insufficiency. *N. Engl. J. Med.* 1999; 341 (14): 1013–1020.

70. Chrousos, G.P. The role of stress and the hypothalamic-pituitary-adrenal axis in the pathogenesis of the metabolic syndrome: neuroendocrine and target tissue-related causes. *Int. J. Obes. Relat. Metab. Disord.* 2000; 24 (Suppl. 2): 50–55.

71. Casson, P.R., K.E. Elkind-Hirsch, J.E. Buster, et al. Effect of postmenopausal estrogen replacement on circulating androgens. *Obstet. Gynecol.* 1997; 90 (6): 995–998.

72. Castelo-Branco, C., E. Casals, F. Figeras, et al. Two-year prospective and comparative study on the effects of tibolone on lipid pattern, behavior of apolipoproteins A1 and B. *Menopause* 1999; 6 (2): 92–97.

73. Smith, R.E., C.R. Taylor, N.A. Rao, et al. Immunohistochemical identification of androgen receptors in human lacrimal glands. *Curr. Eye. Res.* 1999; 18 (4): 300–309.

74. Azzarolo, A.M., R.L. Wood, A.K. Mircheff, et al. Androgen influence on lacrimal gland apoptosis, necrosis, and lymphocytic infiltration. *Invest. Opthalmol. Vis. Sci.* 1999; 40 (3): 592–602.

75. Gao, J., R.W. Lambert, L.A. Wickham, et al. Androgen control of secretory component mRNA levels in the rat lacrimal gland. *J. Steroid Biochem. Mol. Med.* 1995; 52 (3): 239–249.

76. Rocha, F.J., L.A. Wickham, J.D. Pena, et al. Influence of gender and the endocrine environment on the distribution of androgen receptors in the lacrimal gland. *J. Steroid Biochem. Mol. Med.* 1993; 46 (6): 737–749.

77. Vendramini, A.C., C. Soo, and D.A. Sullivan. Testosterone-induced suppression of autoimmune disease in lacrimal tissue of a mouse model (NZB/NZW F1) of Sjogren's syndrome. *Invest. Oppthalmol.* 1991; 32 (11): 3002–3006.

78. Fox, R.I. Sjogren's syndrome: current therapies remain inadequate for a common disease. *Expert Opin. Investig. Drugs* 2000; 9 (9): 2007–2016.

79. Manoussakis, M.N., and H.M. Moutsopoulos. Sjogren's syndrome: autoimmune epithelitis. *Baillieres Best Pract. Res. Clin. Rheumatol.* 2000; 14 (1): 73–95.

80. Sullivan, D.A., L.A. Wickham, E.M. Rocha, et al. Androgens and dry eye in Sjogren's syndrome. *Ann. N.Y. Acad. Sci.* 1999; 876: 312–324.

81. Bizzaro, A., G. Valentini, G. Di Martino, et al. Influence of testosterone therapy on clinical and immunological features of autoimmune diseases associated with Klinefelter's syndrome. *J. Clin. Endocrinol. Metab.* 1987; 64 (1): 32–36.

82. Drosos, A.A., E. van Vliet-Dasclopoulou, A.P. Andonopoulos, et al. Nandrolone decanoate (deca-durabolin) in primary Sjogren's syndrome: a double blind pilot study. *Clin. Exp. Rheumatol.* 1988; 6 (1): 53–57.

83. Nagler, R.M., and S. Pollack. Sjogren's syndrome induced by estrogen therapy. *Semin. Arthritis. Rheum.* 2000; 30 (3): 209–214.

13

Rationale for Anabolic Therapy in Systemic Lupus Erythematosus

Introduction: Sex Hormones and SLE

Systemic lupus erythematosus (SLE) is a chronic, heterogeneous, multiple-organ-system inflammatory disorder with autoimmune dysfunction of unknown etiology in which tissues and cells are damaged by pathogenic autoantibodies and immune complexes.[1] Autoantibodies are produced that react with self-antigens, notably cell membranes, nuclear, and cytoplasmic constituents. The deposition of these autoantibodies and immune complexes often leads to tissue and organ damage. There are many clinical manifestations, including arthritis, arthralgia, myalgia, skin changes, photosensitivity reactions, fever, anemia, thrombocytopenia, proteinuria, and renal, CNS and psychiatric, and cardiopulmonary involvement.[2] The disease characteristically fluctuates between remission and relapse. SLE's complexity, chronicity, and relapsing nature has led to diverse pharmacotherapeutic strategies to combat it based on the organ systems involved.[3]

Over 90 percent of patients with SLE are women who have the onset of the disease prior to menopause. SLE occurs to a much lesser degree in elderly men. These facts clearly demonstrate a strong androgen-dependent gender dimorphism associated with the pathogenesis and disease activity of SLE.[4]

The complete immunopathogenesis of SLE is like a jigsaw puzzle with some pieces of which are missing or have not fallen into place. In predisposed individuals, the initial stimulus is likely to be one or more of the environmental and infectious agents interacting with susceptibility genes. Sex hormones, as well as, physical and psychological stressors, may promote a critical threshold condition for the immune system in response to the initial stimulus (brought about by environmental and infectious agents).[5] Once the critical threshold is breached, there is failure of the immune system to downregulate the ensuing abnormal immune response that involves polyclonal B cell activation and hyperactive T cell help.[6]

In SLE, a role for sex hormones in the etiopathogenesis and disease activity is now recognized and believed to related to the influence that sex hormones have on Th1/Th2 cytokine synthesis and balance.[7, 8, 9, 10, 11] Shifts or imbalances in Th1/Th2 cytokine patterns can play a crucial role in the development of specific immune responses and the modulation of these immune responses in SLE.[12, 13, 14] The cytokine network is a major aspect of the immune regulation and is directly affected by sex steroids. This androgen-dependent gender dimorphism relates to both organ-specific and general synthesis of sex steroids that are affected by and in turn affect cytokine profiles of T helper cells.[15]

SLE is an autoimmune disease with a clear imbalance in the network made up of many different cytokines.[16, 17, 18] Both contributory and contradictory data are available about the dominance of Th1 or Th2 cytokines in the incomplete SLE cytokine puzzle.[19, 20] Recent findings suggest that SLE is characterized by an elevation of both Th1 and Th2 cytokines, such that, the elevation of proinflammatory cytokines (IL-12, IL-17, and IL-18) may trigger the inflammatory process in SLE and an imbalance of cytokine profile (elevation of IL-18/IL-4 ratio) in a mediating response to the initial inflammatory process.[21] Recent evidence also indicates that, during inactive periods of SLE, the Th1/Th2 cytokine secretory balance is normal.[22]

Young and middle-aged men, with normal serum androgen levels, are almost never afflicted with this disease process. However, in women, it has been shown that hypoestrogenemia (due to continuous oral cyclophosphamide therapy that causes ovarian failure)[23] and exogenous androgen administration are both protective against lupus flares and disease activities.

Androgen Deficiency and SLE

Over a decade ago, investigational results suggested that low plasma androgen levels could be a permanent disorder in women SLE patients, especially in the most severe forms of the disease, and could be accentuated by the administration of corticosteroids.[24, 25, 26, 27, 28] Decreased levels of all androgens have been observed in women with SLE, accompanied by increased conversion of androgens to estrogens via increased tissue aromatase activity, giving them hyperestrogenemia and hypoandrogene-mia.[29, 30, 31] In addition, the lowest levels of plasma androgens have been found in female patients who have active disease, as determined by labo-ratory and clinical assessments.[32, 33, 34] Glucocorticoid treatment has been shown to cause a significant decrease in salivary testosterone levels, and testing salivary testosterone levels has been suggested as a method for mon-itoring androgen deficiencies in patients with SLE.[35]

In men patients with SLE who have been shown to have hypoandro-genemia[36] that their conditions:

(1) were associated with a higher prevalence of CNS disease and scrositis than those men with SLE and normal serum androgen levels.[37]

(2) were associated with diminished testis function indicated by reduced response of free testosterone to stimulation with HCG or LHRH.[38, 39, 40]

(3) that hypoandrogenemia rates were at statistically significant prevalence in all men with SLE.[41]

Studies with Androgen Therapy in SLE

Several early European studies, using empirical androgen therapy in patients with SLE, indicated beneficial effects on several aspects of the dis-ease process.[42, 43, 44, 45, 46, 47] In the late 1980s the first American medical study appeared, utilizing androgen therapy in SLE, indicating beneficial results with thrombocytopenia that was SLE-related.[48] In the early 1990s, other studies indicated that androgen therapy for SLE improved specific and general SLE-related conditions.[49, 50] More recent studies with androgen therapy for SLE have shown the following results:

(1) women treated with 19-nortestosterone showed clinical stability for over a year, while men responded less well, indicating that androgen therapy that lowers serum and free testosterone in men may actually worsen some symptoms in male SLE patients. Androgen therapy in men patients with SLE may require the use of androgens that elevate serum testosterone levels.[51]

(2) women treated with the androgen dehydroepiandrosterone (DHEA) showed improvements in physicians' overall assessments and re-duction of corticosteroid requirements.[52]

(3) women treated with DHEA (200mg/day) for three to 12 months, in a double-blind, placebo-controlled, randomized clinical trial showed statistically significant improvements in disease-related symptoms and

reduction in SLE flares. Also, concurrent corticosteroid requirements were reduced. The DHEA therapy was well tolerated with mild acne being the most frequent adverse effect reported.[53, 54]

(4) women treated with DHEA (50–200mg/day) for six months showed statistically significant improvements in all lupus outcomes as judged by the Systemic Lupus Erythematosus Disease Activity Index, Systemic Lupus Activity Measure (SLAM), Health Assessment Questionnaire, and other outcomes. The most common side effect was mild acne.[55]

(5) women treated with DHEA (50–200mg/day) for up to 12 months showed statistically significant improvement in SLE-related symptoms and conditions as measured by SLE Disease Activity Index, patient global assessment, physician global assessment, and concurrent corticosteroid doses. The DHEA therapy was well tolerated in both the premenopausal and postmenopausal women. Mild acne was the most common adverse effect reported.[56]

(6) women treated with DHEA for SLE (in three controlled and several uncontrolled trials, including one large multicenter study comprising nearly 200 patients) have shown a decrease in corticosteroid requirements, improved overall symptomatology, as well as probable bone protective and improved cognition effects.[57, 58]

(7) women successfully treated with androgens (danazol) for SLE-related or rheumatic disease-related refractory autoimmune thrombocytopenia or Evan's syndrome.[59, 60, 61, 62]

(8) women with SLE and low serum androgen levels have a higher incidence of cognitive impairment and clinically overt neuropsychiatric manifestations.[63]

(9) premenopausal women with SLE and low androgen levels have lower bone mineral density (BMD) and greater risk for osteoporosis; this may be due to the down-regulation of endogenous androgen production.[64]

(10) in men with SLE, testosterone administration returned the serum estrogenic/androgenic ratio to the normal range and was associated with decrease in the values of ESR, IL-2, a-DNA, ANF, and CRP titers. Clinical findings and symptoms improved including the degree of expression of lymphadenopathy, polyarthritis, and Raynaud's syndrome.[65]

Androgen Therapy and Cytokine Profiles in SLE

Androgen deficiency in patients with SLE can be associated with dysfunction of the hypothalamic-pituitary-adrenal axis[66, 67] which, in turn, directly affects the immune system in a manner that causes a Th1/Th2 cytokine production imbalance. Recent studies have elucidated some of the correlations of androgen-dependent cytokine levels and functioning in patients with SLE. Among other things, they have shown:

(1) that a positive correlation exists between serum DHEA and soluble immune mediators involved with leukocyte function and leukocyte adhesion in female patients.[68]

(2) that defects of cytokine (interleukin-2, IL-2) synthesis by T cells in vitro are due, in part, to androgen deficiency, which is the case in both murine lupus and human SLE.[69, 70]

(3) that marked adrenal insufficiency further increases the cortisol/DHEA ratios, and that this shift in adrenal steroidogenesis in women with SLE may be due to abnormal Th1/Th2 cytokine balance.[71]

(4) that in a murine model of experimental SLE, the initial active or flaring phases of the disease are associated with an increased production of TH1 cytokines (IL-2 and IFN-gamma) followed by a predominant Th2 cytokine profile and normal or low Th1 cytokine synthesis. This model may help explain the role of androgen therapy in attenuating the active and flaring phases of SLE in women patients via modulating Th1/Th2 cytokine synthesis and balance.[72]

(5) that IL-2 deficiency is a common feature in both murine lupus and human SLE and that exogenous androgen administration for murine lupus dramatically reverses the clinical autoimmune disease conditions by the androgen-induced upregulating of the synthesis of IL-2 by Th cells.[73]

(6) that in murine lupus, androgen therapy (DHEA, danazol, nandrolone decanoate, or testosterone esters) increased longevity and reduced proteinuria and autoimmune T cell imbalance in male and female mice.[74, 75, 76, 77, 78, 79]

(7) that testosterone administration inhibits B cell activity and reduces IL-6 production by monocytes in both women and men, indicating that it exhibits protective and therapeutic effects on human autoimmune diseases.[80]

(8) that testosterone administration directly suppresses anti–DNA antibody production and downregulates IL-6 production in peripheral blood mononuclear cells from patients with SLE, which supports the therapeutic effects of testosterone on SLE.[81]

Summary

The role of androgen deficiency in the etiopathogenesis and disease activity of SLE has been established. Androgen deficiency is associated with an abnormal Th1/Th2 cytokine profile in women patients with SLE. This abnormal cytokine profile has been associated with several aspects of the lupus disease process. Exogenous androgen administration has been shown to improve Th1/Th2 cytokine balance, reduce disease activity, reduce flares, and reduce corticosteroid requirements in women patients afflicted with SLE. This evidence strongly suggests that androgen therapy can be a disease-modifying form of treatment in SLE.

Androgen therapy for SLE patients has been shown to be beneficial in several ways that can improve the outcome of standard rehabilitation protocols. These include:

(1) enhancing neuromuscular strength when combined with rehabilitative and general strength-training programs.

(2) increasing bone mineral density with or without rehabilitative and general strength-training programs, thereby reducing the risk for osteoporosis and osteoporosis-related debilitating fractures.

(3) reducing the disease process and number of flares.

(4) reducing the corticosteroid requirement and reversing the catabolic effects of high-dose or prolonged corticosteroid therapy.

(5) reducing the risk for cognitive deficits associated with the disease.

(6) improving overall neuropsychoendocrine functions including enhanced sense of well-being, energy level, and sexual desire and functions, while reducing mental apathy, fatigue, and depression.

(7) improving pain tolerance and reducing painkiller requirements via elevation of central beta-endorphin levels.

(8) improving all SLE profile ratings and activities of daily living.

(9) probably improving longevity via disease-modifying effects.

Notes

1. Crispin, J.C., and J. Alcocer-Varela. Interleukin-2 and systemic lupus erythematosusfifteen years later. *Lupus* 1998; 7 (4): 214–222.

2. Hutchinson, G.A., J.E. Nehall, and D.T. Simeon. Psychiatric disorders in systemic lupus erythematosus. *West Indian Med. J.* 1996; 45 (2): 48–50.

3. Redford, T.W., and R.E. Small. Update on pharmacotherapy of systemic lupus erythematosus. *Am. J. Health Syst. Pharm.* 1995; 52 (23): 2686–2695.

4. James, W.H. Is hypoandrogenism a cause or a consequence of systemic lupus erythematosus in male patients? *Lupus* 2000; 9 (8): 646.

5. Pawlak, C.R., R. Jacobs, E. Mikeska, et al. Patients with systemic lupus erythematosus differ from healthy controls in their immunological response to acute psychological stress. *Brain Behav. Immun.* 1999; 13 (4): 287–302.

6. Mason, L.J., and D.A. Isenberg. Immunopathogenesis of SLE. *Baillieres Clin. Rheumatol.* 1998; 12 (3): 385–403.

7. Evans, M.J., S. MacLaughlin, R.D. Marvin, et al. Estrogen decreases in vitro apoptosis of peripheral blood mononuclear cells from women with normal menstrual cycles and decreases TNF-alpha production in SLE by not normal cultures. *Clin. Immunol. Immunopathol.* 1997; 82 (3): 258–262.

8. Petty, R.E. Etiology and pathogenesis of rheumatic diseases of adolescence. *Adolesc. Med.* 1998; 9 (1): 11–24.

9. Derksen, R.H. Dehydroepiandrosterone (DHEA) and systemic lupus erythematosus. *Semin. Arthritis Rheum.* 1998; 27 (6): 335–347.

10. Kanda, N, T. Tsuchida, and K. Tamaki. Estrogen enhancement of anti-double-stranded DNA antibody and immunoglobulins G production in peripheral blood mononuclear cells from patients with systemic lupus erythematosus. *Arthritis Rheum.* 1999; 42 (2): 328–337.

11. Wu, W.M., B.F. Lin, Y.C. Su, et al. Tamoxifen decreases renal inflammation and alleviates disease severity in autoimmune NZB/W F1 mice. *Scand. J. Immunol.* 2000; 52 (4): 393–400.

12. Berger, S., H. Ballo, and H.J. Stutte. Distinct antigen-induced cytokine pattern upon stimulation with antibody-complexed antigen consistent with a Th1–>Th2-shift. *Res. Virol.* 1996; 147 (2–3): 103–108.

13. Ostensen, M. Sex hormones and pregnancy in rheumatoid arthritis and systemic lupus erythematosus. *Ann. N.Y. Acad. Sci.* 1999; 876: 131–143.

14. Wong, C.K., E.K. Li, C.Y. Ho, et al. Elevation of plasma interleukin-18 concentration is correlated with disease activity in systemic lupus erythematosus. *Rheumatology (Oxf.)* 2000; 39 (10): 1078–1081.

15. Lahita, R.G. The role of sex hormones in systemic lupus erythematosus. *Curr. Opin. Rheumatol.* 1999; 11 (5): 352–356.

16. Richaud-Patin, Y., J. Alcocer-Alcocer, and L. Liorente. High levels of TH2 cytokine gene expression in systemic lupus erythematosus. *Rev. Invest. Clin.* 1995; 47 (4): 267–272.

17. Lacki, J.K., W. Samborski, and S.H. Mackiewicz. Interleukin-10 and interleukin-6 in lupus erythematosus and rheumatoid arthritis, correlations with acute phase proteins. *Clin. Rheumatol.* 1997; 16 (3): 275–278.

18. Lacki, J.K., P. Leszczynski, P. Kelemen, et al. Cytokine concentration in serum lupus erythematosus patients: the effect on acute phase response. *J. Med.* 1997; 28 (1–2): 99–107.

19. Kirou, K.A., and M.K. Crow. New pieces to the SLE cytokine puzzle. *Clin. Immunol.* 1999; 91 (1): 1–5.

20. Nagy, G., E. Pallinger, P. Antal-Szalmas, et al. Measurement of intracellular interferon-gamma and interleukin-4 in whole blood T lymphocytes from patients with systemic lupus erythematosus. *Immunol. Lett.* 2000; 74 (3): 207–210.

21. Wong, C.K., C.Y. Ho, E.K. Li, et al. Elevation of proinflammatory cytokine (IL-18, IL-17, IL-12) and Th2 cytokine (IL-4) concentrations in patients with systemic lupus erythematosus. *Lupus* 2000; 9 (8): 589–593.

22. Amit, M., A. Mor, J. Weissgarten, et al. Inactive systemic lupus erythematosus is associated with a normal stimulated TH (1)/TH (2) cytokine secretory pattern. *Cytokine* 2000; 12 (9): 1405–1408.

23. Mok, C.C., R.W. Wong, and C.S. Lau. Ovarian failure and flares of systemic lupus erythematosus. *Arthritis Rheum.* 1999; 42 (6): 1274–1280.

24. Jungers, P., K. Nahoul, C. Pelissier, et al. [Plasma androgens in women with disseminated lupus erythematosus.] *Presse. Med.* 1983; 12 (11): 685–688.

25. Feher, K.G., G. Bencze, J. Ujfalussy, et al. Serum steroid hormone levels in systemic lupus erythematosus. *Acta Med. Hung.* 1987; 44 (4): 321–327.

26. Hedman, M., Nilsson, E., and B. del la Torre. Low sulpho-conjugated steroid hormone levels in systemic lupus erythematosus (SLE). *Clin. Exp. Rheumatol.* 1989; 7 (6): 583–588.

27. Williams, W., D. Shah, and O. Parshad. Thyroid-gonad relationship in systemic lupus erythematosus. *West Indian Med. J.* 1991; 40 (3): 124–126.

28. Straub, R.H., M. Seuner, E. Antoniou, et al. Dehydroepiandrosterone sulfate is positively correlated with soluble interleukin 2 receptor and soluble intercellular adhesion molecule in systemic lupus erythematosus. *J. Rheumatol.* 1996; 23 (5): 856–861.

29. Jungers, P., K. Nahoul, C. Pelissier, et al. Low plasma androgens in women with active or quiescent systemic lupus erythematosus. *Arthritis Rheum.* 1982; 25 (4): 454–457.

30. Dougados, M. [Sex hormone metabolism in acute systemic lupus erythematosus.] *Ann. Med. Interne. (Paris)* 1990; 141 (3): 244–246.

31. Wen, C., and L.S. Li. Blood levels of sex hormone in lupus nephritis and their relationship to lupus activity. *Chin. Med. J. (Engl.)* 1993; 106 (1): 49–52.

32. Lahita, R.G., H.L. Bradlow, E. Ginzler, et al. Low plasma androgens in women with systemic lupus erythematosus. *Arthritis Rheum.* 1987; 30 (3): 241–248.

33. Jara-Quezada, L., A. Graef, and C. Lavalle. Prolactin and gonadal hormones during pregnancy in systemic lupus erythematosus. *J. Rheumatol.* 1991; 18 (3): 249–353.

34. Folomeev, M., M. Dougados, J. Beaune, et al. Plasma sex hormones and aromatase activity in tissues of patients with systemic lupus erythematosus. *Lupus.* 1992; 1 (3): 191–195.

35. Navarro, M.A., A. Vidaller, J.B. Ortola, et al. Salivary testosterone levels in women with systemic lupus erythematosus. *Arthritis Rheum.* 1992; 35 (5): 557–559.

36. Mackworth-Young, C.G., A.L. Parke, K.D. Morley, et al. Sex hormones in male patients with systemic lupus erythematosus: a comparison with other disease groups. *Eur. J. Rheumatol. Inflamm.* 1983; 6 (3): 228–232.

37. Mok, C.C. and C.S. Lau. Profile of sex hormones in male patients with systemic lupus erythematosus. *Lupus* 2000; 9 (4): 252–257.

38. Lavalle, C., E. Loyo, R. Paniagua, et al. Correlation study between prolactin and androgens in male patients with systemic lupus erythematosus. *J. Rheumatol.* 1987; 14 (2): 268–272.

39. Carrabba, M., C. Giovine, M. Chevallard, et al. Abnormalities of sex hormones in men with systemic lupus erythematosus. *Clin. Rheumatol.* 1985; 4 (4): 420–425.

40. Vilarinho, S.T., and L.T. Costallat. Evaluation of the hypothalamic-pituitary-gonadal axis in males with systemic lupus erythematosus. *J. Rheumatol.* 1998; 25 (6): 1097–1103.

41. Sequeira, J.F., G. Keser, B. Greenstein, et al. Systemic lupus erythematosus: sex hormones in male patients. *Lupus* 1993; 2 (5): 315–317.

42. Masse, R., P. Youinou, J.C. Dorval, et al. Reversal of lupus-erythematosus-like disease with danazol. *Lancet* 1980; 2 (8195 pt. 1): 651.

43. Donaldson, V.H., and E.V. Hess. Effect of danazol on lupus-erythematosus-like disease in hereditary angioneurotic oedema. *Lancet* 1980; 2 (8204): 1145.

44. Morley, K.D., A. Parke, and G.R. Hughes. Systemic lupus erythematosus: two patients treated with danazol. *Br. Med. J. (Clin. Res. Ed.)* 1982; 284 (6327): 1431–1432.

45. Agnello, V., K. Pariser, J. Gell, et al. Preliminary observations on danazol therapy of systemic lupus erythematosus: effects on DNA antibodies, throbocytopenia and complement. *J. Rheumatol.* 1983; 10 (5): 682–687.

46. David, J. Hyperglucoagonaemia and treatment with danazol for systemic lupus erythematosus. *Br. Med. J. (Clin. Res. Ed.)* 1985; 291 (6503): 1170–1171.

47. Jungers, P., F. Liote, C. Pelissier, et al. [Hormonal modulation in disseminated

lupus erythematosus: the preliminary results with danazol and cyporterone acetate.] *Ann. Med. Interne. (Paris)* 1986; 137 (4): 313–319.

48. West, S.G., and S.C. Johnson. Danazol for the treatment of refractory autoimmune throbocytopenia in systemic lupus erythematosus. *Ann. Internal Med.* 1988; 108 (5): 703–706.

49. Chan, A.C., and K. Sack. Danazol therapy in autoimmune hemolytic anemia associated with systemic lupus erythematosus. *J. Rheumatol.* 1991; 18 (2): 280–282.

50. Wong, K.L. Danazol in treatment of lupus thrombocytopenia. *Asian Pac. J. Allergy Immunol.* 1991; 9 (2): 125–129.

51. Lahita, R.G., C.Y. Cheng, C. Monder, et al. Experience with 19–nortestosterone in the therapy of systemic lupus erythematosus: worsened disease after treatment with 19–nortestosterone in men and lack of improvement of women. *J. Rheumatol.* 1992; 19 (4): 547–555.

52. van Vollenhoven, R.F, E.G. Engleman, and J.L. McGuire. An open study of dehydroepiandrosterone in systemic lupus erythematosus. *Arthritis Rheum.* 1994; 37 (9): 1305–1310.

53. van Vollenhoven, R.F., E.G. Engleman, and J.L. McGuire. Dehydroepiandrosterone in systemic lupus erythematosus. Results of a double-blind, placebo-controlled, randomized clinical trial. *Arthritis Rheum.* 1995; 38 (12): 1826–1831.

54. van Vollenhoven, R.F., and J.L. McGuire. Studies of dehydroepiandrosterone (DHEA) as a therapeutic agent in systemic lupus erythematosus. *Ann. Med. Interne. (Paris)* 1996; 147 (4): 290–296.

55. Barry, N.N, J.L. McGuire, and R.F. van Vollenhoven. Dehydroepiandrosterone in systemic lupus erythematosus: relationship between dosage, serum levels, and clinical response. *J. Rheumatol.* 1998; 25 (12): 2352–2356.

56. van Vollenhoven, R.F., L.M. Morabito, E.G. Engleman, et al. Treatment of systemic lupus erythematosus with dehydroepiandrosterone: 50 patients treated up to 12 months. *J. Rheumatol.* 1998; 25 (2): 285–289.

57. van Vollenhoven, R.F. Dehydroepiandrosterone in systemic lupus erythematosus. *Rheum. Dis. Clin. North. Am.* 2000; 26 (2): 349–262.

58. van Vollenhoven, R.F. Dehydroepiandrosterone in the treatment of systemic lupus erythematosus. *Rheumatol. (Oxf.):* 2000; 39 (8): 929–930.

59. Cervera, H., L.J. L. Jara, S. Pizarro, et al. Danazol for systemic lupus erythematosus with refractory autoimmune thrombocytopenia or Evan's syndrome. *J. Rheumatol.* 1995; 22 (10): 1867–1871.

60. Insiripong, S., T. Chanchairujira, and T. Bumpenboon. Danazol for thrombocytopenia in pregnancy with underlying systemic lupus erythematosus. *J. Med. Assoc. Thai.* 1996; 79 (5): 330–332.

61. M. Petrovsky. Danazol in the treatment of a systemic lupus erythematosus (SLE-like) illness associated with deficiency of the fourth component of complement. *Aust. N. Z. J. Med.* 1997; 27 (2): 189.

62. Blanco, R., V.M. Martinez-Taboada, V. Rodriguez-Valverde, et al. Successful therapy with danazol in refractory autoimmune thrombocytopenia associated with rheumatic diseases. *Br. J. Rheumatol.* 1997; 36 (10): 1095–1099.

63. Hanly, J.G., J.D. Fisk, G. Sherwood, et al. Cognitive impairment in patients with systemic lupus erythematosus. *J. Rheumatol.* 1992; 19 (4): 562–567.

64. Formiga, F., I. Moga, J.M. Nolla, et al. The association of dehydroepiandrosterone sulphate levels with bone mineral density in systemic lupus erythematosus. *Clin. Exp. Rheumatol.* 1997; 15 (4): 387–392.

65. Folomeev, M.I. [Use of androgens in the complex treatment of men with systemic lupus erythematosus.] *Ter. Arkh.* 1986; 58 (7): 112–114.

66. Guiterrez, M.A., M.E. Garcia, J.A. Rodriguez, et al. Hypothalamic-pituitary-adrenal axis function and prolactin secretion in systemic lupus erythematosus. *Lupus* 1998; 7 (6): 404–408.

67. Derksen, R.H. Dehydroepiandrosterone (DHEA) and systemic lupus erythematosus. *Semin. Arthritis. Rheum.* 1998; 27 (6): 335–347.

68. Straub, R.H, M. Zeuner, E. Antoniou, et al. Dehydroepiandrosterone sulfate is positively correlated with soluble interleukin-2 receptor and soluble intercellular adhesion molecule in systemic lupus erythematosus. *J. Rheumatol.* 1996; 23 (5): 856–861.

69. Suzuki, T., N. Suzuki, E.G. Engleman, et al. Low serum levels of dehydroepiandrosterone may cause deficient IL-2 production by lymphocytes in patients with systemic lupus erythematosus (SLE). *Clin. Exp. Immunol.* 1995; 99 (2): 251–255.

70. Suzuki, N, T. Suzuki, and T. Sakane. Hormones and lupus: defective dehydroepiandrosterone activity induces impaired interleukin-2 activity of T lymphocytes in patients with systemic lupus erythematosus. *Ann. Med. Interne. (Paris)* 1996; 147 (4): 248–252.

71. Zietz, B., T. Reber, M. Oertel, et al. Altered function of the hypothalamic stress axes in patients with moderately active systemic lupus erythematosus. II. Dissociation between androstenedione, cortisol, or dehydroepiandrosterone and interleukin 6 and tumor necrosis factor. *J. Rheumatol.* 2000; 27 (4): 911–918.

72. Segal, R., B.L. Bermas, M. Dayan, et al. Kinetics of cytokine production in experimental systemic lupus erythematosus: involvement of T helper cell 1/T helper cell 2–type cytokines in disease. *J. Immunol.* 1997; 158 (6): 3009–3016.

73. Suzuki, T., N. Suzuki, E. G. Engleman, et al. Low serum levels of dehydroepiandrosterone may cause deficient IL-2 production by lymphocytes in patients with systemic lupus erythematosus (SLE). *Clin. Exp. Immunol.* 1995; 99 (2): 251–255.

74. Verheul, H.A., W.H. Stimson, F.C. den Hollander, et al. The effects of nandrolone, testosterone and their esters on murine lupus. *Clin. Exp. Immunol.* 1981; 44 (1): 11–17.

75. Verheul, H.A., G.H. Deckers, and A.H. Schuurs. Effects of nandrolone decanoate or testosterone decanoate on murine lupus: further evidence for a dissociation of autoimmunosuppressive and endocrine effects. *Immunopharmacology* 1986; 11 (2): 93–99.

76. Connolly, K.M., V.J. Stecher, B.W. Synder, et al. The effect of danazol in the MRL/lpr mouse model of autoimmune disease. *Agents Actions* 1988; 25 (1–2): 164–170.

77. Keisler, L.W., A.B. Kier, and S.E. Walker. Effects of prolonged administration of the 19–nor-testosterone derivatives norethindrone and norgestrel to female NZB/W mice: comparison with medroxyprogesterone and ethinyl estradiol. *Autoimmunity* 1991; 9 (1): 21–32.

78. Norton, S.D., L.L. Harrison, R. Yowell, et al. Administration of dehydroepiandrosterone sulfate retards onset but not progression of autoimmune disease in NZB/W mice. *Autoimmunity* 1997; 26 (3): 161–171.

79. Yang, B.C., C.W. Liu, Y.C. Chen, et al. Exogenous dehydroepiandrosterone modified the expression of T-helper-related cytokines in NZB/NZBW F1 mice. *Immunol. Invest.* 1998; 27 (4–5): 291–302.

80. Kanda, N., T. Tsuchida, and T. Tamaki. Testosterone inhibits immunoglobulins production by human peripheral blood mononuclear cells. *Clin. Exp. Immnol.* 1996; 106 (2): 410–415.

81. Kanda, N., T. Tsuchida, and K. Tamaki. Testosterone suppresses anti–DNA antibody production in peripheral blood mononuclear cells from patients with systemic lupus erythematosus. *Arthritis Rheum.* 1997; 40 (9): 1703–1711

14

Rationale for Anabolic Therapy in Systemic Sclerosis

Introduction: Scleroderma and Androgen Deficiency

Systemic sclerosis (SSc), also known as scleroderma, is a complex autoimmune disease that is much more common in women than in men.[1] Its pathology involves endothelial injury, obliterative microvascular lesions, hypercoagulability, and increased wall thickness in the vessels of all involved organs which results in degraded vascular function with increased vasospasm, reduced vasodilatory capacity, and increased adhesiveness of the blood vessels to platelets and lymphocytes.[2]

Initial triggers for the vascular pathology in SSc are not known, but it has been suggested that androgen deficiency plays a role in the pathogenesis and sequelae associated with SSc.[3, 4] It is well recognized that androgens influence and modulate the immune system, cytokine profiles and growth factors in normal, physiologic conditions and autoimmune diseases. Genetic factors have also been shown to have an etiological role in SS.[5]

Considerable research has been conducted to investigate the "downstream" influence of specific cytokines, immunoglobulins, growth factors, growth factor receptors, and their influence on the pathogenesis of SSc.[6, 7, 8, 9, 10, 11, 12, 13, 14, 15, 16, 17, 18, 19, 20, 21, 22] This research has shown that Th2-dominated cytokine profiles play a role in SSc.[23] However, little available science-based information exists regarding the "upstream" regulation of these cytokines brought about by androgen deficiency specifically with SSc. Research with other autoimmune diseases is far ahead of that conducted on SSc with regards to androgen deficiency.

193

Systemic sclerosis is associated with a number of conditions that reflect the well-established conditions associated with hypoandrogenemia, including sarcopenia, osteoporosis, Raynaud's phenomenon, reduced libido, inorgasmia, and erectile dysfunction, depression, cognitive deficits, hyperlipidemia, microvascular thromboembolism, decreased work capacity, fatigability, hypofibrinolysis, and reduced sense of well-being.[24, 25, 26, 27, 28, 29, 30, 31, 32, 33, 34, 35]

Improvements in management of systemic sclerosis have occurred through a growing understanding of pathogenic events, accompanied by advances in diagnosis and assessment, as well as developments in organ-based therapeutics. Unfortunately, disease-modifying therapies of proven efficacy remain elusive.[36] Several recent review articles on updated therapeutics for SSc do not mention androgen therapy or the hypoandrogenemia that can be associated with SSc.[37, 38] Other authors have recommended androgen therapy for the microvascular and organ involvement associated with SSc.[39, 40]

Studies with Androgen Therapy for SSc

Raynaud's phenomenon is the most common sign of vascular involvement in scleroderma and is associated with decreased fibrinolysis and enhanced platelet aggregation that contributes to microvascular thrombosis and damage in involved organs and tissues.[41, 42] Raynaud's phenomenon and reduced fibrinolysis have been documented in patients with hypoandrogenemia and organ involvement.[43] It has been shown that patients with SSc and Raynaud's phenomenon have higher plasma fibrinogen levels and blood viscosity at all shear rates and temperatures.[44] In addition, it has been shown that SSc patients have significantly altered levels of several coagulation and fibrinolysis factors that favor thromboembolism.[45] Therefore, patients with SSc and Raynaud's phenomenon are in a hypercoagulable state that leads to increased risk for microvascular thromboembolism.

Several studies have shown that androgen therapy increases fibrinolysis, reduces Raynaud's phenomenon, and improves microvascular circulation, hand blood flow, and dermal sclerosis.[46, 47, 48] In addition, androgen therapy has been shown to treat refractory and hemolytic anemias associated with SSc.[49, 50] It has been concluded that fibrinolytic enhancement with androgen therapy appears useful in treating the microvascular features of SSc.[51]

Summary

In this chapter, the rationale for anabolic therapy in SSc has been presented. Androgen therapy should be considered as an important therapeutic therapy for patients with SSc, especially those patients who are undergoing traditional rehabilitation modalities. Future studies are warranted and are expected to show that androgen therapy is a disease-modifying modality via its correction in coagulation and cytokine profiles that are associated with progressive disease and increased mortality. In addition, androgen therapy provides neurosteroid effects that can assist with the depression and cognitive defects that can be associated with SSc.

Notes

1. Artlett, C.M., J.B. Smith, and S.A. Jimenez. New perspectives on the etiology of systemic sclerosis. *Mol. Med. Today* 1999; 5 (2): 74–78.

2. Kahaleh, M.B., and E.C. LeRoy. Autoimmunity and vascular involvement in systemic sclerosis (SSc). *Autoimmunity* 1999; 31 (3): 195–214.

3. Nowlin, N.S., S.H. Zwillich, J.E. Brick, et al. Male hypogonadism and scleroderma. *J. Rheumatol.* 1985; 12 (3): 606–606.

4. Straub, R.H., M. Zeuner, G. Lock, et al. High prolactin and low dehydroepiandrosterone sulfate serum levels in patients with severe systemic sclerosis. *Br. J. Rheumatol.* 1997; 36 (4): 426–432.

5. Tan, F.K., and F.C. Arnett. Genetic factors in the etiology of systemic sclerosis and Raynaud phenomenon. *Curr. Opin. Rheumatol.* 2000; 12 (6): 511–519.

6. Kantor, T.V., D. Friberg, T.A. Medsger, et al. Cytokine production and serum levels in systemic sclerosis. *Clin. Immunol. Immunopathol.* 1992; 65 (3): 278–285.

7. Bruns, M., K. Herrmann, and U.F. Haustein. Immunologic parameters in systemic sclerosis. *Int. J. Dermatol.* 1994; 33 (1): 25–32.

8. Uziel, Y., B.R. Krafshik, B. Feldman, et al. Serum levels of soluble interleukin-2 receptor. A marker of disease activity in localized scleroderma. *Arthritis Rheum.* 1994; 37 (6): 898–901.

9. Bruns, M., K. Herrmann, and U.F. Haustein. Immunologic parameters in systemic sclerosis. *Int. J. Dermatol.* 1994; 33 (1): 25–32.

10. Patrick, M.R., B.W. Kirkham, M. Graham, et al. Circulating interleukin 1 beta and soluble interleukin 2 receptor: evaluation as markers of disease activity in scleroderma. *J. Rheumatol.* 1995; 22 (4): 654–658.

11. Ihn, H., S. Sato, M. Fujimoto, et al. Clinical significance of serum levels of soluble interleukin-2 receptor in patients with localized scleroderma. *Br. J. Dermatol.* 1996; 134 (5): 843–847.

12. Steen, V.D., E.E. Engel, M.R. Charley, et al. Soluble serum interleukin 2 receptors in patients with systemic sclerosis. *J. Rheumatol.* 1996; 23 (4): 646–649.

13. Lis, A., L. Brzezinska-Wcislo, J. Rubisz-Brzezinska, et al. Serum levels of soluble interleukin-2 receptor — a possible index of disease prognosis in systemic sclerosis. *Clin. Exp. Dermatol.* 1997; 22 (1): 60–61.

14. Kucharz, E.J., L. Brzezinska-Weislo, A. Kotusksa, et al. Elevated serum level of interleukin-10 in patients with systemic sclerosis. *Clin. Rheumatol.* 1997; 16 (6): 638–639.

15. Hasegawa, M., S. Sato, M. Fujimoto, et al. Serum levels of interleukin 6 (IL-6), oncostatin M, soluble IL-6 receptor, and soluble gp 130 in patients with systemic sclerosis. *J. Rheumatol.* 1998; 25 (2): 308–313.

16. Majewski, S., A. Wojas-Pelc, M. Malejczyk, et al. Serum levels of soluble TNF

alpha receptor type 1 and the severity of systemic sclerosis. *Acta Derm. Venereol.* 1999; 79 (3): 207–210.

17. Dalkilic, E., K. Dilek, M. Gullulu, et al. Lymphocyte phenotype in systemic sclerosis. *Ann. Rheum. Dis.* 1999; 58 (11): 719–720.

18. Kurasawa, K., K. Hirose, H. Sano, et al. Increased interleukin-17 production in patients with systemic sclerosis. *Arthritis Rheum.* 2000; 43 (11): 2455–2463.

19. Sato, S., T. Nagakoka, M. Hasegawa, et al. Elevated serum KL-6 levels in patients with systemic sclerosis: association with the severity of pulmonary fibrosis. *Dermatology* 2000; 200 (3): 196–201.

20. Sato, S., T. Nagaoka, M. Hasegawa, et al. Serum levels of connective tissue growth factor are elevated in patients with systemic sclerosis: association with extent of skin sclerosis and severity of pulmonary fibrosis. *J. Rheumatol.* 2000; 27 (1): 149–154.

21. Yuhara, T., H. Takemura, T. Akama, et al. The relationship between serum immunoglobulins levels and pulmonary involvement in systemic sclerosis. *J. Rheumatol.* 2000; 27 (5): 1207–1214.

22. Kucharz, E.J., E. Grucka-Mamczar, A. Mamczar, et al. *Clin. Rheumatol.* 2000; 19 (2): 165–166.

23. Romangnani, S. T-cell subsets (Th1 versus Th2). *Ann. Allergy Asthma Immunol.* 2000; 85 (1): 9–18.

24. Lally, E.V., and S.A. Jimenez. Impotence in progressively systemic sclerosis. *Ann. Intern. Med.* 1981; 95 (2): 150–153.

25. Blom-Bulow, B., B. Jonson, and K. Bauer. Factors limiting exercise performance in progressive systemic sclerosis. *Semin. Arthritis Rheum.* 1983; 13 (2): 174–181.

26. Chausow, A.M., T. Kane, D. Levinson, et al. Reversible hypercapnic respiratory insufficiency in scleroderma caused by respiratory muscle weakness. *Am. Rev. Respir. Dis.* 1984; 130 (1): 142–144.

27. Rothschild, B., L.D. Thompson, M. Chesney, et al. Perturbation of fibrinolysis in progressive systemic sclerosis. *Med. Hypotheses* 1985; 16 (3): 253–260.

28. Nowlin, N.S., J.E. Brick, D.J. Weaver, et al. Impotence in scleroderma. *Ann. Intern. Med.* 1986; 104 (6): 794–798.

29. Di Munno, O., M. Mazzantini, P. Massei, et al. Reduced bone mass and normal calcium metabolism in systemic sclerosis with and without calcinosis. *Clin. Rheumatol.* 1994; 14 (4): 407–412.

30. Wigley, F.M. Clinical aspects of systemic and localized scleroderma. *Curr. Opin. Rheumatol.* 1994; 6 (6): 628–636.

31. Sauer, I., W. Ries, M. Mittag, et al. [Biological age in patients with progressive scleroderma.] *Z. Gerontol. Geriatr.* 1996; 29 (3): 223–232.

32. Roca, R.P., F.M. Wigley, and B. White. Depressive symptoms associated with scleroderma. *Arthritis Rheum.* 1996; 39 (6): 1035–1040.

33. Vaillant, P., O. Menard, J.M. Vignaud, et al. The role of cytokines in human lung fibrosis. *Monaldi. Arch. Chest. Dis.* 1996; 51 (2): 145–152.

34. Noboli, F., M. Cutolo, A. Sulli, et al. Impaired quantitative cerebral blood flow in scleroderma patients. *J. Neurol. Sci.* 1997; 152 (1): 63–71.

35. Ihata, A., A Shirai, T. Okubo, et al. Severity of seropositive isolated Raynaud's phenomenon is associated with serological profile. *J. Rheumatol.* 2000; 27 (7): 1686–1692.

36. Denton, C.P., and C.M. Black. Scleroderma and related disorders: therapeutic aspects. *Baillieres Best Pract. Res. Clin. Rheumatol.* 2000; 14 (1): 17–35.

37. Denton, C.P., and C.M. Black. Novel therapeutic strategies in scleroderma. *Curr. Rheumatol. Rep.* 1999; 1 (1): 22–27.

38. Furst, D.E. Rational therapy in the treatment of systemic sclerosis. *Curr. Opin. Rheumatol.* 2000; 12 (6): 540–544.

39. Steen, V. Treatment of systemic sclerosis. *Curr. Opin. Rheumatol.* 1991; 3 (6): 979–985.

40. Muller-Ladner, U., K. Benning, and B. Lang. Current therapy of systemic sclerosis (scleroderma). *Clin. Investig.* 1993; 71 (4): 257–263.

41. Kahaleh, M.B. Raynaud's phenomenon and vascular disease in scleroderma. *Curr. Opin. Rheumatol.* 1994; 6 (6): 621–627.

42. Maeda, M., H. Kachi, and S. Mori. Plasma levels of molecular markers of blood coagulation and fibrinolysis in progressive systemic sclerosis (PSS). *J. Dermatol. Sci.* 1996; 11 (3): 223–227.

43. Straub, R.H., M. Zeuner, G. Lock, et al. High prolactin and low dehydroepiandrosterone sulphate serum levels in patients with severe systemic sclerosis. *Br. J. Rheumatol.* 1997; 36 (4): 426–432.

44. Ayres, M.L., P.E. Jarrett, and N.L. Browse. Blood viscosity, Raynaud's phenomenon and the effect of fibrinolytic enhancement. *Br. J. Surg.* 1981; 68 (1): 51–54.

45. Ames, P.R., S. Lupoli, J. Alves, et al. The coagulation/fibrinolysis balance in systemic sclerosis: evidence for a hematological stress syndrome. *Br. J. Rheumatol.* 1997; 36 (10): 1045–1050.

46. Jarrett, P.E., M. Morland, and N.L. Browse. Treatment of Raynaud's phenomenon by fibrinolytic enhancement. *Br. Med. J.* 1978; 2 (6136): 523–525.

47. Ayres, M.L., P.E. Jarrett, and N.L. Browse. Blood viscosity, Raynaud's phenomenon and the effect of fibrinolytic enhancement. *Br. J. Surg.* 1981; 68 (1): 51–54.

48. Jayson, M.I., C.D. Holland, A. Keegan, et al. A controlled study of stanozolol in primary Raynaud's phenomenon and systemic sclerosis. *Ann. Rheum. Dis.* 1991; 50 (1): 41–47.

49. Lugassy, G., T. Reitblatt, A. Ducach, et al. Severe autoimmune hemolytic anemia with cold agglutinin and sclerodermic features—favorable response to danazol. *Ann. Hematol.* 1993; 67 (3): 143–144.

50. Hamamoto, K., T. Ohno, and H. Ogawa. [Myelodysplastic syndrome with CREST syndrome successfully treated with metenolone—A case report.] *Rinsho Ketseuki* 1996; 37 (4): 362–365.

51. Jayson, M.I., C.D. Holland, A. Keegan, et al. A controlled study of stanozolol in primary Raynaud's phenomenon and systemic sclerosis. *Ann. Rheum. Dis.* 1991; 50 (1): 41–47.

Part 4

Anabolic Therapy for Other Catabolic Diseases and Conditions

15

Rationale for Anabolic Therapy in AIDS and HIV Infection

Introduction: Hypoandrogenemia and AIDS Wasting

Body wasting and sarcopenia have been associated with increased mortality, disease progression, and reduced quality of life in patients with human immunodeficiency virus (HIV) infection and full-blown acquired immunodeficiency syndrome (AIDS). The failure of nutritional therapies and effective viral suppression to consistently restore lean body mass has prompted investigation of pharmacologic use of a number of anabolic agents including androgens, recombinant human growth hormone (rhGH), growth hormone (GH) secretagogues, and recombinant insulin-like growth factor-1 (rhIGF-1).[1, 2, 3]

Although weight loss and wasting associated with HIV infection is multifaceted in its pathogenesis, it has been shown that hypoandrogenemia is a common occurrence in HIV disease and contributes significantly to depletion of lean tissue and muscle dysfunction in both men and women.[4, 5, 6] Hypoandrogenemia has been shown to occur in as many as half of patients with the acquired immunodeficiency syndrome (AIDS) wasting.[7] Low serum levels of several androgens have been shown to be involved with HIV-infection, including total testosterone, free testosterone, dehydroepiandrosterone (DHEA), dehydroepiandrosterone sulfate (DHEAS), and dihydrotestosterone (DHT).[8]

The etiology of hypoandrogenemia in HIV-infected men has been shown to be a combination of nonspecific changes from acute and chronic illness, and specific effects due to HIV infection. Depressed serum androgen levels have been associated with viral or infectious invasion of the

201

endocrine organs in both men and women and with medications commonly used for the treatment of HIV infection.[9] Specific mechanisms for hypoandrogenemia in HIV-infected patients have been identified and include:

(1) alterations of the hypothalamic-pituitary-gonadal axis indicative of primary hypogonadism in men.[10]

(2) alterations of the hypothalamic-pituitary-adrenal axis that results in increased adrenal secretion of cortisol and decreased secretion of androgens in both men and women.[11, 12, 13]

Hypoandrogenemia has been shown to have negative implications on morbidity and mortality in HIV-infected patients. Significantly low androgen levels have been associated with a greater prevalence of opportunistic infections and malignancies, lower T-lymphocyte counts, increased viral load, HIV illness markers, and catabolic cytokine profiles, and death.[14, 15, 16, 17] Most importantly, hypoandrogenemia has been found to play a pathogenic role in the progression of HIV infection to full-blown AIDS wasting.[18, 19, 20, 21, 22, 23, 24]

Along with hypoandrogenemia, HIV infection is associated with reductions in other anabolic hormones and potentials. Low circulating levels of IGF (hyposomatomedinemia) are common in HIV infected individuals and contribute to wasting. It has been shown that hyposomatomedinemia associated with HIV infection tends to primarily stem from endogenous GH resistance and a blunted response to GH stimulation.[25, 26] Therefore, many HIV-infected patients have both hypoandrogenemia and hyposomatomedinemia, which significantly contributes to a major loss of anabolic potentials, subsequent wasting, and disease progression.

Studies of Anabolic Therapy for HIV-Infected Patients

Several recent investigational studies have shown that anabolic therapy can have a major impact on the health and well-being of HIV-infected individuals. The results of these studies have indicated that:

(1) androgen therapy, in the absence of an exercise program, in HIV-infected men and women with hypoandrogenemia, causes substantial increases in nitrogen retention, lean body mass, muscle mass, and quality of life.[27, 28, 29, 30]

(2) androgen therapy, in the absence of an exercise program, in

borderline hypogonadal men with HIV-associated weight loss, causes substantial increases in nitrogen retention, lean body mass, and treadmill exercise performance.[31]

(3) the majority of HIV-positive men who presented with fatigue responded to androgen therapy with much improved levels of energy, elevated mood, and increased muscle mass.[32, 33, 34]

(4) sustained androgen therapy increases lean body mass during 12 months of treatment in hypogonadal men with AIDS wasting.[35]

(5) pharmacologic androgen therapy can be effective in treating andropause symptoms in *eugonadal* symptomatic HIV-infected individuals.[36]

(6) pharmacologic androgen therapy in both hypogonadal and eugonadal HIV-infected men produces statistically significant improvements in mood (as determined by Beck Depression Inventory scores), which correlates (statistically significant) with weight control, viral load, and circulating T-lymphocyte levels.[37]

(7) progressive exercise programs may be an important adjunct to androgen therapy in the treatment of psychological distress and wasting symptoms in symptomatic HIV illness.[38, 39, 40, 41]

(8) progressive strength training and pharmacologic androgen therapy in *eugonadal* men with AIDS wasting can be an effective treatment to increase muscle mass and improve overall health.[42, 43, 44]

(9) pharmacologic androgen therapy has beneficial impacts on immune system functions[45] without interference with the antiviral effects of other drugs commonly used to treat HIV infection, such as zidovudine (ZDV), dideoxyinosine (ddI), and dideoxycytidine (ddC).[46]

(10) administration of rhGH or rhIGF-1 improves lean body mass and body composition, modulates the marrow suppressive effects of antiviral therapy, improves immune system function, and enhances exercise work output.[47, 48, 49]

These studies have indicated that the short-term use of anabolic agents can halt or reverse the progression of HIV-associated wasting. Improved metabolic outcomes, increased lean body mass, improved survival rates, enhanced physical and social functioning, enriched quality of life, and enhanced immune system function have resulted from anabolic therapy in men and women patients with HIV infection.[50, 51, 52, 53] Longer-term studies are under way and should be published in the near future.[54]

Summary

In this chapter the rationale for using anabolic therapy for patients with HIV infection has been presented. Therapy with anabolic agents, in the absence of a concomitant exercise program, has been shown to have several beneficial effects in HIV-infected patients. Concomitant exercise and anabolic therapy have been shown to have additive and beneficial effects on muscle mass, viral markers, immune responses, mood, and all quality of life measurements.

Although recent investigational studies have reported on short-term anabolic therapy, it has become evident that anabolic therapies for HIV-infected patients should be considered as "standard of care" for patients undergoing conventional rehabilitative modalities. Maintaining the quality of health in these patients with anabolic therapy is justified and it may increase longevity for those patients while potential therapeutic cures are being developed. Therapy with replacement doses or pharmacologic doses has been utilized in investigational studies with beneficial results.

Notes

1. Mulligan, K., V.W. Tai, and M. Schambelan. Use of growth hormone and other anabolic agents in AIDS wasting. *J. Parenter. Enteral Nutr.* 1999; 23 (6 Suppl): S202–209.

2. Segal, D.M., M. Perez, and P. Shapshak. Oxandrolone, used for treatment of wasting disease in HIV-1–infected patients, does not diminish the antiviral activity of deoxymucleoside analogues in lymphocyte and macrophage cell cultures. *J. Acquir. Immune. Defic. Syndr. Hum. Retrovirol.* 1999; 20 (3): 215–219.

3. Nemechek, P.M., B. Polsky, and M.S. Gottlieb. Treatment guidelines for HIV-associated wasting. *Mayo Clin. Proc.* 2000; 75 (4): 386–394.

4. Grinspoon, S., C. Corcoran, K. Miller, et al. Body composition and endocrine function in women with acquired immunodeficiency syndrome wasting. *J. Clin. Endocrinol. Metab.* 1997; 82 (5): 1332–1337.

5. Bhasin, S., T.W. Storer, N. Asbel-Sethi, et al. Effects of testosterone replacement with a nongenital, transdermal system, Androderm, in human immunodeficiency virus–infected men with low testosterone levels. *J. Clin. Endocrinol. Metab.* 1998; 83 (9): 3155–3162.

6. Miller, K., C. Corcoran, C. Armstrong, et al. Transdermal testosterone administration in women with acquired immunodeficiency syndrome wasting: a pilot study. *J. Clin. Endocrinol. Metab.* 1998; 83 (3): 2717–2725.

7. Grinspoon, S., C. Corcoran, K. Lee, et al. Loss of lean body and muscle mass correlates with androgen levels in hypogonadal men with acquired immunodeficiency syndrome and wasting. *J. Clin. Endocrinol. Metab.* 1997; 81 (11): 4051–4058.

8. Sattler, F., W. Briggs, I. Antonipillai, et al. Low dihydrotestosterone and weight loss in the AIDS wasting syndrome. *J. Acquir. Immune. Defic. Syndr. Hum. Retrovirol.* 1998; 18 (3): 246–251.

9. Dobs, A.S. Androgen therapy in AIDS wasting. *Baillieres Clin. Endocrinol. Metab.* 1998; 12 (3): 379–390.

10. Croxson, T.S., W.E. Chapman, L.K. Miller, et al. Changes in the hypothalamic-pituitary-gonadal axis in human immunodeficiency virus–infected homosexual men. *J. Clin. Endocrinol. Metab.* 1989; 68 (2): 317–321.

11. Christeff, N., S. Gharakhanian, N. Thobie, et al. Evidence for changes in adrenal and testicular steroids during HIV infection. *J. Acquir. Immune. Defic. Syndr.* 1992; 5 (8): 841–846.

12. Honour, J.W., M.A. Schneider, and R.F. Miller. Low adrenal androgens in men with HIV infection and the acquired immunodeficiency syndrome. *Horm. Res.* 1995; 44 (1): 35–39.

13. Christeff, N., N. Gherbi, O. Mammes, et al. Serum cortisol and DHEA concentrations during HIV infection. *Psychoneuroendocrinology* 1997; 22 (Suppl. 1): S11–S18.

14. Laudat, A., L. Blum, J. Geuchot, et al. Changes in systemic gonadal and adrenal steroids in asymptomatic human immunodeficiency virus–infected men: relationship with the CD4 cell counts. *Eur. J. Endocrinol.* 1995; 133 (4): 418–424.

15. Kopicko, J.J., I. Momodu, A. Adedokun, et al. Characteristics of HIV-infected men with low serum testosterone levels. *Int. J. STD AIDS* 1999; 19 (12): 817–820.

16. Ferrando, S.J., J.G. Rabkin, and L. Poretsky. Dehydroepiandrosterone sulfate (DHEAS) and testosterone: relation to HIV illness stage and progression over one year. *J. Acquir. Immune. Defic. Syndr.* 1999; 22 (2): 146–154.

17. Schiffito, G., M.P. McDermott, T. Evans, et al. Autonomic performance and dehydroepiandrosterone sulfate levels in HIV-1–infected individuals: relationship to TH1 and TH2 cytokine profile. *Arch. Neurol.* 2000; 57 (7): 1027–1032.

18. Jacobson, M.A., R.E. Fusaro, M. Galmarini, et al. Decreased serum dehydroepiandrosterone is associated with an increased progression of human immunodeficiency virus infection in men with CD4 cell counts of 200–499. *J. Infect. Dis.* 1991; 164 (5): 864–868.

19. Mulder, J.W., P.H. Frissen, P.l. Krijnen, et al. Dehydroepiandrosterone as a predictor for progression to AIDS in asymptomatic human immunodeficiency virus–infected men. *J. Infect. Dis.* 1992; 165 (3): 413–418.

20. Yang, J.Y., A. Schwartz, and E.E. Henderson. Inhibition of HIV-1 latency reactivation by dehydroepiandrosterone (DHEA) and an analogue of DHEA. *AIDS Res. Hum. Retroviruses* 1993; 9 (8): 747–754.

21. Laudat, A., L. Blum, J. Geuchot, et al. Changes in systemic gonadal and adrenal steroids in asymptomatic human immunodeficiency virus–infected men: relationship with the DC4 cell counts. *Eur. J. Endocrinol.* 1995; 133 (4): 418–424.

22. Christeff, N., O. Lortholary, P. Casassus, et al. Relationship between sex steroid hormone levels and CD4 lymphocytes in HIV infected men. *Exp. Clin. Endocrinol. Diabetes* 1996; 104 (2): 130–136.

23. Cofrancesco, J., J.J. Whalen, and A.S. Dobs. Testosterone replacement treatment options for HIV-infected men. *J. Acquir. Immune. Defic. Syndr. Hum. Retrovirol.* 1997; 16 (4): 254–265.

24. Schifitto, G., M.P. McDermott, T. Evans, et al. Autonomic performance and dehydroepiandrosterone sulfate levels in HIV-1–infected individuals: relationship to TH1 and TH2 cytokine profile. *Arch. Neurol.* 2000; 57 (7): 1027–1032.

25. Grinspoon, S., C. Corcoran, K. Lee, et al. Loss of lean body and muscle mass correlates androgen levels in hypogonadal men with acquired immunodeficiency syndrome and wasting. *J. Clin. Endocrinol. Metab.* 1996; 81 (11): 4051–4058.

26. Grinspoon, S., C. Corcoran, T. Stanley, et al. Effects of androgen administration on the growth hormone-insulin-like growth factor 1 axis in men with acquired immunodeficiency syndrome wasting. *J. Clin. Endocrinol. Metab.* 1998; 83 (12): 4251–4256.

27. Bhasin, S., T.W. Storer, N. Asbel-Sethi, et al. Effects of testosterone replacement with a nongenital, transdermal system, Androderm, in human immunodeficiency virus–infected men with low testosterone levels. *J. Clin. Endocrinol. Metab.* 1998; 83 (9): 3155–3162.

28. Grinspoon, S., C. Corcoran, H. Askari, et al. Effects of androgen administration in men with the AIDS wasting syndrome. A randomized, double-blind, placebo-controlled trial. *Ann. Intern. Med.* 1998; 129 (1): 18–26.

29. Miller, K., C. Corcoran, C. Armstrong, et al. Transdermal testosterone administration in women with acquired immunodeficiency syndrome wasting: a pilot study. *J. Clin. Endocrinol. Metab.* 1998; 83 (8): 2717–2725.

30. Van Loan, M.D., A. Strawford, M. Jacob, et al. Monitoring changes in fat-free mass in HIV-positive men with hypotestosteronemia and AIDS wasting syndrome treated with gonadal hormone replacement therapy. *AIDS* 1999; 13 (2): 241–248.

31. Strawford, A., T. Barbieri, R. Neeze, et al. Effects of nandrolone decanoate therapy in borderline hypogonadal men with HIV-associated weight loss. *J. Acquir. Immune. Defic. Syndr. Hum. Retrovirol.* 1999; 20 (2): 137–146.

32. Wagner, G.J., J.G. Rabkin, and R. Rabkin. Testosterone and a treatment for fatigue in HIV+ men. *Gen. Hosp. Psychiatry* 1998; 20 (4): 209–213.

33. Rabkin, J.C., G.J. Wagner, and R. Rabkin. A double-blind, placebo-controlled trial of testosterone therapy for HIV-positive men with hypogonadal symptoms. *Arch. Gen. Psychiatry* 2000; 57 (2): 141–147.

34. Rabkin, J.G., S.J. Ferando, G.J. Wagner, et al. DHEA treatment for HIV+ patients: effects on mood, androgenic and anabolic parameters. *Psychoneuroendocrinology* 2000; 25 (1): 53–68.

35. Grinspoon, S., C. Corcoran, E. Anderson, et al. Sustained anabolic effects of long-term androgen administration in men with AIDS wasting. *Clin. Infect. Dis.* 1999; 28 (3): 634–636.

36. Wagner, G.J., and J.G. Rabkin. Testosterone therapy for clinical symptoms of hypogonadism in eugonadal men with AIDS. *Int. J. STD AIDS* 1998; 9 (1): 41–44.

37. Grinspoon, S., C. Corcoran, T. Stanley, et al. Effects of hypogonadism and testosterone administration on depression indices in HIV-infected men. *J. Clin. Endocrinol. Metab.* 2000; 85 (1): 60–65.

38. Wagner, G., J. Rabkin, and R. Rabkin. Exercise as a mediator of psychological and nutritional effects of testosterone therapy in HIV+ men. *Med. Sci. Sports Exerc.* 1998; 30 (6): 811–817.

39. Romeyn, M., and N. Gunn. Resistance exercise and oxandrolone for men with HIV-related weight loss. *JAMA* 2000; 284 (2): 176.

40. Berger, J.R. Resistance exercise and oxandrolone for men with HIV-related weight loss. *JAMA* 2000; 284 (2): 176.

41. Bhasin, S., T.W. Storer, M. Javanbakht, et al. Testosterone replacement and resistance exercise in HIV-infected men with weight loss and low testosterone levels. *JAMA* 2000; 283 (6): 763–770.

42. Strawford, A., T. Barbieri, M. Van Loan, et al. Resistance exercise and supraphysiologic androgen therapy in eugonadal men with HIV-related weight loss: a randomized controlled trial. *JAMA* 1999; 281 (14): 1282–1290.

43. Sattler, F.R., S.V. Jaque, E.T. Schroeder, et al. Effects of pharmacological doses of nandrolone decanoate and progressive resistance training in immunodeficient patients infected with human immunodeficiency virus. *J. Clin. Endocrinol. Metab.* 1999; 84 (4): 1268–1276.

44. Grinspoon, S., C. Corcoran, K. Parlman, et al. Effects of testosterone and progressive resistance training in eugonadal men with AIDS wasting. A randomized, controlled trial. *Ann. Intern. Med.* 2000; 133 (5): 348–355.

45. Calabrese, L.H., S.M. Kleiner, B.P. Barna, et al. The effects of anabolic steroids and strength training on the human immune response. *Med. Sci. Sports Exerc.* 1989; 21 (4): 386–392.

46. Segal, D.M., M. Perez, and P. Shapshak. Oxandrolone, used for treatment of wasting disease in HIV-1–infected patients, does not diminish the antiviral activity of deoxyneucleoside analogues in lymphocyte and macrophage cell cultures. *J. Acquir. Immune. Defic. Syndr. Hum. Retrovirol.* 1999; 20 (3): 215–219.

47. Crist, D.M., G.T. Peake, L.T. Mackinnon, et al. Exogenous growth hormone treatment alters body composition and increases natural killer cell activity in women with impaired endogenous growth hormone secretion. *Metabolism* 1987; 36 (12): 1115–1117.

48. Schambelan, M., K. Mulligan, C. Grunfeld, et al. Recombinant human growth hormone in patients with HIV-associated wasting. A randomized, placebo-controlled trial. Serostim Study Group. *Ann. Intern. Med.* 1996; 125 (11): 873–882.

49. S. Hirschfeld. Use of human recombinant growth hormone and human recombinant insulin-like growth factor-1 in patients with human immunodeficiency virus infection. *Horm. Res.* 1996; 46 (4–5): 215–221.

50. Cofrancesco, J., J.J. Whalen, and A.S. Dobs. Testosterone replacement treatment options for HIV-infected men. *J. Acquir. Immune. Defic. Syndr. Hum. Retrovirol.* 1997; 16 (4): 254–265.

51. Dobs, A.S. Androgen therapy in AIDS wasting. *Baillieres Clin. Endocrinol. Metab.* 1998; 12 (3): 379–390.

52. Schwenk, A. HIV infection and malnutrition. *Curr. Opin. Clin. Nutr. Metab. Care* 1998; 1 (4): 375–380.

53. Nemechek, P.M., B. Polsky, M.S. Gottlieb. Treatment guidelines for HIV-associated wasting. *Mayo Clin. Proc.* 2000; 75 (4): 386–394.

54. Mulligan, K., V.W. Tai, and M. Schambelan. Use of growth hormone and other anabolic agents in AIDS wasting. *J. Parenter. Enteral. Nutr.* 1999; 23 (6 Suppl.): S202–209.

16

Rationale for Anabolic Therapy in Burns and Major Thermal Injuries

Introduction: A Prolonged Major Catabolic Condition

Endocrine responses to major thermal injuries can result in a major catabolic state associated with losses in lean body mass and compromised wound healing potentials. It has been shown that with proper nutrition, reduction of stress, use of resistance exercise, and the addition of pharmacologic anabolic agents, lean body mass can be restored and wound healing promoted and hastened.[1] Pharmacologic anabolic therapy attenuates and reverses net catabolism and sarcopenia, reduces the associated psychiatric effects, hastens and improves wound healing, improves rehabilitation index and outcomes, and reduces inpatient rehabilitation periods after major burn injures.[2, 3, 4, 5]

Hypoandrogenemia and Hyposomatomedinemia in Major Burns

Hypoandrogenemia associated with major thermal injuries has been well established for over two decades. Reduced androgen production has been attributed to dysfunction of both the hypothalamic-pituitary-gonadal axis and the hypothalamic-pituitary-adrenal axis in both genders.[6, 7, 8, 9, 10, 11, 12, 13, 14, 15] In burned men, it has been shown that the more severe the burns, the lower the androgen levels, and that luteinizing hormone (LH) and testosterone levels are below normal in the days post burn and remain in the low to midnormal range thereafter.[16] In both genders, major burns have been shown to significantly reduce adrenal androgen production acutely and during the postburn period and weeks thereafter.[17, 18]

Besides the reduction in anabolic potentials that occurs directly with hypoandrogenemia, patients who survive major thermal injuries have other reductions in anabolic potentials. Low circulating levels of insulin-like growth factor-1 (IGF-1) (hyposomatomedinemia) has been shown to be associated with thermal injuries[19, 20, 21] both acutely and for several weeks during the postburn period.[22] Thermal injury-induced hyposomatomedinemia has been shown to occur with low or elevated growth hormone (GH) levels.[23]

Hypoandrogenemia contributes to the hyposomatomedinemia in patients who have sustained significant burn injuries. It has been shown that growth hormone-releasing hormone (GHRH) action is reduced during severe illness (usually greater in men than women) that accompanies profound hypoandrogenemia.[24] Moreover, it has been shown that androgens directly stimulate the GHRH-GH-IGF-IGFBP axis by increasing GH secretion and elevating circulating IGF-1, free IGF-1, and IGFBP (insulin-like growth factor binding protein) levels in normal, hypogonadal, and aging individuals[25, 26, 27, 28, 29, 30] by a direct stimulatory effect on the hypothalamus that increases GHRH pulse amplitudes.[31, 32]

Complications and Sequelae of Thermal Injury-Induced Hypoandrogenemia and Hyposomatomedinemia

Survivors of major thermal injuries have a number of complications and sequelae that are associated with hypoandrogenemia and hyposomatomedinemia acutely, during the postburn rehabilitation period, and beyond. These include sarcopenia, osteoporosis, depression, reduced fibrinolysis, infection, anemia, pathologic cytokine profile, and depressed immune system function.[33, 34, 35, 36, 37, 38, 39, 40, 41, 42, 43, 44, 45, 46]

Studies of Anabolic Therapy for Major Thermal Injuries

Patients who have survived major burn injuries are in an extreme and prolonged catabolic state. Therefore, pharmacologic anabolic therapies should be considered in the medical management of these patients during all phases of postburn therapy. Numerous studies have shown that anabolic therapies (with androgens, GH, and IGF-1) have multifaceted and beneficial influences on the survival, healing rates, and rehabilitation of patients with substantial thermal injuries. The results from the available studies on anabolic therapy in burn victims, obtained from experimental animal models and human studies, have shown that:

(1) androgen therapy has a beneficial effect on the immune system and cytokine balance.[47, 48, 49]

(2) androgen therapy prevents further postburn tissue destruction caused by progressive ischemia.[50]

(3) androgen therapy hastens the healing processes of and oxygen delivery to dermal, conjunctival, and other damaged tissues.[51, 52, 53, 54, 55, 56, 57, 58]

(4) androgen therapy enhances the synthesis of dermal, synovial, muscle, and bone tissues.[59, 60, 61, 62, 63]

(5) androgen therapy normalizes fibrinolysis and reduces the incidence of superficial and deep vein thrombosis, arterial occlusions, and cutaneous vasculitis.[64, 65, 66, 67, 68, 69, 70, 71, 72, 73, 74, 75, 76, 77, 78, 79]

(6) androgen therapy enhances collagen synthesis via local growth factor stimulation.[80, 81]

(7) androgen therapy restores appetite, restores nitrogen balance, and increases lean body mass and enhances wound healing.[82, 83, 84]

(8) androgen therapy hastens recovery, decreases rehabilitation time, and improves physical therapy modalities in burn patients over and above nutritional optimization alone.[85]

(9) androgen therapy is equal or superior to GH in the safety, cost, and efficacy parameters for the treatment of severe burn injuries.[86]

(10) androgen therapy modulates depression and dysthymia associated with major thermal injuries.[87]

(11) androgen therapy results in a 30 percent decrease in length of stay in the burn rehabilitation unit regardless of the age of the patient.[88]

(12) anabolic therapy with recombinant human growth hormone (rhGH) or recombinant human insulin-like growth factor-1 (rhIGF-1) provides an anabolic stimulus, reduces healing times, and improves mortality rates of severely burned patients over and above nutritional therapies alone.[89, 90, 91, 92, 93]

Summary

In this chapter, the rationale and supportive scientific evidence for the use of anabolic therapy in patients who have sustained major thermal injures has been presented. The use of anabolic agents should be considered as an appropriate, safe, and effective method to counteract and reverse the pronounced catabolic state that accompanies major burns.

Androgen therapy should be considered the cornerstone of anabolic therapy for severely burned patients. The regimen that has been routinely studied has been oxandrolone (20 mg/day) in both genders. Other logical choices could include stanozolol (10–20 mg/day), nandrolone decanoate (100–200mg IM weekly), or various testosterone preparations.

Other anabolic agents (rhGH and rhIGF-1) have also been shown to reverse catabolism and induce anabolism in patients after major thermal injuries. It is likely that other anabolic agents may be investigated for this purpose, including GH secretagogues, GHRH analogues, and other anabolic and trophic agents.

Perhaps the best regimen for anabolic therapy in life-threatening thermal injuries would be a combination of anabolic agents, such as androgens combined with one or more of the recombinant anabolic agents that drive the GHRH-GH-IGF-IGFBP axis. Future research is warranted to delineate the best use of these anabolic therapies in severely burned patients.

In summary, anabolic therapy has been shown to increase survival rates, reduce infection risks, hasten and promote the healing of burned tissues, reduce postburn rehabilitation times and complications, modulate postburn mental depression, modulate cytokine profiles, normalize fibrinolysis, and improve physical therapy indices in patients who have sustained major thermal injuries. Androgen therapy alone, or in combination with other anabolic agents, should become a substantial part of the standard of care for patients in all phases of postburn recovery.

Notes

1. Demling, R.H., and L. DeSanti. Involuntary weight loss and the nonhealing wound: the role of anabolic agents. *Adv. Wound Care* 1999; 12 (1 Suppl.): 1–14.

2. Demling, R.H., and L. DeSanti. Oxandrolone, an anabolic steroid, significantly increases the rate of weight gain in the recovery phase after major burns. *J. Trauma* 1997; 43 (1): 47–51.

3. Demling, R.H. Comparison of the anabolic effects and complications of human growth hormone and the testosterone analogue, oxandrolone, after severe burn injury. *Burns* 1999; 25 (3): 215–221.

4. Morton, R., O. Gleason, and W. Yates. Psychiatric effects of anabolic steroids after burn injuries. *Psychosomatics* 2000; 41 (1): 66–68.

5. Demling, R.H., and D.P. Orgill. The anticatabolic and wound healing effects of the testosterone analogue oxandrolone after severe burn injury. *J. Crit. Care* 2000; 15 (1): 12–17.

6. Dolecek, R., M. Adamkaova, T. Sorornikova, et al. Syndrome of afterburn peripheral endocrine gland involvement — very low plasma testosterone levels in burned male patients. *Acta Chir. Plast.* 1979; 21 (2): 114–119.

7. Diem, E., R. Schmid, W.H. Schneider, et al. The influence of burn trauma on the hypothalamus-pituitary axis in normal female subjects. *Scand. J. Plast. Reconstr. Surg.* 1979; 13 (1): 17–20.

8. Dolecek, R., M. Adamkova, T. Sotornikova, et al. Endocrine response after burn. *Scand. J. Plast. Reconstr. Surg.* 1979; 13 (1): 9–16.

9. Dolecek, R., C. Dvoracek, M. Jezek, et al. Very low serum testosterone levels and severe impairment of spermatogenesis in burned male patients. Correlations with basal levels and levels of FSH, LH, and PRL after LHRH + TRH. *Endocrinol. Exp.* 1983; 33–45.

10. Balogh, D., R. Moncayo, and M. Bauer. Hormonal dysregulations in severe burns. *Burns Incl. Therm. Inj.* 1984; 10 (4): 257–263.

11. Vogel, A.V., G.T. Peake, and R.T. Rada. Pituitary-testicular axis dysfunction in burned men. *J. Clin. Endocrinol. Metab.* 1985; 60 (4): 658–665.

12. Semple, C.G., W.R. Robertson, R. Mitchell, et al. Mechanisms leading to hypogonadism in men with burn injuries. *Br. Med. J. (Clin. Res. Ed.)* 1987; 295 (6595): 403–407.

13. Semple, C.G., R. Mitchell, S. Hollis, et al. An investigation of LH pulsatility in burned men by bioassay and radioimmunoassay. *Acta Endocrinol. (Copen.)* 1992; 126 (5): 404–409.

14. Baker, H.W. Reproductive effects of nontesticular illness. *Endocrinol. Metab. Clin. North Am.* 1998; 27 (4): 831–850.

15. Gambineri, A., and R. Pasquali. Testosterone therapy in men: clinical and pharmacological perspectives. *J. Endocrinol. Invest.* 2000; 23 (3): 196–214.

16. Vogel, A.V., G.T. Peake, and R.T. Rada. Pituitary-testicular axis dysfunction in burned men. *J. Clin. Endocrinol. Metab.* 1985; 60 (4): 658–665.

17. Parker, C.R., and C.R. Baxter. Divergence in adrenal secretory pattern after thermal injury in adult patients. *J. Trauma* 1985; 25 (6): 508–510.

18. Semple, C.G., C.E. Gray, and G.H. Beastall. Adrenal androgens and illness. *Acta Endocrinol. (Copenh.)* 1987; 116 (1): 155–160.

19. Girard, J. [Growth hormone and its significance beyond growth. Current aspects of the effects of this model anabolic hormone.] *Schweiz Rundsch. Med. Prax.* 1993; 82 (32): 845–850.

20. Lal, S.O., S.E. Wolf, and D.N. Herndon. Growth hormone, burns and tissue healing. *Growth Horm. IGF Res.* 2000 (10 Suppl. B): S39–S43.

21. Lang, C.H., X. Liu, G.J. Nystrom, et al. Acute response of IGF-1 and IGF binding proteins induced by thermal injury. *Am. J. Physiol. Endocrinol. Metab.* 2000; 278 (6): E1087–E1096.

22. Abribat, T., B. Nedelec, N. Jobin, et al. Decreased serum insulin-like growth factor-1 in burn patients: relationship with serum insulin-like growth factor binding protein-3 proteolysis and the influence of lipid composition in nutritional support. *Crit. Care Med.* 2000; 28 (7): 2366–2372.

23. Gianotti, L., F. Broglio, G. Aimaretti, et al. Low IGF-1 levels are often uncoupled with elevated GH levels in catabolic conditions. *J. Endocrinol. Invest.* 1998; 21 (2): 115–121.

24. Van den Berghe, G., R.C. Baxter, F. Weeks, et al. A paradoxical gender dissociation within the growth hormone/insulin-like growth factor 1 axis during protracted critical illness. *J. Clin. Endocrinol. Metab.* 2000; 85 (1): 183–192.

25. Hobbs, C.J., S.R. Plymate, C.J. Rosen, et al. Testosterone administration

increases insulin-like growth factor-1 levels in normal men. *J. Clin. Endocrinol. Metab.* 1994; 78 (6): 1360–1367.

26. Morales, A.J., J.J. Nolan, J.C. Nelson, et al. Effects of replacement dose of dehydroepiandrosterone in men and women of advancing age. *J. Clin. Endocrinol. Metab.* 1994; 78 (6): 1360–1367.

27. Gelato, M.C., and R.A. Frost. IGFBP. Functional and structural implications in aging and wasting syndromes. *Endocrine* 1997; 7 (1): 81–85.

28. Casson, P.R., N. Santoro, K. Elkind-Hirch, et al. Postmenopausal dehydroepiandrosterone administration increases free insulin-like growth factor-1 and decreases high-density lipoprotein: a six month trial. *Fertil. Steril.* 1998; 70 (1): 107–110.

29. Jorgensen, J.O., N. Vahl, T.B. Hansen, et al. Determinants of serum insulin-like growth factor 1 in growth hormone deficient adults as compared to healthy subjects. *Clin. Endocrinol. (Oxf.)* 2000; 48 (4): 479–486.

30. Span, J.P., G.F. Pieters, C.G. Sweep, et al. Gender difference in insulin-like growth factor 1 response to growth hormone (GH) treatment and GH-deficient adults: role of sex hormone replacement. *J. Clin. Endocrinol. Metab.* 2000; 85 (3): 1121–1125.

31. Eakman, G.D., J.S. Dallas, S.W. Ponder, et al. The effects of testosterone and dihydrotestosterone on hypothalamic regulation of growth hormone secretion. *J. Clin. Endocrinol. Metab.* 1996; 81 (3): 1217–1223.

32. Fryberg, D.A., A. Weltman, L.A. Jahn, et al. Short-term modulation of the androgen milieu alters pulsatile, but not exercise- or growth hormone (GH)-releasing hormone-stimulated GH secretion in health men: impact of gonadal steroid and GH secretory changes on metabolic outcomes. *J. Clin. Endocrinol. Metab.* 1997; 82 (11): 3710–3719.

33. Andes, W.A., P.W. Rogers, J.W. Beason, et al. The erythropoietin response to the anemia of thermal injury. *J. Lab. Clin. Med.* 1976; 88 (4): 584–592.

34. Wallner, S.F., and R. Vautrin. The anemia of thermal injury: mechanism of inhibition of erythropoiesis. *Proc. Soc. Exp. Biol. Med.* 1986; 181 (1): 144–150.

35. Vasko, S.D., J.J. Burdge, R.L. Ruberg, et al. Evaluation of erythropoietin levels in the anemia of thermal injury. *J. Burn Care Rehabil.* 1991; 12 (5): 437–441.

36. Kowal-Vern, A., R.L. Gamelli, J.M. Walenga, et al. The effect of burn wound size on hemostasis: a correlation of the hemostatic changes to the clinical state. *J. Trauma* 1992; 33 (1): 50–56.

37. Pandit, S.K., C.N. Malla, H.U. Zarger, et al. A study of bone and joint changes secondary to burns. *Burns* 1993; 19 (3): 227–228.

38. Araneo, B., and R. Daynes. Dehydroepiandrosterone functions as more than an antiglucocorticoid in preserving immunocompetence after thermal injury. *Endocrinology* 1995; 136 (2): 393–401.

39. Still, J.M., K. Belcher, E.J. Law, et al. A double-blind prospective evaluation of recombinant human erythropoietin in acutely burned patients. *J. Trauma* 1995; 38 (2): 233–236.

40. Frost, H.M. Osteoporosis treatment: quo vadis? (A brief overview). *Medicina (B. Aires)* 1997; 57 (Suppl. 1): 119–126.

41. Kowal-Vern, A., M.M. Sharp-Pucci, J.M. Valenga, et al. Trauma and thermal injury: comparison of hemostatic and cytokine changes in the acute phase of injury. *J. Trauma* 1998; 44 (2): 325–329.

42. Garcia-Avello, A., J.A. Lorente, J. Cesar-Perez, et al. Degree of hypercoagulability and hyperfibrinolysis is related to organ failure and prognosis after burn trauma. *Thromb. Res.* 1998; 89 (2): 59–64.

43. Peteiro-Cartelle, F.J., and A. Alvarez-Jorge. Dynamic profiles of interleukin-6 and the soluble form of CD25 in burned patients. *Burns* 1999; 25 (6): 487–491.

44. Fauerbach, J.A., L.J. Heinberg, J.W. Lawrence, et al. Effect of early body image dissatisfaction on subsequent psychological and physical adjustment after disfiguring injury. *Psychosom. Med.* 2000; 62 (4): 576–582.

45. Menzies, V. Depression and burn wounds. *Arch. Psychiatr. Nurs.* 2000; 14 (4): 199–206.

46. Van Loey, N.E., A.W. Faber, and L.A. Taal. A European hospital survey to determine the extent of psychological services offered to patients with severe burns. *Burns* 2001; 27 (1): 23–31.

47. Araneo, B.A., J. Shelby, G.Z. Li, et al. Administration of dehydroepiandrosterone to burned mice preserves normal immunologic competence. *Arch. Surg.* 1993; 128 (3): 318–325.

48. Araneo, B., and R. Daynes. Dehydroepiandrosterone functions as more than an antiglucocorticoid in preserving immunocompetence after thermal injury. *Endocrinology* 1995; 136 (2): 393–401.

49. Zofkova, I., R.L. Kancheva, and R. Hampl. A decreasing CD4+/CD8+ ratio after one month of treatment of stanozolol in postmenopausal women. *Steroids* 1995; 60 (7): 430–433.

50. Araneo, B.A., S.Y. Ryu, S. Barton, et al. Dehydroepiandrosterone reduces progressive dermal ischemia caused by thermal injury. *J. Surg. Res.* 1995; 59 (2): 250–262.

51. Fittipaldi, L., F. Giacomini, and B. Rizzi. [Topical action on anabolic steroid (methandrostenolone) on the healing process of non extensive second and third degree burns.] *Biol. Lat.* 1965; 18 (1): 59–75.

52. Giacomini, F., B Rizzi, and E. Terni. [Research on the action of methandrostenolone in experimental third degree burns.] *Biol. Lat.* 1965; 18 (1): 45–57.

53. Roman Calderon, J. [Studies of the effect of a new anabolic agent in burned patients.] *Prensa Med. Mex.* 1968; 33 (1): 51–53.

54. Marpillero, P., and F. Dani. [On the local activity of an anabolizing agent in the repair processes of cutaneous lesions. Clinical study.] *Minerva Dermatol.* 1968; 43 (4): 182–184.

55. Kowalewski, K., and S. Yong. Dermal collagen response to experimental thermal injury in normal and in steroid hormone-treated rats. *Can. J. Surg.* 1969; 12 (3): 342–350.

56. Falanga, V., and W.H. Eaglstein. A therapeutic approach to venous ulcers. *J. Am. Acad. Dermatol.* 1986; 14 (5 Pt.1): 777–784.

57. Davletov, E.G., R.M. Saliakhova, and F.K. Kamilov. [Effect of retabol and oxymetacyl on protein metabolism in experimental burns in immature rats.] *Vopr. Med. Khim.* 1987; 33 (6): 51–56.

58. Stacey, M.C., K.G. Burnand, G.T. Layer, et al. Transcutaneous oxygen tensions in assessing the treatment of healed venous ulcers. *Br. J. Surg.* 1990; 77 (9): 1050–1054.

59. Vaishnav, R., J.N. Beresford, J.A. Gallagher, et al. Effects of the anabolic steroid stanozolol on cells derived from human bone. *Clin. Sci. (Colch.):* 1988; 74 (5): 455–460.

60. Ellis, A.J., J.K. Wright, T.E. Cawston, et al. The differential responses of human skin and synovial fibroblasts to stanozolol in vitro: production of prostaglandin E2 and matrix metalloproteinases. *Agents Actions* 1992; 35 (3–4): 232–237.

61. Wolfe, R., A. Ferrando, M. Sheffield-Moore, et al. Testosterone and muscle protein metabolism. *Mayo Clin. Proc.* 2000; 75 (Suppl.): S55–S59.

62. Sheffield-Moore, M. Androgens and the control of skeletal muscle protein synthesis. *Ann. Med.* 2000; 32 (3): 181–186.

63. Sheffield-Moore, M., R.R. Wolfe, D.C. Gore, et al. Combined effects of hyperaminoacidemia and oxandrolone on skeletal muscle protein synthesis. *Am. J. Physiol. Endocrinol. Metab.* 2000; 278 (2): E273–279.

64. Davidson, J.F., M. Lochhead, G.A. McDonald, et al. Fibrinolytic enhancement by stanozolol: a double blind trial. *Br. J. Haematol.* 1972; 22 (5): 543–559.

65. Davidson, J.F., G.A. McDonald, and J.A. Conkie. Fibrinolytic enhancement by stanozolol — a two year study. *Br. J. Haematol.* 1972; 22 (5): 639–640.

66. Walker, I.D., J.F Davidson, P. Young, et al. Plasma antithrombin III levels and plasma fibrinolytic activity following oral anabolic steroid therapy. *Monograph* 1976; 4: 85–95.

67. Cunliffe, W.J., B. Dodman, B.E. Roberts, et al. Clinical and laboratory double-blind investigation of fibrinolytic therapy of cutaneous vasculitis. *Monograph* 1976; 4: 325–333.

68. Jarrett, P.E., M. Morland, and N.L. Browse. Idiopathic recurrent superficial thrombophlebitis: treatment with fibrinolytic enhancement. *Br. Med.* 1977; 1 (6066): 933–934.

69. Burnand, K., G. Clemenson, M. Morland, et al. Venous lipodermatosclerosis: treatment by fibrinolytic enhancement and elastic compression. *Br. Med. J.* 1980; 280 (6206): 7–11.

70. Small, M., B.M. McArdle, G.D. Lowe, et al. The effect of intramuscular stanozolol on fibrinolysis and blood lipids. *Thromb. Res.* 1982; 28 (1): 27–36.

71. Kluft, C., F.E. Preston, R.G. Malia, et al. Stanozolol-induced changes in fibrinolysis and coagulation in healthy adults. *Thromb. Haemost.* 1984; 51 (2): 157–164.

72. Verheijen, J.H., D.C. Rijken, G.T. Chang, et al. Modulation of rapid plasminogen activator inhibitor in plasma by stanozolol. *Thromb. Haemost.* 1984; 51 (3): 396–397.

73. Noll, G., B. Lammle, and F. Duckert. Treatment with stanozolol before thrombolysis in patients with arterial occlusions. *Thromb. Res.* 1985; 37 (4): 529–532.

74. Sue-Ling, H.M., J.A. Davies, C.R. Prentice, et al. Effects of oral stanozolol in the prevention of postoperative deep vein thrombosis on fibrinolytic activity. *Thromb. Haemost.* 1985; 53 (1): 141–142.

75. Hessel, L.W., and C. Kluft. Advances in clinical fibrinolysis. *Clin. Haematol.* 1986; 15 (2): 443–463.

76. Small, M., C. Kluft, A.C. MacCuish, et al. Tissue plasminogen activator inhibition in diabetes mellitus. *Diabetes Care* 1989; 12 (9): 655–658.

77. McMullin, G.M., G.T. Watkin, P.D. Coleridge Smith, et al. Efficacy of fibrinolytic enhancement with stanozolol in the treatment of venous insufficiency. *Aust. N.Z. J. Surg.* 1991; 61 (4): 306–309.

78. Colgan, M.P., D.J. Moore, and D.G. Shanik. New approaches in the medical management of venous ulceration. *Angiology* 1993; 44 (2): 138–142.

79. Helfman, T., and V. Falanga. Stanozolol as a novel therapeutic agent in dermatology. *J. Am. Acad. Dermatol.* 1995; 33 (2 Pt. 1): 254–258.

80. Falanga, V., A.S. Greenberg, L. Zhou, et al. Stimulation of collagen synthesis by the anabolic steroid stanozolol. *J. Invest. Dermatol.* 1998; 111 (6): 1193–1197.

81. Falabella, A.F. American Academy of Dermatology 1998 Awards for Young Investigators in Dermatology. The anabolic steroid stanozolol upregulates collagen synthesis through the action of transforming growth factor-beta 1. *J. Am. Acad. Dermatol.* 1998; 39 (2 Pt.1): 272–273.

82. Demling, R., and L. DeSanti. Closure of the "non-healing wound" corresponds with correction of weight loss using the anabolic agent oxandrolone. *Ostomy Wound Manage.* 1998; 44 (10): 58–62.

83. Krasner, D.L., and A.E. Belcher. Oxandrolone restores appetite. An increase in weight helps heal wounds. *Am. J. Nurs.* 2000; 100 (11): 53.

84. Demling, R.H., and D.P. Orgill. The anticatabolic and wound healing effects

of the testosterone analogue oxandrolone after severe burn injury. *J. Crit. Care* 2000; 15 (1): 12–17.

85. Demling, R.H., and L. DeSanti. Oxandrolone, an anabolic steroid, significantly increases the rate of weight gain in the recovery phase after major burns. *J. Trauma* 1997; 43 (1): 47–51.

86. Demling, R.H. Comparison of the anabolic effects and complications of human growth hormone and the testosterone analogue, oxandrolone, after severe burn injury. *Burns* 1999; 25 (3): 215–221.

87. Morton, R., O. Gleason, and W. Yates. Psychiatric effects of anabolic steroids after burn injuries. *Psychosomatics* 2000; 41 (1): 66–68.

88. Demling, R.H., and L. DeSanti. The rate of restoration of body weight after burn injury, using the anabolic agent oxandrolone, is not age dependent. *Burns* 2001; 27 (1): 46–51.

89. Ziegler, T.R., L.S. Young, E. Ferrari-Baliviera, et al. Use of human growth hormone combined with nutritional support in a critical care unit. *J. Pareter. Enteral Nutr.* 1990; 14 (6): 574–581.

90. Knox, J., R. Demling, D. Wilmore, et al. Increased survival after major thermal injury: the effect of growth hormone therapy in adults. *J. Trauma* 1995; 39 (3): 526–530.

91. Jarrar, D., S.E. Wolf, M.G. Jeschke, et al. Growth hormone attenuates the acute-phase response to thermal injury. *Arch. Surg.* 1997; 132 (11): 1171–1175.

92. Singh, K.P., R. Prasad, P.S. Chari, et al. Effect of growth hormone therapy in burn patients on conservative treatment. *Burns* 1998; 24 (8): 733–738.

93. Lal, S.O., S.E. Wolf, and D.N. Herndon. Growth hormone, burns and tissue healing. *Growth Horm. IGF Res.* 2000; 10 (Suppl. B): S39–S43.

17

Rationale for Anabolic Therapy in Cancer Patients

Introduction: The Anorexia/Cachexia Syndrome: Description and Pharmacologic Management

Anorexia (reduced or loss of appetite) is a primary symptom seen in the majority of patients with cancer. It is frequently not seen as a symptom requiring management in the same proactive manner as pain, nausea, or constipation. Anorexia, progressive wasting, weakness, fatigue, poor performance status, and impaired immune function are fundamental components of the complex phenomenon known as the anorexia/cachexia syndrome (ACS).[1] Diminished nutritional intake, maladaptive metabolic, endocrine, and catabolic processes, and increased metabolic expenditure all play roles in the development of this syndrome.[2] ACS can be seen in the full spectrum of cancer patient care settings: as a presenting complaint, defining condition, treatment-related toxicity, or as a hallmark of impending death.

The anorexia/cachexia syndrome may result from pain, depression or anxiety, taste and food aversions, chronic nausea, vomiting, early satiety, malfunction of the gastrointestinal system (delayed digestion, malabsorption, gastric stasis and associated emptying, or atrophic changes of the mucosa), metabolic shifts, cytokine action, production of substances by tumor cells, or iatrogenic causes such as chemotherapy and radiotherapy. The syndrome also involves metabolic and immune changes mediated by either the pathophysiological process of the tumor, or host-derived chemical factors such as peptides, neurotransmitters, cytokines, and lipid-mobilizing factors. The result is an acceleration of protein turnover, loss of body fat, and loss of body protein. Increased resting energy expenditure and constant negative energy balance in ACS can occur despite reduced dietary intake, indicating a systemic dysregulation of metabolism.[3]

ACS has a metabolic profile that is significantly different from that observed during simple starvation. Cytokines are proposed to participate in the development or progression of ACS and these include interleukin-1, interleukin-6, interferon-gamma, tumor necrosis factor-alpha, and brain-derived neurotrophic factor. The interactions of these cytokines with the neuroendocrine system, immune system, and neurotransmitters in various brain mechanisms merit significant attention for managing ACS.[4]

Treatment of ACS is not entirely satisfactory and should be directed toward improving the quality of life of the patient and should often include nutritional counseling.[5] Primary pharmacologic management of ACS includes use of orexigenic agents (appetite stimulants), anticatabolic agents (antimetabolic and anticytokine), and anabolic agents (primarily hormonal).[6] Numerous drugs (growth hormone, megestrol, cyproheptadine, tetrahydrocannabinol, androgens and anabolic steroids, prokinetic agents, and antidepressants) have been utilized with some success in treating ACS.[7] The anabolic agents that provide for a benefit to many of the aspects of ACS (orexigenic, antimetabolic, cytokine modulation, and anabolic) are androgens and anabolic steroids.

Hypoandrogenemia and Hyposomatomedinemia in Cancer Patients

Hypoandrogenemia and hyposomatomedinemia are associated with a number of cancer types and contribute to ACS. It has been shown that hypoandrogenemia:

(1) can be a preexisting condition associated with the development of certain cancers or subclinical subtypes of cancer, such as adult T-cell leukemia (ATL).[8]

(2) can be an acquired condition associated with certain cancers, including all types of leukemia[9, 10] and lung cancer.[11]

(3) can be an acquired condition associated with chemotherapy,[12, 13, 14, 15] radiation therapy, or a combination of both chemotherapy and radiation therapies.[16, 17, 18, 19]

(4) can be an acquired condition of corticosteroid therapy in cancer patients, especially after bone marrow transplantation.[20]

(5) can become a permanent condition in long-term cancer survivors, especially in those patients who were treated for cancer during childhood or adolescence.[21][22,23] Many of these patients require androgen therapy to induce delayed puberty and throughout life.[24][25,26,27,28]

Studies with Androgen Therapy for Cancer Patients

Androgen therapy has been considered by some physicians to be an important part of the overall treatment of cancer patients for decades.[29][30, 31, 32, 33, 34, 35, 36, 37, 38, 39, 40, 41, 42, 43, 44, 45, 46, 47, 48, 49, 50, 51, 52, 53, 54, 55] Some, but not all of these studies, have shown beneficial effects with androgen therapy in cancer patients, including:

(1) management of ACS and improved quality of life.

(2) prolonged remission periods in some studies.

(3) moderate increases in longevity in some studies.

(4) improved recovery from the catabolic sequelae of cytotoxic chemotherapy and corticosteroid therapy, including hematological parameters such as anemia, neutropenia, and thrombocytopenia. Androgen therapy remains a justified adjuvant therapy in selected cases.[56]

(5) enhanced fibrinolysis. Cancer patients show an increased susceptibility to develop thromboembolic diseases. Multiple risk factors associated with malignant disease contribute to a hypercoagulability state, including stasis induced by prolonged bed rest, vascular invasion by tumor, and iatrogenic complications including the use of central vein catheters and chemotherapy. Clinical manifestations vary from localized deep venous thrombosis and pulmonary embolism to disseminated intravascular coagulation.[57] It is well known that androgen therapy provides enhanced fibrinolysis through several mechanisms.

(6) correction of hypoandrogenemia and hyposomatomedinemia and their associated conditions such as sarcopenia, osteopenia, fatigue, weakness, depression, cognitive defects, pathologic cytokine profiles, reduced libido, sexual dysfunction, and reduced sense of well-being.

Summary

The evidence-based rationale for androgen therapy in cancer patients has been presented. Androgen therapy affords a multifaceted adjunctive therapy for patients with a variety of cancers. A substantial number of patients who become long-term survivors of cancer with chemotherapeutic and radiotherapeutic treatments will suffer from prolonged hypoandrogenemia and sexual dysfunction and may require prolonged androgen therapy.

Cancer patients make up a significant population of patients who can benefit from rehabilitation modalities. These modalities can be hastened and enhanced with androgen therapy in order to prevent or reverse the catabolic alterations brought about by the malignancy and the catabolic events brought about by various cancer treatments.

Notes

1. Ottery, F.D., D. Walsh, and A. Strawford. Pharmacologic management of anorexia/cachexia. *Semin. Oncol.* 1998; 25 (2 Suppl. 6): 35–44.

2. Puccio, M., and L. Nathanson. The cancer cachexia syndrome. *Semin. Oncol.* 1997; 24 (3): 277–287.

3. Plata-Salaman, C.R. Central nervous system mechanisms contributing to the cachexia-anorexia syndrome. *Nutrition* 2000; 16 (10): 1009–1012.

4. Plata-Salaman, C.R. Central nervous system mechanisms contributing to the cachexia-anorexia syndrome. *Nutrition* 2000; 16 (10): 1009–1012.

5. Puccio, M., and L. Nathanson. The cancer cachexia syndrome. *Semin. Oncol.* 1997; 24 (3): 277–287.

6. Ottery, F.D., D. Walsh, and A. Strawford. Pharmacologic management of anorexia/cachexia. *Semin. Oncol.* 1998; 25 (2 Suppl. 6): 35–44.

7. Morley, J.E. Anorexia in older persons: epidemiology and optimal treatment. *Drugs Aging* 1996; 8 (2): 134–155.

8. Uozumi, K., T. Uematsu, M. Otsuka, et al. Serum dehydroepiandrosterone and DHEA-sulfate in patients with adult T-cell leukemia and human T-lymphotropic virus type 1 carriers. *Am. J. Hematol.* 1996; 53 (3): 165–168.

9. Goncharova, N.D., and N.P. Goncharov. [Hormonal function of adrenal glands and gonads in patients with leukemia.] *Vopr. Onkol.* 1985; 31 (11): 54–59.

10. Uozumi, K., T. Uematsu, M. Otsuka, et al. Serum dehydroepiandrosterone and DHEA-sulfate in patients with adult T-cell leukemia and human T-lymphotropic virus type 1 carriers. *Am. J. Hematol.* 1996; 53 (3): 165–168.

11. Simons, J.P., A.M. Schols, W.A. Buurman, et al. Weight loss and low body cell mass in males with lung cancer: relationship with systemic inflammation, acute-phase response, resting energy expenditure, and catabolic and anabolic hormones. *Clin. Sci. (Colch.)* 1999; 97 (2): 215–223.

12. Wang, C., R.P. Ng, T.K. Chan, et al. Effect of combination chemotherapy on pituitary-gonadal function in patients with lymphoma and leukemia. *Cancer* 1980; 45 (8): 2030–2037.

13. Ise, T., K. Kishi, S. Imashuku, et al. Testicular histology and function following long-term chemotherapy of acute leukemia in children and outcome of the patients who received testicular biopsy. *Am. J. Pediatr. Hematol. Oncol.* 1986; 8 (4): 288–293.

14. Kreuser, E.D., W.D. Hetzel, D.O. Billia, et al. Gonadal toxicity following cancer therapy in adults: significance, diagnosis, prevention and treatment. *Cancer Treat. Rev.* 1990; 17 (2–3): 169–175.

15. Chatterjee, R., G.A. Haines, D.M. Perera, et al. Testicular and sperm DNA damage after treatment with fludarabine for chronic lymphocytic leukemia. *Hum. Reprod.* 2000; 15 (4): 762–766.

16. Carrascosa, A., L. Audi, J.J. Ortega. Hypothalamo-hypophyseal-testicular function in prepubertal boys with acute lymphoblastic leukemia following chemotherapy and testicular radiotherapy. *Acta Paediatr. Scand.* 1984; 73 (3): 364–371.

17. Kreuser, E.D., W.D. Hetzel, D.O. Billia, et al. Gonadal toxicity following cancer therapy in adults: significance, diagnosis, prevention, and treatment. *Cancer Treat. Rev.* 1990; 17 (2–3): 169–175.

18. Siimes, M.A., S.O. Lie, O. Andersen, et al. Prophylactic cranial irradiation increases the risk of testicular damage in adult males surviving ALL in childhood. *Med. Pediatr. Oncol.* 1993; 21 (2): 117–121.

19. Siimes, M.A., J. Rautonen, A. Makipernaa, et al. Testicular function in adult males surviving childhood malignancy. *Pediatr. Hematol. Oncol.* 1995; 12 (3): 231–241.

20. Bolme, P., B. Borgstrom, and K. Carlstrom. Longitudinal study of adrenocortical function following allogeneic bone marrow transplantation in children. *Horm. Res.* 1995; 43 (6): 279–285.

21. Siimes, M.A., and J. Rautonen. Small testicles with impaired production of sperm in adult male survivors of childhood malignancies. *Cancer* 1990; 65 (6): 1303–1306.

22. Siimes, M.A., S.O. Lie, O. Andersen, et al. Prophylactic cranial irradiation increases the risk of testicular damage in adult males surviving ALL in childhood. *Med. Pediatr. Oncol.* 1993; 21 (2): 117–121.

23. Relander, T., E. Cavallin-Stahl, S. Garwicz, et al. Gonadal and sexual function in men treated for childhood cancer. *Med. Pediatr. Oncol.* 2000; 35 (1): 52–63.

24. Didi, M., P.H. Morris–Jones, H.R. Gattamaneni, et al. Pubertal growth in response to testosterone replacement therapy for radiation-induced Leydig cell failure. *Med. Pediatr. Oncol.* 1994; 22 (4): 250–254.

25. Siimes, M.A., J. Routenen, A. Makipernaa, et al. Testicular function in adult males surviving childhood malignancy. *Pediatr. Hematol. Oncol.* 1995; 12 (3): 231–241.

26. Grundy, R.G., A.D. Leiper, R. Stanhope, et al. Survival and endocrine outcome after testicular relapse in acute lymphoblastic leukemia. *Arch. Dis. Child.* 1997; 76 (3): 190–196.

27. Mayer, E.I., R.E. Dopfer, T. Klingebiel, et al. Longitudinal gonadal function after bone marrow transplantation for acute lymphoblastic leukemia during childhood. *Pediatr. Transplant.* 1999; 3 (1): 38–44.

28. Humpl. T, P. Schramm, and P. Gutjahr. Male fertility in long-term survivors of childhood ALL. *Arch. Androl.* 1999; 43 (2): 123–129.

29. Jenkin, R.D. Androgens in metastatic renal adenocarcinoma. *Br. Med. J.* 1967; 1 (536): 361.

30. Host, H. [The place of anabolic steroids in cancer therapy.] *Tidsskr. Nor. Laegeforen* 1969; 89 (6): 417–418.

31. Sotto, J.J., D. Hollard, R. Schaerer, et al. [Androgens and prolonged complete remissions in acute non lymphoblastic leukemias. Results of a systematic treatment with stanozolol associated with chemotherapy. *Nouv. Rev. Fr. Hematol.* 1975; 15 (1): 57–72.

32. Hollard, D., J.J. Sotto, C. Bachelot, et al. [Trial of androgen therapy in the treatment of non-lymphoblastic acute leukemia. First results.] *Nouv. Presse. Med.* 1976; 5 (20): 1289–1293.

33. Perloff, M., R.D. Hart, and J.F. Holland. Vinblastin, adriamycin, thiotepa, and halotestin (VATH): therapy for advanced breast cancer refractory to prior chemotherapy. *Cancer* 1978; 42 (6): 2534–2537.

34. Hollard, D., J.J. Sotto, R. Berthier, et al. High rate of long-term survivals in AML treated by chemotherapy and androgen therapy: a pilot study. *Cancer.* 1980; 45 (7): 1540–1548.

35. Westberg, H. Tamoxifen and fluoxymesterone in advanced breast cancer: a controlled clinical trial. *Cancer Treat. Rep.* 1980; 64 (1): 117–121.

36. Spiers, A.S., S.F. DeVita, M.J. Allar, et al. Beneficial effects of an anabolic steroid during cytotoxic chemotherapy for metastatic cancer. *J. Med.* 1981; 12 (6): 433–435.

37. Hart, R.D., M. Perloff, and J.F. Holland. One-day VATH (vinblastine, adriamycin, thiotepa, and halotestin) therapy for advanced breast cancer refractory to chemotherapy. *Cancer* 1981; 48 (7): 1522–1527.

38. Mandelli, F., S. Amadori, E. Dini, et al. Randomized clinical trial of immunotherapy and androgentherapy for remission maintenance in acute non-lymphocytic leukemia. *Leuk. Res.* 1981; 5 (6): 447–452.

39. Feffer, S.E., D.W. Westring, A.C. Lee, et al. A case of leukemia reticuloendotheliosis responding to oxymetholone. *Cancer* 1982; 50 (3): 396–400.

40. Muss, H.B., D. Case, M.R. Cooper, et al. Cytotoxic chemotherapy and androgen priming in patients with advanced carcinoma of the prostate. A phase II trial of the Piedmont Oncology Association. *Am. J. Clin. Oncol.* 1985; 8 (5): 396–400.

41. Chlebowski, R.T., H. Herrold, I. Ali, et al. Influence of nandrolone decanoate on weight loss in advanced non-small cell lung cancer. *Cancer* 1986; 58 (1): 183–186.

42. Hayat, M., U. Jehn, R. Willemze, et al. A randomized comparison of maintenance treatment with androgens, immunotherapy, and chemotherapy in adult acute myelogenous leukemia. A Leukemia-Lymphoma Group Trial of the EORTC. *Cancer* 1986; 58 (3): 617–623.

43. Kellokumpu-Lehtinen, P., R. Houvinen, and R. Johansson, et al. Hormonal treatment of advanced breast cancer. A randomized trial of tamoxifen versus nandrolone decanoate. *Cancer* 1987; 60 (10): 2376–2381.

44. Kavanagh, J.J., J.T. Wharton, and W.S. Roberts. Androgen therapy in the treatment of refractory epithelial ovarian cancer. *Cancer Treat. Rep.* 1987; 71 (5): 537–538.

45. Swain, S.M., S.M. Steinberg, C. Bagley, et al. Tamoxifen and fluoxymesterone versus tamoxifen and danazol in metastatic breast cancer — a randomized study. *Breast Cancer Res. Treat.* 1988; 12 (1): 51–57.

46. Ingle, J.N., D.I. Twito, D.J. Schaid, et al. Randomized clinical trial of tamoxifen alone or combined with fluoxymesterone in postmenopausal women with metastatic breast cancer. *J. Clin. Oncol.* 1988; 6 (5): 825–831.

47. Pain, J.A., S.S. Wickresinghe, and J.W. Bradbeer. Combined tamoxifen and anabolic steroid as primary treatment for breast carcinoma in the elderly. *Eur. J. Surg. Oncol.* 1990; 16 (3): 225–228.

48. Daniel, F., D.G. Rao, and C.J. Tyrrell. A pilot study of stanozolol for advanced breast carcinoma. *Cancer* 1991; 67 (12): 2966–2968.

49. Ingle, J.N., D.I. Twito, D.J. Schaid, et al. Combination hormonal therapy with tamoxifen plus fluoxymesterone versus tamoxifen alone in postmenopausal women with metastatic breast cancer. An updated analysis. *Cancer* 1991; 67 (4): 886–891.

50. Schifeling, D.J., D.V. Jackson, P.J. Zekan, et al. Fluoxymesterone as third line endocrine therapy for advanced breast cancer. A phase II trial of the Piedmont Oncology Association. *Am. J. Clin. Oncol.* 1992; 15 (3): 233–235.

51. Quaglino, D., G. Di Leonardo, N. Furia, et al. Therapeutic management of hematological malignancies in elderly patients. Biological and clinical considerations. Part III. The chronic leukemias and myelfibrosis. *Aging (Milano)* 1997; 9 (6): 383–390.

52. Colleoni, M., A. Coates, O. Pagni, et al. Combined chemo-endocrine adjuvant

therapy for patients with operable breast cancer: still a question? *Cancer Treat. Res.* 1998; 24 (1): 15–26.

53. Darnton, S.J., B. Zgainski, I. Grenier, et al. The use of an anabolic steroid (nandrolone decanoate) to improve nutritional status after esophageal resection for carcinoma. *Dis. Esophagus* 1999; 12 (4): 283–288.

54. Loprinzi, C.L., J.W. Kugler, J.A. Sloan, et al. Randomized comparison of megestrol acetate versus dexamethasone versus fluoxymesterone for the treatment of cancer anorexia/cachexia. *J. Clin. Oncol.* 1999; 17 (10): 3299–3306.

55. Sledge, G.W., P. Hu, G. Falkson, et al. Comparison of chemotherapy with chemohormonal therapy as first-line therapy for metastatic, hormone-sensitive breast cancer: An Eastern Cooperative Oncology Group study. *J. Clin. Oncol.* 2000; 18 (2): 262–266.

56. Heimpel, H. Aplastic anemia before bone marrow transplantation and antilymphocyte globulin. *Acta Haematol.* 2000; 103 (1): 11–15

57. Corsi, M.P., M. De Martinis, G. Di Leonardo, et al. [Blood coagulation changes and neoplastic pathology.] *Recenti Prog. Med.* 2000; 91 (10): 532–537.

18

Rationale for Anabolic Therapy in Cardiovascular Diseases and Cardiac Rehabilitation

Introduction: Hypoandrogenemia Is a Multifaceted Risk Factor for Heart Disease

The association between circulating endogenous sex steroids and cardiovascular disease in both genders has been a longstanding topic of debate. The long-held view by most physicians has been that elevated or normal circulating androgen levels promote atherogenic lipid profiles, atherogenesis, and cardiovascular disease. Furthermore, elevated or normal androgen levels have been suspected in the gender-related and age-related differences in the incidence of heart disease, since the rates of myocardial infarction (MI) are elevated at an early age in men.

The traditional view of androgens and heart disease seems to be valid for athletes who use huge androgen doses over prolonged periods of time for boosting muscle mass, strength, and athletic performance. Conversely, these long-held views of the role of endogenous androgens in the pathogenesis of heart disease are not only incorrect but are diametrically opposed to the true role that these anabolic agents play.

It is now well understood that the available evidence-based studies support the modern concept that age-related hypoandrogenemia is closely linked with the incidence of CHD in both genders. Recent studies have linked hypoandrogenemia and hyposomatomedinemia with coronary heart disease (CHD), congestive heart failure (CHF), angina pectoris (AP), hypertension, and increased risks for these diseases. Recent studies, supported by older studies, have also indicated that correcting hypoandrogenemia and hyposomatomedinemia with anabolic therapies has protective and beneficial effects. Therefore, it has become more apparent that anabolic therapy should be considered as cardioprotective and therapeutic for a number of cardiovascular-related conditions, including cardiac rehabilitation.

Hypoandrogenemia Promotes Cardiovascular Disease

Hypoandrogenemia promotes CHD in both genders via a number of mechanisms that involve general and specific catabolic mechanisms, and by several interrelated endocrine, neuroendocrine, neuroimmune, and neuropsychiatric alterations. In men, perhaps the best investigation that illustrates this point is a large, recently published, nested case-control study of healthy men (matched by age and ethnic origin). This study showed that men who had low plasma total testosterone levels had significantly increased risk for cardiovascular disease as indicated by[1]:

(1) higher body mass index (P<0.01).
(2) higher waist/hip ratio (P<0.001).
(3) higher systolic blood pressures (P<0.05).
(4) higher fasting and two-hour plasma glucose levels (P<0.04 and P<0.02 respectively).
(5) higher serum triglyceride levels (P<0.001).
(6) higher total cholesterol levels (P<0.04).
(7) higher low density lipoprotein cholesterol (LDL-C) levels (P<0.01).
(8) higher apolipoprotein B levels (P<0.01).
(9) higher fasting and two-hour plasma insulin levels (P<0.0001).
(10) lower serum high density lipoprotein cholesterol (HDL-C) levels (P<0.01).
(11) lower apolipoprotein A1 levels (P<0.05).
(12) markedly lower sex hormone binding globulin (SHBG) levels (P<0.0001).

Besides these effects, hypoandrogenemia has been shown to be associated with pathologic coagulation indices that increase the risks of thromboembolic events, including[2]:

(1) increased fibrinogen levels (P=0.004).
(2) reduced plasminogen activator activity levels (P=0.02).

The importance of these hypoandrogenemia-associated coagulation disorders for predicting cardiovascular mortality rates has been shown by a recent ten-year longitudinal study. This study concludes that hypoandrogenemia correlates statistically with two elevated clotting factors (elevated von Willebrand's factor, vWF, and tissue plasminogen activator antigen, t-PA) that are both independent clinical risk factors for CHD.[3]

Other evidence-based information has associated pathologic immunologic alterations with the pathogenesis of CHD. Elevated estrogenic/androgenic ratios have been shown to increase CHD risks[4] and CHF in men via altered circulating cytokine profiles that are induced by hypoandrogenemia.[5]

An extensive review of the relationship of endogenous circulating androgens to CHD in men has concluded that serum androgens have a favorable or neutral effect on CHD in men.[6] Taken in total, from all of the available evidence-based information, hypoandrogenemia emerges as the most prominent pathogenic, multifaceted risk factor for CHD in men.

Hypoandrogenemia in women is one of the most common biochemical alterations associated with a wide range of diseases, including CHD. Low circulating androgen levels is a common biochemical finding in perimenopausal, menopausal, and postmenopausal women that may be responsible for significantly more morbidity and mortality than is currently known.[7] The incidence rates for CHD in women closely parallel the incidence rates of hypoandrogenemia, although definitive longitudinal studies on the subject have not been published to date.

Incidence of Hypoandrogenemia and Coronary Heart Disease in Men

Both the incidence of hypoandrogenemia and its contribution to CHD risks and mortality in men have been vastly underestimated historically. Numerous cross-sectional studies have demonstrated lower concentrations of circulating total and/or free androgen levels in aging men.[8, 9, 10, 11, 12, 13, 14, 15, 16] Two small-scale investigations have reported that androgen levels decrease in otherwise healthy aging men.[17, 18] The most definitive longitudinal study (the Baltimore Longitudinal Study of Aging from Johns Hopkins University School of Medicine) published to date illustrates that hypoandrogenemia occurs, in otherwise healthy men (as defined by total serum testosterone levels or "free" serum testosterone levels), in a progressive age-related manner[19]:

(1) as measured as total serum testosterone levels in men in their 50s, 60s, 70s and 80s at 12 percent, 19 percent, 28 percent, and 49 percent rates respectively.

(2) as measured as "free" serum testosterone levels in men in their 50s, 60s, 70s and 80s at 9 percent, 34 percent, 68 percent, and 91 percent rates respectively.

The incidence rates for hypoandrogenemia and CHD in men closely parallel each other; however, the definitive longitudinal studies to correlate these conditions have not been published to date.

Hypoandrogenemia Contributes to Hyposomatomedinemia and Heart Disease

It is well recognized that hypoandrogenemia contributes to hyposomatomedinemia in both genders and induces a low anabolic potential that has been attributed to an increased incidence of CHD and other cardiac conditions, such as CHF. Hypoandrogenemia can result in a depressed GHRH-GH-IGF-IGFBP axis.

Androgens have been shown to directly stimulate the GHRH-GH-IGF-IGFBP axis at the hypothalamic level by a direct stimulatory effect that increases GHRH pulse amplitudes.[20, 21] Also, androgen receptors have been identified in GH secreting cells in the anterior pituitary gland that suggests that androgens can act directly on the pituitary gland to stimulate GH secretion.[22] Androgen stimulation has been shown to elevate circulating IGF-1, free IGF-1, and IGFBP levels in normal, hypogonadal, hyposomatotrophic, and aging individuals of both genders.[23, 24, 25, 26, 27, 28, 29]

Androgens have been shown to drive the GHRH-GH-IGF-IGFBP axis at both the hypothalamic and pituitary levels and result in an improved overall anabolic state. GH-deficient adults have been shown to have an increased cardiovascular mortality and markers for cardiovascular disease.[30, 31] Anabolic IGF-1 levels have been shown to be an important contributor to cardiovascular health. Accumulating evidence has indicated that IGF-1 plays an important role in the intricate cascade of events in cardiovascular function, in addition to its well-established anabolic effects. It has been shown that IGF-1 promotes cardiac growth and cardiac tissue remodeling, and improves myocardial contractility, cardiac output, stroke volume, and ejection fraction.[32] Hyposomatomedinemia (which can result from hypoandrogenemia)[33, 34] has been implicated in the pathogenesis of certain cardiac diseases.[35, 36, 37]

Androgens Are Beneficial Cardiovascular Agents

Androgens have been shown to have protective and beneficial effects in both healthy and diseased cardiovascular systems. The mechanisms by which androgens accomplish these effects are both independent of and interrelated with other factors, and include:

(1) actions via direct androgen receptor binding in myocardial tissues[38, 39] which results in beneficial effects on healthy and deteriorated myocardial tissues.[40] It has been suggested that androgen binding to the myocardial androgen receptors plays a role in optimum cardiac functioning.[41, 42, 43] Surprisingly, it has been found that androgen concentrations and androgen receptors are higher in healthy cardiac muscle than in skeletal muscle. It has also been shown that androgen and androgen receptor concentrations in cardiac and pulmonary tissues declines (statistically significant) with age.[44] It follows that age-related decreases in circulating androgen levels reflect reduced myocardial androgen and androgen receptor concentrations which results in decreased myocardial function.

(2) actions via elevating and normalizing the serum IGF-1 level that promotes cardiac growth and remodeling, improves cardiac contractility, cardiac output, stroke volume, and ejection fraction, especially after myocardial infarction. Furthermore, IGF-1 facilitates glucose metabolism, lowers insulin levels, increases insulin sensitivity, and improves lipid and cytokine profiles.[45, 46]

(3) actions as a direct neurosteroid by correcting hypoandrogenemia and treating depression and dysthymia that are well-known to be risks for CHD.[47, 48]

(4) actions on systemic lipid metabolism which reduce plasma lipoprotein a, LP(a), an independent risk factor for atherogenesis.[49, 50, 51]

(5) actions on systemic lipid metabolism which reduce elevated total cholesterol, LDL-cholesterol, and triglyceride levels.[52, 53, 54]

(6) actions that augment the systemic fibrinolytic system[55] and antithrombin III activity[56] while decreasing fibrinogen, tissue plasminogen activator antigen, and von Willebrand factor levels.[57, 58, 59, 60, 61]

(7) actions via the neuroimmunoendocrine system that modulate and correct pathologic inflammatory cytokine and lymphocyte profiles.[62, 63]

(8) actions via the hematological system that elevate hemoglobin concentrations, correct anemic states, and improve the oxygen-carrying capacity to and by the cardiovascular system.[64]

(9) actions that dilate the coronary arteries, increase coronary blood

flow, and reduce angina, nitrate requirement, and signs of myocardial ischemia (ECG and Holter monitoring) for cardiac patients.[65, 66, 67, 68, 69]

(10) actions that dilate systemic arteries and arterioles via androgen receptors located in the smooth muscle of these tissues,[70] and reduce hypertension and afterload, thereby reducing cardiac work load requirements.[71]

Summary

The rationale for the use of androgens as cardiovascular drugs and for the prevention of CHD, has been presented in this chapter. It appears that androgen and other anabolic therapies have recently been supported by the available evidence-based information.

The earliest studies (from the 1930s and 1940s) had previously indicated that androgen therapy for advanced-aged men and women had powerful effects on the cardiovascular system, such as increasing the angina threshold, reducing hypertension, increasing exercise tolerance, and improving ischemic ECG findings and cardiac rehabilitation.[72, 73, 74, 75, 76, 77, 78, 79, 80, 81, 82, 83, 84] Recent studies have confirmed these earlier findings and defined many of the mechanisms of action that androgen therapy has on the cardiovascular system. Continued research and clinical use of androgen therapy for cardiovascular disease is warranted.

The available science-based information regarding the beneficial use of other anabolic therapies (GH and IGF-1) has also been presented. However, many of these effects can be produced with androgen therapy acting via the GHRH-GH-IGF-IGFBP axis. The cost-effectiveness of anabolic therapy with androgens strongly favors it over the other recombinant anabolic therapies. Androgen therapy also offers a greater range of benefits including positive effects on mood, libido, cognition, and immune system modulation.

Androgen therapy should be considered as an adjunctive pharmacologic therapy for patients undergoing cardiopulmonary rehabilitation. Besides the protective, preventive, and cardiovascular benefits, androgen therapy can treat and reverse musculoskeletal weakness, sarcopenia, and osteoporosis, and increase aerobic capacity in conjunction with traditional cardiopulmonary rehabilitation methods.

Notes

1. Simon, D., M.A. Charles, K. Nahoul, et al. Association between plasma total testosterone and cardiovascular risk factors in healthy adult men: The Telecom Study. *J. Clin. Endocrinol. Metab.* 1997; 82 (2): 682–685.

2. Glueck, C.J., H.I. Glueck, D. Stroop, et al. Endogenous testosterone, fibrinolysis, and coronary heart disease in hyperlipidemic men. *J. Lab. Clin. Med.* 1993; 122 (4): 412–420.

3. Jansson, J.H., T.K. Nilsson, and O. Johnson. Von Willebrand factor, tissue plasminogen activator, and dehydroepiandrosterone sulphate predict cardiovascular death in a 10 year follow up of survivors of acute myocardial infarction. *Heart* 1998; 80 (4): 334–337.

4. Wu, S.Z., and X.Z. Weng. Therapeutic effects of an androgenic preparation on myocardial ischemia and cardiac function in 62 elderly male coronary heart disease patients. *Clin. Med. J. (Engl.)* 1993; 10 (96): 425–418.

5. Anker, S.D., P.P. Ponikowski, A.L. Clark, et al. Cytokines and neurohormones relating to body composition alterations in the wasting syndrome of chronic heart failure. *Eur. Heart J.* 1999; 20 (9): 683–693.

6. Alexanderson, P., J. Haarbo, and C. Christiansen. The relationship of natural androgens to coronary heart disease in males: a review. *Atherosclerosis* 1996; 125 (1): 1–13.

7. Rako, S. Testosterone supplemental therapy after hysterectomy with or without concomitant oophorectomy: estrogen alone is not enough. *J. Women's Health Gend. Based Med.* 2000; 9 (8): 917–923.

8. Vermeulen, R., R. Rubens, and L. Verndock. Testosterone secretion and metabolism in male senescence. *J. Clin. Endocrinol. Metab.* 1972; 34: 730–735.

9. Rubens, R., M. Dhont, and A. Vermeulen. Further studies on Leydig cell function in old age. *J. Clin. Endocrinol. Metab.* 1974; 39: 40–45.

10. Baker, H.W., H.G. Burger, D.M. de Kretser, et al. Changes in the pituitary-testicular system with age. *Clin. Endocrinol. (Oxf.):* 1976; 5: 349–372.

11. Pirke, K.M., and P. Doerr. Age related changes in free plasma testosterone, dihydrotestosterone and oestradiol. *Acta Endocrinol. (Copenh.)* 1975; 80: 171–178.

12. Purifoy, F.E., L.H. Koopmans, and D.M. Mays. Age differences in serum androgen levels in normal male adults. *Hum. Biol.* 1981; 53: 499–511.

13. Bremner, W.J., and P.N. Prinz. A loss of circadian rhythmicity in blood testosterone levels with aging normal men. *J. Clin. Endocrinol. Metab.* 1983; 56: 1278–1281.

14. Tenover, J.S., A.M. Matsumoto, S.R. Plymate, et al. The effects of aging in normal men on bioavailable testosterone and luteinizing hormone secretion: Response to clomiphene citrate. *J. Clin. Endocrinol. Metab.* 1987; 65: 1118–1126.

15. Gray, A., J.A. Berlin, J.B. McKinlay, et al. An examination of research design effects on the association of testosterone and male aging: results of a meta-analysis. *J. Clin. Epidemiol.* 1991; 44: 671–684.

16. Gerrini, R.L., and E. Barret-Conner. Sex hormones and age: a cross–sectional study of testosterone and estradiol and their bioavailable fractions in community-dwelling men. *Am. J. Epidemiol.* 1998; 147: 750–754.

17. Zmuda, J.M., J.A. Cauley, A. Kriska, et al. Longitudinal relation between endogenous testosterone and cardiovascular disease risk factors in middle-aged men. A 13–year follow-up of former Multiple Risk Factor Intervention Trial participants. *Am. J. Epidemiol.* 1997; 146: 609–617.

18. Morley, J.E., F.E. Kaiser, H.M. Perry, et al. Longitudinal changes in testosterone, luteinizing hormone, and follicle-stimulating hormone in healthy older men. *Metabolism* 1997; 46: 410–413.

19. Mitchell, S., E. Harman, E.J. Metter, et al. Longitudinal effects of aging on serum and free testosterone levels in healthy men. *J. Clin. Endocrinol. Metab.* 2001; 86 (2): 724–731.

20. Eakman, G.D., J.S. Dallas, S.W. Ponder, et al. The effects of testosterone and dihydrotestosterone on hypothalamic regulation of growth hormone secretion. *J. Clin. Endocrinol. Metab.* 1996; 81 (3): 1212–1223.

21. Genazzani, A.D., O. Gamba, L. Nappi, et al. Modulatory effects of synthetic steroid (tibolone) and estradiol on spontaneous and GHRH-induced GH secretion in postmenopausal women. *Maturitas* 1997; 28 (1): 27–33.

22. Kimura, N., A. Mizokami, T. Oonuma, et al. Immunocytochemical localization of androgen receptor with polyclonal antibody in paraffin-embedded human tissue. *J. Histochem. Cytochem.* 1993; 41 (5): 671–678.

23. Hobbs, C.J., S.R. Plymate, C.J. Rosen, et al. Testosterone administration increases insulin-like growth factor-1 levels in normal men. *J. Clin. Endocrinol. Metab.* 1993; 77 (3): 776–779.

24. Morales, A.J., J.J. Nolen, J.C. Nelson, et al. Effects of replacement dose of dehydroepiandrosterone in men and women of advancing age. *J. Clin. Endocrinol. Metab.* 1994; 78 (6): 1360–1367.

25. Gelato, M.C., and R.A. Frost. IGFBP-3. Functional and structural implications in aging and wasting syndromes. *Endocrine* 1997; 7 (1): 81–85.

26. Casson, P.R., N. Santoro, K. Elkin-Hirsch, et al. Postmenopausal dehydroepiandrosterone administration increases free insulin-like growth factor-1 and decreases high-density lipoprotein: a six month trial. *Fertil. Steril.* 1998; 70 (1): 107–110.

27. Jorgensen, J.O., N. Vahl, T.B. Hansen, et al. Determinants of serum insulin-like growth factor-1 in growth hormone deficient adults as compared to healthy adults. *Clin. Endocrinol. (Oxf.)* 1998; 48 (4): 479–486.

28. Morales, A.J., R.H. Haubrich, J.Y. Hwang, et al. The effects of six months treatment with 100mg daily dose of dehydroepiandrosterone (DHEA) on circulating sex steroids, body composition, and muscle strength in age-advance men and women. *Clin. Endocrinol. (Oxf.)* 1998; 49 (4): 421–434.

29. Span, J.P., G.F. Pieters, C.G. Sweep, et al. Gender difference in insulin-like growth factor-1 response to growth hormone (GH) treatment and GH-deficient adults: role of sex hormone replacement. *J. Clin. Endocrinol. Metab.* 2000; 85 (3): 1121–1125.

30. Weaver, J.U., J.P. Monson, K. Noonan, et al. The effect of low dose recombinant human growth hormone replacement on regional fat distribution, insulin sensitivity, and cardiovascular risk factors in hypopituitary adults. *J. Clin. Endocrinol. Metab.* 1995; 80 (1): 153–159.

31. Sesmilo, G., B.M. Biller, J. Lievadot, et al. Effects of growth hormone administration on inflammatory and other cardiovascular risk markers in men with growth hormone deficiency. A randomized, controlled trial. *Ann. Intern. Med.* 2000; 133 (2): 111–122.

32. Ren, J., W.K. Samson, and J.R. Sowers. Insulin-like growth factor 1 as a cardiac hormone: physiological and pathophysiological implications in heart disease. *J. Mol. Cell. Cardiol.* 1999; 31 (11): 2049–2061.

33. Anker, S.D., P.P. Ponikowski, A.L. Clark, et al. Cytokines and neurohormones relating to body composition alterations in the wasting syndrome of chronic heart failure. *Eur. Heart J.* 1999; 20 (9): 683–693.

34. Moriyama, Y., H. Hasue, M. Yoshimura, et al. The plasma levels of dehydroepiandrosterone sulfate are decreased in patients with chronic heart failure in proportion to the severity. *J. Clin. Endocrinol. Metab.* 2000; 85 (5): 1834–1840.

35. Niebauer, J., C.D. Pflaum, A.L. Clark, et al. Deficient insulin-like growth factor 1 in chronic heart failure predicts altered body composition, anabolic deficiency, cytokine and neurohormonal activation. *J. Am. Coll. Cardio.* 1998; 32 (2): 393–397.

36. Ren, J., W.K. Samson, and J.R. Sowers. Insulin-like growth factor 1 as a cardiac hormone: physiological and pathophysiological implications in heart disease. *J. Mol. Cell. Cardiol.* 1999; 31 (11): 2049–2061.

37. Osteriziel, K.J., M.B. Ranke, O. Strohm, et al. The somatotrophic system in

patients with dilated cardiomyopathy: relation of insulin-like growth factor-1 and its alterations during growth hormone therapy to cardiac function. *Clin. Endocrinol. (Oxf.)* 2000; 53 (1): 61–68.

38. Kimura, N.A., Misokami, T. Oonuma, et al. Immunocytochemical localization of androgen receptor with polyclonal antibody in paraffin-embedded human tissues. *J. Histochem. Cytochem.* 1993; 41 (5): 671–678.

39. Marsh, J.D., M.H. Lehmann, R.H. Ritchie, et al. Androgen receptors mediate hypertrophy in cardiac monocytes. *Circulation* 1998; 98 (2): 256–261.

40. Tomoda, H. Effect of oxymetholone on left ventricular dimensions in heart failure secondary to idiopathic dilated cardiomyopathy or to mitral or aortic regurgitation. *Am. J. Cardiol.* 1999; 83 (1): 123–125.

41. Deslypere, J.P., and A. Vermeulen. Aging and tissue androgens. *J. Clin. Endocrinol. Metab.* 1981; 53: 430–463.

42. Deslypere, J.P., A. Sayad, L. Verdonc, et al. Androgen concentrations in sexual and non-sexual skins as well as in striated muscle in man. *J. Steroid Biochem.* 1980; 13: 1455–1460.

43. Marsh, J.D., M.H. Lehmann, R.H. Ritchie, et al. Androgen receptors mediate hypertrophy in cardiac monocytes. *Circulation* 1998; 98 (3): 256–261.

44. Deslypere, J.P., and A. Vermeulen. Influence of age on steroid concentrations in skin and striated muscle in women and cardiac muscle and lung tissue in men. *J. Clin. Endocrinol. Metab.* 1985; 61: 648–653.

45. Ren, J., W.K. Samson, and J.R. Sowers. Insulin-like growth factor 1 as a cardiac hormone: physiological and pathophysiological implications in heart disease. *J. Mol. Cell. Cardiol.* 1999; 31 (11): 2049–61.

46. Sesmilo, G., B.M. Biller, J. Llevadot, et al. Effects of growth hormone administration on inflammatory and other cardiovascular risk markers in men with growth hormone deficiency. A randomized, controlled clinical trial. *Ann. Intern. Med.* 2000; 133 (2): 111–122.

47. Rabijewski, M., M. Adamkiewicz, and S. Zgliczynski. [The influence of testosterone replacement therapy on well-being, bone mineral density and lipids in elderly men.] *Pol. Arch. Med. Wewn.* 1998; 100 (3): 212–221.

48. Bloch, M., P.J. Schmidt, M.A. Danaceau, et al. Dehydroepiandrosterone treatment in midlife dysthymia. *Soc. Biol. Psychiatry* 1999; 45; 1533–1541.

49. Davidoff, P. [LP (a) lipoprotein: a new independent risk factor for atherogenesis.] *Rev. Med. Chil.* 1991; 119 (1): 64–68.

50. Soma, M.R., M. Meschia, F. Bruschi, et al. Hormonal agents used in lowering lipoprotein (a). *Chem. Phys. Lipids* 1994; 67–68: 345–350.

51. Li, X., S. Zhao, Y. Li, et al. [Changes of plasma testosterone level in male patients with coronary heart disease.] *Hunan I. Ko. Hsueh. Hsueh. Pao.* 1998; 23 (1): 53–56.

52. Wu, S.Z., X.Z. Weng, and X.X. Yao. [Antianginal and lipid lowering effects of oral androgenic preparation (Andriol) on elderly male patients with coronary heart disease.] *Chung Hua. Nei. Ko. Tsa. Chih.* 1993; 32 (4): 235–238.

53. Glueck, C.J., H.I. Gleuck, D. Stroop, et al. Endogenous testosterone, fibrinolysis, and coronary heart disease risk in hyperlipidemic men. *J. Lab. Clin. Med.* 1993; 122 (4): 412–420.

54. Rabijewski, M., M. Adamkiewicz, and S. Zgliczynski. [The influence of testosterone replacement therapy on well-being, bone mineral density, and lipids in elderly men.] *Pol. Arch. Med. Wewn.* 1998; 100 (3): 212–221.

55. Hessel, L.W., and C. Kluft. Advances in clinical fibrinolysis. *Clin. Haematol.* 1986; 15 (2): 443–463.

56. Kluft, C., F.E. Preston, R.G. Malia, et al. Stanozolol-induced changes in fibrinolysis and coagulation in healthy adults. *Thromb. Haemost.* 1984; 51 (2): 157–164.

57. Verheijen, J.H., D.C. Rijken, G.T. Chang, et al. Modulation of rapid plasminogen activator inhibitor in plasma by stanozolol. *Thromb. Haemost.* 1984; 51 (3): 396–397.

58. Small, M., C. Kluft, A.C. MacCuish, et al. Tissue plasminogen activator inhibition in diabetes mellitus. *Diabetes Care*1989; 12 (9): 655–658.

59. Glueck, C.J., H.I. Gleuck, D. Stroop, et al. Endogenous testosterone, fibrinolysis, and coronary heart disease risk in hyperlipemic men. *J. Lab. Clin. Med.* 1993; 122 (4): 412–420.

60. Jansson, J.H., T.K. Nilsson, and O. Johnson. Von Willebrand factor, tissue plasminogen activator, and dehydroepiandrosterone sulphate predict cardiovascular death in a 10 year follow up of survivors of acute myocardial infarction. *Heart* 1998; 80 (4): 334–337.

61. Shapiro, J., J. Christiana, and W.H. Frishman. Testosterone and other anabolic steroids as cardiovascular drugs. *Am. J. Ther.* 1999; 6 (3): 167–174.

62. Zofkova, I., R.L. Kancheva, and R. Hampl. A decreasing CD4+/CD8+ ratio after one month of treatment with stanozolol in postmenopausal women. *Steroids* 1995; 60 (7): 430–433.

63. Anker, S.D., P.P. Ponikowski, A.L. Clark, et al. Cytokines and neurohormones relating to body compositions in wasting syndrome of chronic heart failure. *Eur. Heart J.* 1999; 20 (9): 683–693.

64. Rabinjewski, M., M. Adamkiewicz, and S. Zgliczynski. [The influence of testosterone replacement therapy on well-being, bone mineral density, and lipids in elderly men.] *Pol. Arch. Med. Wewn.* 1998; 100 (3): 212–221.

65. Wu, S.Z. and X.Z. Weng. Therapeutic effects of an androgenic preparation on myocardial ischemia and cardiac function in 62 elderly male coronary heart disease patients. *Chin. Med. J. (Engl.)* 1993; 106 (6): 415–418.

66. Wu, S.Z., X.Z. Weng, and X.X. Yao. [Antianginal and lipid lowering effects of oral androgenic preparation (Andriol) on elderly male patients with coronary artery disease.] *Chung Hua. Nei. Ko. Tsa Chih.* 1993; 32 (4): 235–238.

67. Rablijewski, M., M. Adamkiewicz, and S. Zgliczynksi. [The influence of testosterone replacement therapy on well-being, bone mineral density, and lipids in elderly men.] *Pol. Arch. Med. Wewn.* 1998; 100 (3): 212–221.

68. Webb, C.M., J.G. McNeill, C.S. Hayward, et al. Effects of testosterone on coronary vasomotor regulation in men with coronary artery disease. *Circulation* 1999; 100 (16): 1690–1696.

69. English, K.M., R.P. Steeds, T.H. Jones, et al. Low-dose transdermal testosterone therapy improves angina threshold in men with chronic stable angina: A randomized, double-blind, placebo-controlled study. *Circulation* 2000; 102 (16): 1096–1911.

70. Kimura, N., A. Mizokami, T. Oonuma, et al. Immunocytochemical localization of androgen receptor with polyclonal antibody in paraffin-embedded human tissues. *J. Histochem. Cytochem.* 1993; 41 (5): 671–678.

71. Shapiro, J., J. Christiana, and W.H. Frishman. Testosterone and other anabolic steroids as cardiovascular drugs. *Am. J. Ther.* 1999; 6 (3): 167–174.

72. Edwards, E.A., J.B. Hamilton, and S.Q. Duntley. Testosterone propionate as a therapeutic agent in patients with organic disease of the peripheral vessels: a preliminary report. *N. Engl. J. Med.* 1939; 220: 865–870.

73. Bonnell, R.W., C.P. Prichett, and T.E. Rardin. Treatment of angina pectoris and coronary artery disease with sex hormones. *Ohio State Med. J.* 1940; 37 (6): 554–556.

74. Lesser, M.A. The treatment of angina pectoris with testosterone propionate. *N. Engl. J. Med.* 1942; 226 (2): 51–54.

75. Hamm, L. Testosterone propionate in the treatment of angina pectoris. *J. Clin. Endocrinol.* 1942; 2: 325–328.

76. Walker, T.C. The use of testosterone propionate and estrogenic substance in the treatment of essential hypertension, angina pectoris and peripheral vascular disease. *J. Clin. Endocrinol.* 1942; 2: 560–568.

77. Lesser, M.A. The treatment of angina pectoris with testosterone propionate: further observations. *N. Engl. J. Med.* 1943; 228 (6): 185–188.

78. Levine, S.A., and W.B. Likoff. The therapeutic use of testosterone propionate in angina pectoris. *N. Engl. J. Med.* 1943; 229: 770–772.

79. McGavack, T.H. Angina-like pain; a manifestation of the male climacterium. *J. Clin. Endocrinol.* 1943; 3: 71–80.

80. Opit, L. The treatment of angina pectoris by testosterone. *Med. J. Australia* 1943; 1: 546.

81. Sigler, L.H., and J. Tulgan. Treatment of angina pectoris by testosterone. *N.Y. State J. Med.* 1943; 43: 1424–1428.

82. Opit, L. The treatment of angina pectoris and peripheral vascular disease by testosterone propionate. *Med. J. Australia* 1943; 2: 173.

83. Strong, G.F., and A.W. Wallace. Treatment of angina pectoris and peripheral vascular disease with sex hormones. *Canad. Med. Assoc. J.* 1944; 50: 30–33.

84. Waldman, S. The treatment of angina pectoris with testosterone propionate. *J. Clin. Endocrinol.* 1945; 5: 305–317.

19

Rationale for Anabolic Therapy in Chronic Obstructive Pulmonary Disease

Introduction: A Major Catabolic Condition

Chronic obstructive pulmonary disease (COPD) afflicts millions of people and is severely disabling.[1] Exercise intolerance and shortness of breath with little or no exertion are usually the chief complaints of patients with COPD. Long-term smoking is the major contributor to the disease.

Many patients with COPD acquire the anorexia/cachexia syndrome (ACS) and are in a prolonged and constant catabolic state.[2] Weight and lean body mass losses are primary factors in determining the COPD patient's functional capacity, health status, and mortality risk.[3, 4]

Recently, several lines of evidence have associated sarcopenia, diaphragmatic muscle weakness, and diminished strength in the accessory muscles of respiration to potentially reversible contributory factors in COPD. Mechanisms involved with sarcopenia, skeletal muscle weakness, and respiratory muscle weakness in COPD patients include overall physical deconditioning and low levels of anabolic hormones.[5] Accumulating evidence has suggested and supported the rationale for the use of anabolic hormones, along with rehabilitative modalities, as anabolic therapy for COPD patients.[6]

Hypoandrogenemia in COPD Patients

After being controversial for a long time, the age-associated decline in serum androgens in both genders has been generally accepted and well recognized.[7] Hypoandrogenemia has been shown to be inherent to the aging gonadal and adrenal biochemical processes. These aging processes may be worsened in patients with chronic diseases, corticosteroid therapy, prolonged smoking history, and physical inactivity.[8, 9, 10]

Several studies have shown that COPD is associated with hypoandrogenemia both with and without previous or concurrent corticosteroid therapy.[11, 12, 13, 14, 15] However, it has also been shown that corticosteroid therapy aggravates the hypoandrogenemia that is associated with COPD.[16, 17, 18] Most importantly, the degree of hypoandrogenemia has been shown to correlate with the severity of arterial hypoxia in COPD patients.[19]

Androgen concentrations and androgen receptors have been located and studied in pulmonary tissues.[20, 21, 22, 23] Both androgen and androgen receptor concentrations have been shown to decrease with age[24, 25] suggesting a role for reduced androgen receptor binding as part of the age-related decline in pulmonary function. It has also been shown that androgen administration is associated with an upregulation of androgen receptors in certain tissues (androgen-induced androgen-receptor augmentation) that results in[26]:

(1) an increase in androgen receptor half-life.
(2) an increased rate of synthesis of androgen receptors.

These mechanisms may be involved with androgen therapy on strengthening the skeletal muscle, and the diaphragmatic and other respiratory muscles.

Studies with Anabolic Therapy in COPD

Recent studies in both animals[27, 28, 29, 30] and in humans[31, 32, 33] have demonstrated a distinct impact of androgen therapy on strengthening respiratory and skeletal muscles. In animal models, it has been shown that androgen therapy improves both isometric and isotonic contractile function of the diaphragm.[34, 35, 36] Also, anabolic therapy with recombinant growth hormone (GH) has been shown to improve pulmonary function and to allow ventilator weaning and decreased mortality of patients in intensive care who failed traditional ventilator weaning protocols.[37, 38]

The available studies with androgen therapy in COPD patients have shown that:

(1) nutritional supplementation in combination with a short-course androgen therapy (women 25mg nandrolone decanoate on days 1, 15, 29,

and 43; men 50mg nandrolone decanoate on days 1, 15, 29, and 43) and an exercise protocol, in a placebo-controlled randomized trial, resulted in gains in fat-free mass and respiratory muscle function without causing adverse effects.[39]

(2) androgen therapy (250 mg testosterone cypionate IM at baseline and 12mg oral stanozolol daily for 27 weeks) combined with a pulmonary rehabilitation program, in a placebo-controlled trial of men with COPD, resulted in significant increases in maximum inspiratory pressure (PI max), and increases (statistically significant) in lean body mass, body mass index, and anthropometric measures of arm and thigh circumference.[40]

These findings suggest that anabolic therapy for patients with COPD augments the effects of pulmonary rehabilitation protocols by increasing overall muscle mass and strength and by increasing the strength of the muscles involved with respiration.

It has been proposed that anabolic hormone therapy may find a permanent place in COPD therapy, especially when combined with pulmonary rehabilitation modalities.[41] Further research should help refine these therapies.

Summary

In this chapter the available evidence-based rationale has been presented to support the use of anabolic therapy in patients with COPD. It has been shown that hypoandrogenemia is often associated with COPD. It has also been shown that hypoandrogenemia may play a major role in ACS and disability in patients with COPD. Anabolic therapy to correct these conditions has been shown to translate into improved respiratory function and quality of life in these patients.

Few effective therapies exist for patients with COPD. Rehabilitative therapy should be aimed at reversing sarcopenia and enhancing skeletal and respiratory muscle strength and function in order to return the patient to the highest possible level of health. To date, therapies for COPD have been unable to reverse the underlying intrinsic pulmonary damages.

Accumulating evidence shows that anabolic therapies (androgens and GH) can manage ACS, reverse sarcopenia, and increase skeletal and respiratory muscle strength, especially in combination with optimized nutrition and pulmonary rehabilitation protocols. It is expected that anabolic therapies will become part of the standard of care for COPD patients. Certainly, further research in this area is warranted.

Notes

1. Casaburi, R. Rationale for anabolic therapy to facilitate rehabilitation in chronic obstructive pulmonary disease. *Baillieres Clin. Endocrinol. Metab.* 1998; 12 (3): 407–418.

2. Plata-Salaman, C.R. Central nervous system mechanisms contributing to the cachexia-anorexia syndrome. *Nutrition* 2000; 16 (10): 1009–1012.

3. Schols, A.M., P.B. Soeters, R. Mostert, et al. Physiologic effects of nutritional support and anabolic steroids in patients with chronic obstructive pulmonary disease. A placebo-controlled randomized trial. *Am. J. Respir. Crit. Care Med.* 1995; 152 (4 Pt. 1): 1268–1274.

4. Schols, A.M. Nutrition in chronic obstructive pulmonary disease. *Curr. Opin. Pulm. Med.* 2000; 6 (2): 110–115.

5. Casaburi, R. Skeletal muscle function in COPD. *Chest* 2000; 117 (5 Suppl. 1): 267S–271S.

6. Casaburi, R. Rationale for anabolic therapy to facilitate rehabilitation in chronic obstructive pulmonary disease. *Baillieres Clin. Endocrinol. Metab.* 1998; 12 (3): 407–418.

7. Vermeulen, A., J.P. Deslypere, and K. De Mierlier. A new look to the andropause: altered functions of the gonadotrophs. *J. Steroid Biochem.* 1989; 32 (1B): 163–165.

8. Vermeulen, A., J.P. Desylpere, W. Schelfhout, et al. Adrenocortical function in old age: response to acute adrenocorticotropin stimulation. *J. Clin. Endocrinol. Metab.* 1982; 54 (1): 187–191.

9. Vermeulen, A., and J.P. Deslypere. Testicular endocrine function in the age-ing male. *Maturitas* 1985; 7 (3): 273–279.

10. Contreras, L.N., A.M. Masini, M.M. Danna, et al. Glucocorticoids: their role on gonadal function and LH secretion. *Minerva Endocrinol.* 1996; 21 (2): 43–46.

11. Semple, P.D., G.H. Beastall, W.S. Watson, et al. Hypothalamic-pituitary dysfunction in respiratory hypoxia. *Thorax* 1981; 36 (8): 605–609.

12. Fletcher, E.C., and R.J. Martin. Sexual dysfunction and erectile impotence in chronic obstructive pulmonary disease. *Chest* 1982; 81 (4): 413–421.

13. Gow, S.M., J. Seth, G.J. Beckett, et al. Thyroid function and endocrine abnormalities in elderly patients with severe chronic obstructive lung disease. *Thorax* 1987; 42 (7): 520–525.

14. Aasebo, U., A. Gyltnes, R.M. Bremnes, et al. Reversal of sexual impotence in males with chronic obstructive pulmonary disease and hypoxemia with long-term oxygen therapy. *J. Steroid Biochem. Mol. Biol.* 1993; 46 (6): 799–803.

15. Kamischke, A., D.E. Kemper, M.A. Castel, et al. Testosterone levels in men with chronic obstructive pulmonary disease with or without glucocorticoid therapy. *Eur. Respir. J.* 1998; 11 (1): 41–45.

16. MacAdams, M.R., R.H. White, and B.E. Chipps. Reduction of serum testosterone levels during chronic glucocorticoid therapy. *Ann. Intern. Med.* 1986; 104 (5): 648–651.

17. Contreras, L.N., A.M. Masini, M.M. Danna, et al. Glucocorticoids: their role on gonadal function and LH secretion. *Minerva Endocrinol.* 1996; 21 (2): 43–46.

18. Kamischke, A., D.E. Kemper, M.A. Castel, et al. Testosterone levels in men with chronic obstructive pulmonary disease with or without glucocorticoid therapy. *Eur. Respir. J.* 1998; 11 (1): 41–45.

19. Semple, P.D., G.H. Beastall, W.S. Watson, et al. Serum testosterone depression associated with hypoxia in respiratory failure. *Clin Sci. (Colch.)* 1980; 58 (1): 105–106.

20. Deslypere, J.P., A. Sayed, L. Verdonck, et al. Androgen concentrations in sexual

and non-sexual skin as well as striated muscle in man. *J. Steroid Biochem.* 1980; 13 (12): 1455–1458.

21. Morishige, W.K. Endocrine influences on aspects of lung biochemistry. *Ciba Found. Symp.* 1980; 78: 239–250.

22. Kimura, N., A. Mizokami, T. Oonuma, et al. Immunocytochemical localization of androgen receptor with polyclonal antibody in paraffin-embedded human tissues. *J. Histochem. Cytochem.* 1993; 41 (5): 671–678.

23. Provost, P.R., C.H. Blomquist, C. Godin, et al. Androgen formation and metabolism in the pulmonary epithelial cell line A549: expression of 17beta-hydroxysteroid dehydrogenase type 5 and 3alpha-hydroxysteroid dehydrogenase type 3. *Endocrinology* 2000; 141 (8): 2786–2794.

24. Deslypere, J.P., and A. Vermeulen. Aging and tissue androgens. *J. Clin. Endocrinol. Metab.* 1981; 53 (2): 430–434.

25. Deslypere, J.P., and A. Vermeulen. Influence of age on steroid concentrations in skin and striated muscle in women and cardiac muscle and lung tissue in men. *J. Clin. Endocrionol. Metab.* 1985; 61 (4): 648–653.

26. Syms, A.J., J.S. Norris, W.B. Panko, et al. Mechanism of androgen-receptor augmentation. Analysis of receptor synthesis and degradation by the density-shift technique. *J. Biol. Chem.* 1985; 260 (1): 455–461.

27. Prezant, D.J., D.E. Valentine, E.I. Gentry, et al. Effects of short-term and long-term androgen treatment on the diaphragm in male and female rats. *J. Appl. Physiol.* 1993; 1140–1149.

28. Bisschop, A., G. Gayan-Ramirez, H. Rollier, et al. Effects of nandrolone decanoate on respiratory and peripheral muscles in male and female rats. *J. Appl. Physiol.* 1997; 82: 1112–1118.

29. Prezant, D.J., M.L. Karwa, H.H. Kim, et al. Short- and long-term effects of testosterone on diaphragm in castrated and normal male rats. *J. Appl. Physiol.* 1997; 82: 134–143.

30. van Balkom, R.H., P.N. Dekhuijzen, H.F. van der Heijden, et al. Effects of anabolic steroids on diaphragm impairment induced by methylprednisolone in emphysematous hamsters. *Eur. Respir. J.* 1999; 13 (5): 1062–1069.

31. Schols, A.M., P.B. Soeters, R. Mostert, et al. Physiologic effects of nutritional support and anabolic-androgenic steroids in patients with chronic obstructive pulmonary disease: a placebo-controlled randomized trial. *Am.J. Respir. Crit. Care Med.* 1995; 152 (4 Pt. 1): 1268–1274.

32. Bhasin, S., and W.J. Bremmer. The effects of supraphysiologic doses of testosterone on muscle size and strength in normal men. *N. Engl. J. Med.* 1996; 335: 1–7.

33. Ferreira, I.M., I.T. Verreschi, L.E. Nery, et al. The influence of 6 months oral anabolic steroids on body mass and respiratory muscles in undernourished COPD patients. *Chest* 1998; 114 (1): 19–28.

34. DeLilly, J., T. LoRusso, M. Founier, et al. Effects of anabolic-androgenic steroids on diaphragm structure and function. *Am. J. Respir. Crit. Care Med.* 1995; 151: 813.

35. Yeh, A.Y., M. Fournier, P.E. Micevych, et al. Impact of nandrolone treatment on hamster diaphragm structure and function. *Am. J. Respir. Crit. Care Med.* 1996; 153: 686.

36. Lewis, M.I., M. Fournier, A.Y. Yey, et al. Alterations in diaphragm contractility after nandrolone administration: an analysis of potential mechanisms. *J. Appl. Physiol.* 1999; 86 (3): 985–992.

37. Knox, J.B., D.W. Wilmore, R.H. Demling, et al. Use of growth hormone for postoperative respiratory failure. *Am. J. Surg.* 1996; 171 (6): 576–580.

38. Merola, B., S. Longobardi, M. Sofia, et al. Lung volumes and respiratory muscle strength in adult patients with childhood- or adult-onset growth hormone deficiency: effect of 12 month's growth hormone replacement therapy. *Eur. J. Endocrinol.* 1996; 135 (5): 553–558.

39. Schols, A.M., P.B. Soeters, R. Mostert, et al. Physiologic effects of nutritional support and anabolic steroids in patients with chronic obstructive pulmonary disease. A placebo-controlled randomized trial. *Am. J. Respir. Crit. Care Med.* 1995; 152 (4 Pt. 1): 1268–1274.

40. Ferriera, I.M., I.T. Verreschi, L.E. Nery, et al. The influence of 6 months of oral anabolic steroids on body mass and respiratory muscles in undernourished COPD patients. *Chest* 1998; 114 (1): 19–28.

41. Casaburi, R. Skeletal muscle function in COPD. *Chest* 2000; 117 (5 Suppl. 1): 267S–271S.

20

Rationale for Anabolic Therapy in Stroke Treatment and Rehabilitation

Introduction: A Lack of Clinical Use of Anabolic Agents for Stroke Patients

Despite much progress in stroke prevention and acute intervention, the recovery and rehabilitation phases have traditionally received relatively little scientific attention. However, within the past few years there has been increasing interest in the development of recovery drugs and innovative rehabilitation techniques to promote or enhance functional recovery after a completed stroke.

Experimental work over the past two decades indicates that pharmacologic intervention ("rehabilitative pharmacology") to enhance recovery has become possible in the subacute stages, days to weeks poststroke, after previously perceived, irreversible injury has occurred.[1, 2] Several review articles have summarized combinations of thrombolytic and neuroprotective drugs that may be used to attempt maximum rates of recovery after acute ischemic stroke.[3, 4] However, a recent study has pointed out 20 barriers, perceived by health professionals working within the field of stroke rehabilitation, to the use of such drugs in the care of their daily patients.[5] Support for such performance-enhancing pharmacology from the latest editions of the major textbooks that deal with physical medicine and rehabilitation has not been forthcoming. Little or no mention is made of therapy with these anabolic and recovery agents in these books. However, this is not a unique situation in clinical medicine, for in most cases, the clinical use of anabolic agents has lagged far behind the supportive science that recommends anabolic modalities in disease prevention and therapeutic intervention.

Over the past decade, it has become clear that the brain is a steroidogenic organ. These steroids, including androgens, synthesized in the central and peripheral nervous system and given the name neurosteroids, have a wide variety of diverse functions.[6, 7] Some of these functions, derived from human and animal model studies, attributed to androgens, include modulation of several neurotransmitters via binding with neuroreceptors (GABA[A], NMDA, 5HT, opioid, sigma, substance P, and others), regulation of myelinization, neuroprotection, modulation of brain cytokines, and stimulation of the growth of axons and dendrites.[8, 9, 10, 11, 12, 13, 14, 15, 16, 17]

In animal models, androgens have been shown to alter neuronal outgrowth, synaptic organization, interneural communications, and cell survival in various portions of the brain and spinal cord, through androgen receptor (AR) binding in AR-containing cells, and through upregulating and increasing the number of AR when androgens are administered.[18, 19] Androgens also have been shown to regulate and upregulate several neurotrophins and growth factors (brain-derived neurotrophic factor, BDNF, nerve growth factor, NGF, basic fibroblast growth factor, bFGF, and transforming growth factor-beta, TGF-beta) which assist in neuronal survival and regeneration.[20, 21, 22, 23, 24, 25, 26]

Numerous authors of scientific reports have recommended the use of androgens for patients undergoing rehabilitation to provide an appropriate anabolic stimulus to prevent or reverse disease and age-related catabolism, sarcopenia, osteoporosis, and body composition alterations.[27, 28, 29, 30, 31, 32, 33, 34, 35, 36, 37, 38] Androgen therapy has been shown to increase muscle mass and strength, reverse catabolism, and improve sense of well-being.[39, 40, 41, 42, 43, 44, 45, 46]

Loss of anabolic stimuli and lean body mass compromises the patient's ability to handle acute complications of disease states and impairs efforts towards rehabilitation.[47] Androgen therapy has been shown to provide an appropriate and multifaceted anabolic stimulus for patients undergoing conventional rehabilitation techniques. A double-blind trial of stanozolol therapy for elderly disabled men and women has shown significant increased levels of physical activity and speed of rehabilitation.[48] It has also been shown, in a randomized, placebo-controlled, double-blind study, that androgen replacement improves the rehabilitation outcomes in ill older men who are undergoing conventional rehabilitative modalities.[49]

Androgen therapy has been proved to be safe and effective treatment for elderly patients (60- to 80-year-old men and women).[50, 51] A large double-blind, placebo-controlled study, androgen therapy (DHEA 50mg/day for one year in aging men and women) confirmed that low-dose androgen therapy lacks harmful consequences and does not create "supermen or superwomen" as seen with androgen abuse by bodybuilders.[52] These findings have provided the physiological evidence that androgen therapy can be efficacious in the clinical area as a pharmacological intervention against losses of lean body mass associated with age, disease, stroke, trauma, and burn injury.[53]

Androgen Deficiency and Low Anabolic Stimuli in Stroke Patients

Several recent studies have shown that stroke patients are low on anabolic hormones and growth factors prior to and during stroke, and for a significant period poststroke. Androgen deficiency has been well recognized in stroke patients[54, 55] and has been associated with both gonadal and hypothalamic-pituitary-gonadal dysfunction.[56] This state of hypoandrogenemia can be further exacerbated by hypothalamic-pituitary-adrenal dysfunction in stroke patients where there is a significant hypersecretion by the adrenal gland of cortisol relative to androgens.[57]

In postmenopausal women, androgen deficiency can be even further exacerbated by estrogen monotherapy that raises SHBG and reduces circulating total and free androgen levels. In these women, bioavailable testosterone has been shown to be reduced even more profoundly by estrogen monotherapy, because SHBG is increased by 160 percent, and by the reduction of remaining ovarian and adrenal androgen production, which creates sufficient rationale for androgen therapy.[58] Moreover, numerous studies have also shown that the age-related changes in the adrenal gland, especially in women, can cause hypercortisolemia and hypoandrogenemia, when the adrenal glands are activated from internal and external stressors and chronic disease states.[59, 60, 61] Postmenopausal women, who are generally androgen-deficient due to ovarian involution, who have a family history of stroke, who have a history of thrombosis (such as DVT), who are on estrogen monotherapy, who are under stressful life circumstances,[62] and who have age-related insufficient adrenal androgen production, can have profound androgen deficiency and have a marked elevation in the risk for stroke.

Investigational studies have shown that the hypothalamic-GH-IGF-1-IGFPB-3 axis can be significantly depressed, due to age-related alterations in that axis, which leads to the reduction in levels of available IGF-1.[63, 64, 65] According to the pertinent literature, plasma IGF-1and IFGPB-3 concentrations in patients who have suffered acute cerebral ischemia are strikingly lower than those in control subjects and healthy age-matched individuals. After an acute ischemic stroke, increased demand for growth factors, altered tissue distribution, accelerated metabolic clearance rate or central inhibition of the GHRH-GH-IGF axis, and androgen deficiency may contribute to the significant reduction in plasma IGF-1 concentrations.[66] It has been shown that IGF-1 may be part of an endogenous neuroprotective and neuronal rescue systems,[67] and that, in animal models, the early intravenous administration of IGF-1 (within two hours post injury) reduces the phase of secondary neuronal loss.[68] Androgen therapy has been shown to elevate both GH and IGF-1 levels in normal, hypogonadal, and aging individuals[69, 70, 71, 72, 73] and decrease IGFBP-3 levels, thus increasing bioavailable IGF-1 levels.[74] It has been proved that androgens enhance GH release via increased GHRH pulse amplitude.[75]

The combination of hypogonadism and hyposomatomedinemia causes a severe loss of anabolic stimuli in many stroke patients.[76] This phenomenon places most stroke patients into a catabolic and hypoandrogenemic hormonal imbalance that has been shown to be associated with the acute pathogenesis of the stroke, accelerated stroke severity, greater infarct size, and increased six-month mortality rates.[77] The lack of an adequate anabolic stimulus also impedes the regeneration of nervous tissues and general recovery of functional capacity during the rehabilitation period and beyond. Androgens and growth factors play an important role in the pathophysiology of acute cerebral ischemia and may have a considerable effect of future therapeutic regimens.[78] Moreover, because correction of androgen and IGF-1 deficiencies improves muscle strength, work capacity, and quality of life, treatment with androgens, human growth hormone, and IFG-1 may be a useful adjunct to physical measures in the rehabilitation of stroke survivors.[79]

Despite the strong scientific evidence that supports the use of anabolic agents during the acute, subacute, and poststroke phases, no controlled human studies on the specific use of these agents have been published to date. However, the available animal studies on stroke models have shown promising results with the administration of androgens (DHEA and herbal androgens), biosynthetic GH, biosynthetic IGF-1, and IGF-1 enhancing agents.[80, 81, 82, 83, 84]

Androgen Deficiency, Atherogenesis, Fibrinolysis, and Thromboembolic Events

It is well recognized that androgen deficiency is associated with an increased incidence of cardiovascular disease and thromboembolic events, including stroke.[85] Androgens can interfere with the atherogenic process by several mechanisms. They influence enzymes such as glucose-6-phosphate dehydrogenase, which can modify the lipid spectrum. Furthermore, androgens can inhibit human platelet aggregation, enhance fibrinolysis, reduce cell proliferation in an accumulating thrombus, and lower plasma levels of plasminogen activator inhibitor type 1 (PAI-1) and tissue plasminogen activator antigen.[86] High PAI-1 and high tissue plasminogen activator antigen have been shown to be independent risk factors for an initial thromboembolic event.[87] Moreover, it has been shown that there is a negative correlation between central nervous system androgen levels and the neurological disorders in men and women.[88]

Serum androgen levels have been correlated with the major stimulator of fibrinolysis, tissue plasminogen activator activity, and inversely correlated with two independent atherogenic factors, PAI-1 and fibrinogen levels. Serum testosterone levels have also been shown to be an independent inverse predictor of tissue plasminogen activator antigen (statistically significant)[89] and PAI-1 (statistically significant)[90] in men. Moreover, serum testosterone levels have been negatively correlated with factor VII activity and alpha 2-antiplasmin, the major inhibitor of fibrinolysis.[91] These findings have suggested that low circulating androgen levels are associated with a hypercoagulability state that contributes to an increased risk of thromboembolic events. Androgen therapy in men has been shown to have significant fibrinolytic effects.[92, 93, 94, 95, 96, 97, 98, 99]

Androgen therapy in women, such as stanozolol, danazol, and others, has shown to reduce PAI-1 and is associated with and increased fibrinolytic activity.[100, 101, 102, 103, 104, 105, 106] Also, in hormone replacement therapy (HRT) for postmenopausal women, androgens and androgenic progesterones have been shown to cause a marked reduction of PAI-1 and an improved fibrinolytic activity. Thus, these profibrinolytic effects of androgens may be of particular interest in relation to the beneficial effects of HRT in decreasing atherogenesis and thromboembolism.[107, 108]

Androgens Are Neuroprotective Neurosteroids and Neuroendocrine Modulators of the Cytokine System

In recent years investigations have shown that androgens belong to the group of neurosteroids synthesized and metabolized in a variety of brain tissues.[109] Androgens are also made available to the brain via the general circulation after they are synthesized by the endocrine system or introduced via exogenous routes. There is evidence that androgens exhibit their neuroprotective and neuroregenerative effects by a number of mechanisms. There is:

(1) evidence from cell culture experiments that suggests that androgens increase the survival, differentiation, and regeneration of neurons, glial cells, and Schwann cells, and that they can be synthesized from cholesterol within both the central and peripheral nervous systems.[110, 111, 112, 113]

(2) evidence from immunocytochemistry that androgens may serve as precursors for other steroids in a biosynthetic pathway in the oligodendrocytes and glial cells which subsequently stimulate myelin synthesis.[114, 115, 116]

(3) evidence indicating that androgens are synthesized by pyramidal neurons and stimulate the hippocampal neurons which play an important role in memory and learning.[117]

(4) evidence that androgens exhibit neurotransmitter modulation effects by receptor-mediated binding to ligand-gated ion channels resulting in repolarization of the plasma membrane, and inhibit further neuronal firing via GABA(A), NMDA, BDNF, and sigma receptors resulting in neuroprotective, neuromodulatory, anxiolytic, antiepileptic, and analgesic effects.[118, 119, 120, 121, 122, 123, 124, 125, 126, 127, 128]

(5) strong evidence that androgens increase the serum and tissue levels of a number of the anabolic and neurotrophic polypeptide growth factors that may limit the extent of acute ischemic neuronal injury, stimulate neovascularization, and enhance functional neurorecovery following stroke.[129, 130, 131, 132, 133, 134, 135, 136, 137, 138, 139, 140]

(6) very strong evidence that androgens promote anabolic influences on cytokines and modulate or correct inflammatory and autoimmune cytokine imbalances.[141, 142, 143, 144, 145, 146, 147, 148, 149, 150, 151] Many cytokines have been identified and found to play a role either in the pathogenesis and acceleration of stroke or the neuroprotection, recovery, and neuroregeneration from it.[152, 153, 154, 155, 156, 157, 158, 159, 160, 161, 162, 163, 164, 165, 166, 167] Androgens have been found to inhibit many of the pathogenic, inflammatory, and catabolic cytokines while stimulating immunoprotective and anabolic cytokines.[168, 169, 170]

Conclusion: Androgens Play a Key Role in the Entire Constellation of Stroke Pathogenesis, Recovery, and Rehabilitation

It has been proved that androgens play a key role in stroke: in the prestroke period, the acute stroke phase, the subacute stroke phase, and the rehabilitation phases. These roles are summarized below.

(1) *The prestroke period*. Androgen deficiency has been shown to be very common in men and women patients who suffer a stroke. Androgen deficiency causes an imbalance in the immune system, resulting in a pathological imbalance in the cytokines which play a role in the inflammatory aspect of cerebrovascular disease. Androgens have a beneficial modulating role on the cytokine balance and overall cytokine functions. Androgen deficiency causes the neuroimmunoendocrine system to become unbalanced in a manner that allows for a pathologic inflammatory process to accelerate the atherogenic processes that can lead to embolic or thrombotic strokes.

Androgen deficiency can be due to a number of factors in stroke patients. These include:

a) the age-related reduction in gonadal androgen production due to a decline in the hypothalamic-pituitary-gonadal axis or gonadal involution.

b) the age-related reduction in adrenal androgen production and a shift towards an increased cortisol to androgen ratio when the adrenal gland is stimulated by acute illness, chronic illness, physical exertion, or stress. This shift alters the cytokine profiles that are conducive to atherogenesis.

c) the age-related decline in the hypothalamic-pituitary-adrenal axis, which reduces adrenal androgen production.

d) the use of postmenopausal estrogen monotherapy as HRT, which significantly increases SHBG and further reduces androgen levels and bioavailability.

e) the existence of a concurrent chronic illness, especially one which is associated with autoimmune disorders or immune deficiency syndromes (see the full discussion in other chapters).

f) the therapeutic use of corticosteroids, which reduces adrenal androgen production.

g) the presence of secondary hypogonadism from immobilization or a variety of disabling conditions (see other chapters for a full discussion).

Androgen deficiency during the prestroke period can place an individual in a chronic catabolic state that can induce atherogenesis, influence the pathogenesis of a stroke and impede the immediate recovery mechanisms. Androgen therapy results in:

a) a reversal of sarcopenia (discussion presented in another chapter).

b) a reversal of osteoporosis (discussion presented in another chapter).

c) an androgen-mediated increase in GH secretion and IGF-1 levels and elevated IGFBP-3 levels causing a significant reduction in available IGF-1 for repair and regeneration. Studies have shown that during the acute phase of a stroke, available IGF-1 is recruited to the ischemic brain tissue and that low availability of IGF-1 may limit the body's endogenous immediate repair and regenerative processes. Androgen therapy has been shown to increase GH secretion, elevate IGF-1 levels, and reduce IGFBP-3 levels that combine to increase bioavailable IGF-1.

d) an androgen-mediated increase in neurotrophin and growth factor levels. Scientific studies have shown that androgen levels play an important role in the stimulation and modulation of a number of the neurotrophins including BDNF, NGF, TGF-beta, and bFGF that play important roles in the maintenance, repair, and regeneration of neural tissues. It could be postulated that decreased levels of these important neurotrophins, due to androgen deficiency, could reduce an individual's biochemical responses to an acute ischemic brain insult.

e) a modulation of brain cytokine balance, assuring an appropriate cytokine-mediated inflammatory response to hypoxia or injury.

f) a role in alleviating mental depression[171] and anxiety and in improving the sense of well-being.[172] Depression plays a role in the pathogenesis and rehabilitation phases of stroke patients. It has been shown that many patients felt exhausted or depressed before an acute thromboembolic event and that this mental state is positively associated with serological markers of inflammation. There is a growing body of evidence that has suggested that infection and inflammation have interactive roles in the pathogenesis of thromboembolism.[173, 174] It remains to be seen whether the inflammation causes feelings of exhaustion, whether exhaustion and depression set the stage for inflammation, or whether existing feelings of exhaustion and depression are amplified by the inflammation.[175] However, androgens have been shown to be potent neurosteroids that bind directly to AR and other receptors that modulate and stimulate several neurotransmitters. Androgen deficiency has been associated with mental depression and anxiety,[176, 177] and androgens have been proved to be antidepression and neurosteroids by their binding to opioid receptors and elevating beta-endorphin levels[178] (full discussion in another chapter).

g) a correction of the hypercoagulable state associated with the reduced fibrinolysis activity that is an independent risk factor for thromboembolism.

h) a correction of the down-regulation of AR and androgen deficiency-related reduction in AR concentrations in brain tissues and neurons.

(2) *The acute and subacute stroke periods.* In an ideal situation, the pharmacological goal in treating thromboembolic stroke should be to re-open the occluded vessels involved and administer an appropriate anabolic stimulus in order to preserve brain tissue and begin the regeneration processes. Since most patients who present with stroke are low on anabolic stimuli, it makes sense to administer drugs that provide for anabolism. These anabolic drugs could include androgens, GH, IGF-1, and specific neurotrophins. Although the research and clinical trials on the more exotic and expensive neurotrophins are ongoing and will continue, it seems obvious that androgen therapy should be the cornerstone of providing the appropriate and necessary anabolic stimuli for the majority of these patients. Androgen therapy provides:

a) a corrective effect for hypoandrogenemia and provides for an up-regulation of AR activity and AR receptor concentrations, which stimulates the regeneration of neural tissues.

b) an overall stimulus to the important neurotransmitters that play roles in brain metabolism and homeostasis.

c) an overall anabolic stimulus that counteracts the catabolic situation of stroke patients.

d) an overall anabolic stimulus that elevates GH, IGF-1, and specific neurotrophins responsible for the preservation and regeneration of neural tissues.

e) an overall balance to the cytokine system that down-regulates pathogenic levels of catabolic cytokines and up-regulates levels of anabolic and neuroprotective cytokines.

f) an important fibrinolytic effect that assists in dissolving current emboli or thrombi and inhibits further concomitant thromboembolic events.

g) an important mental and psychological stimulus to elevate mood and combat depression, anxiety, and improve sense of well-being.

h) an overall anabolic stimulus to prepare the patient for the lengthy rehabilitative processes.

(3) *The Rehabilitative Phase.* A stroke is an acute catabolic, neuroendocrine, neuroimmune, and inflammatory event that is often preceded by chronic catabolic, neuroendocrine, neuroimmune, and inflammatory factors. It is often accelerated by a sedentary lifestyle, chronic diseases, and alterations in the biochemistry that are associated with aging. Therefore, it seems prudent to administer the appropriate pharmacologic anabolic stimulus to maximize the effects of conventional rehabilitation. To date,

little scientific and medical attention has been paid to the anabolic pharmacology relating to the rehabilitation of stroke patients.

For many reasons, an appropriate place to start is with androgen therapy. Androgen therapy, combined with conventional physical, occupational, and speech therapy is an inexpensive, cost-effective, safe, and efficacious measure that provides:

a) a correction to the hypoandrogenemia and hyposomatomedinemia that most stroke patients present with or incur during the acute and subacute stroke phases.

b) a multifaceted anabolic stimulus that assists the progress made via conventional rehabilitation therapy.

c) a multifaceted anabolic stimulus that helps reverse sarcopenia, osteoporosis, and loss of neuromuscular strength and neuronal function, and facilitates conventional rehabilitation efforts in these areas.

d) an improved mental outlook toward the rehabilitation process, including an enhanced sense of well-being and mood, and increased energy levels, all of which facilitate rehabilitation efforts.

e) an acceleration of the rehabilitation process with an improved outcome, which assists in the patient's return to activities of daily living (ADLs).

Recommendations for Anabolic Therapy

Anabolic therapy for stroke patients should start immediately since an acute stroke represents a catastrophic and catabolic event. It is reasonable and prudent to administer the following androgens in pharmacological doses during the acute and subacute stroke phases:

(1) a testosterone ester given intramuscularly regardless of the gender of the patient. Testosterone cypionate, enanthate, or propionate can be administered at 200–400mg IM.

(2) a nandrolone ester given intramuscularly regardless of the gender of the patient. Nandrolone phenpropionate (Durabolin) or nandrolone decanoate (Deca-Durabolin) can be administered at 100–400mg IM.

(3) stanozolol (Winstrol) 6–20mg regardless of the gender of the patient provided orally on a daily basis for the first few days if the patient can swallow.

During the early rehabilitation period, gender may play a role in androgen selection and dosage and the recommendations vary accordingly.

The following recommendations are made for men during the first few weeks of stroke rehabilitation:

(1) testosterone cypionate can be administered at 200–400mg IM bi-weekly.

(2) nandrolone decanoate can be administered at 100–400mg IM bi-weekly.

(3) stanozolol can be prescribed at 10–20mg orally on a daily basis.

For women undergoing rehabilitation during the first few weeks poststroke:

(1) nandrolone decanoate can be administered IM at 50–100mg on a biweekly basis.

(2) stanozolol can be prescribed at 4–10mg orally on a daily basis.

(3) DHEA can be prescribed or recommended at 50–200mg orally on a daily basis. For both men and women undergoing rehabilitation from a stroke, after one month androgen therapy may need to be re-evaluated: the potential for adverse effects should be weighed against the benefit of the therapy on a case-by-case basis.

The adverse effects most common in prudent androgen therapy, in both genders, include mild acne and mild alterations in lipoprotein profiles. Women patients may experience hoarseness of the voice and oily skin. However, it should be noted that if androgen therapy is discontinued at this point, then the progress gained with conventional rehabilitation protocols is likely to be temporarily set back.

Generally speaking, over the longer term, androgen therapy is beneficial poststroke, and could be considered HRT, either for men or women. While specific recommendations would have to be made for individual patients, continued androgen therapy, perhaps at lower doses, is encouraged, provided there is medical follow-up.

Notes

1. Jean, W.C., S.R. Spellman, E.S Nussbaum, et al. Reperfusion injury after focal cerebral ischemia: role of inflammation and the therapeutic horizon. *Neurosurgery* 1998; 43 (6): 1382–1396.

2. Gladstone, D.J., and S.E. Black. Enhancing recovery after stroke with noradrenergic pharmacotherapy: a new frontier? *Can. J. Neurol. Sci.* 2000; 27 (2): 97–105.

3. Silver, B., J. Weber, and M. Fisher. Medical therapy for ischemic stroke. *Clin. Neuropharmacol.* 1996; 19 (2): 101–128.

4. Fisher, M., and J. Bogousslavaksy. Further evolution toward effective therapy for acute ischemic stroke. *JAMA* 1998; 279 (16): 1298–1303.

5. Pollock, A.S., L. Legg, P. Langhorne, et al. Barriers to achieving evidence-based stroke rehabilitation. *Cllin. Rehabil.* 2000; 14 (6): 611–617.

6. Baulieu, E.E. Neurosteroids: a novel function of the brain. *Psychoneuroendocrinology* 1998; 23 (8): 963–987.

7. Genazzani, A.R., F. Bernardi, P. Monteleone, et al. Neuropeptides, neurotransmitters, neurosteroids, and the onset of puberty. *Ann. N.Y. Acad. Sci.* 2000; 900: 1–9.

8. Masonis, A.E., and M.P. McCarthy. Direct effects of the anabolic/androgenic steroids, stanozolol and 17alpha-methyltestosterone, on benzodiazepine binding to the gamma-aminobutyric acid (a) receptor. *Neurosci. Lett.* 1996; 189 (1): 35–38.

9. Bitran, D., R.J. Hilvers, C.A. Frye, et al. Chronic anabolic-androgenic steroid treatment affects brain GABA (A) receptor-gated chloride ion transport. *Life Sci.* 1996; 58 (7): 573–583.

10. Masonis, A.E., and M.P. McCarthy. Effects of the androgenic/anabolic steroid stanozolol on GABA (A) receptor function: GABA-stimulated 36Cl–influx and [35S] TBPS binding. *J. Pharmacol. Exp. Ther.* 1996; 279 (1): 186–193.

11. Bebo, B.F., J.C. Schuster, A.A. Vandenbark, et al. Androgens alter the cytokine profile and reduce encephalogenicity of myelin-reactive T cells. *J. Immunol.* 1999; 162 (1): 35–40.

12. Le Greves, P., W. Huang, P. Johansson, et al. Effects of an anabolic-androgenic steroid on the regulation of NMDA receptor NR1, NR2a, and NR2b subunit mRNAs in brain regions of the male rat. *Neurosci. Lett.* 1997; 226 (1): 61–64.

13. Wang, L.H., and C.L. Tsai. Effects of gonadal steroids on the GABA and glutamate contents of the early developing tilapia brain. *Brain Res. Dev. Brain Res.* 1999; 114 (2): 273–276.

14. Stomati, M., S. Rubino, A. Spinetti, et al. Endocrine, neuroendocrine and behavioral effects of oral dehydroepiandrosterone sulfate supplementation in postmenopausal women. *Gynecol. Endocrinol.* 1999; 13 (1): 15–25.

15. Thiblin, I., A. Finn, S.B. Ross, et al. Increased dopaminergic and 5–hydroxytryptamergic activities in male rat brain following long-term treatment with anabolic androgenic steroids. *Br. J. Pharmacol.* 1999; 126 (6): 1301–1306.

16. Compagnone, N.A., and S.H. Mellon. Neurosteroids: biosynthesis and function of these novel neuromodulators. *Front. Neuroendocrinol.* 2000; 21 (1): 1–56.

17. Hallberg, M., P. Johansson, A.M. Kindlundh, et al. Anabolic-androgenic steroids affect the content of substance P and substance P (1–7) in the rat brain. *Peptides* 2000; 21 (6): 845–852.

18. Menard, C.S., and R.E. Harlan. Up-regulating of androgen receptor immunoreactivity in the rat brain by anabolic-androgenic steroids. *Brain Res.* 1993; 622 (1–2): 226–236.

19. Lustig, R.H., P. Hua, L.S. Smith, et al. An in vitro model for the effects of androgen on neurons employing androgen receptor-transfected PC12 cells. *Mol. Cell. Neurosci.* 1994; 5 (6): 587–596.

20. Katoh-Semba, R. Semba, S. Kashiwamata, et al. Influences of neonatal and adult exposures to testosterone on the levels of the beta-subunit of nerve growth factor in the neural tissue of mice. *Brain Res.* 1990; 522 (1): 112–117.

21. Yoshimura, K., H. Kaji, S. Kamindono, et al. Expression of basic fibroblast growth factor (FGF-2) messenger ribonucleic acid is regulated by testosterone in the rat anterior pituitary. *Growth Factors* 1994; 10 (4): 253–258.

22. Kotoh-Semba, R. Semba, H. Kato, et al. Regulation by androgen levels of the

beta subunit of nerve growth factor and its mRNA in selected regions of the mouse brain. *J. Neurochem.* 1994; 62 (6): 2141–2147.

23. Tirassa, P., I Thiblin, G. Agren, et al. High-dose anabolic androgenic steroids modulate concentrations of nerve growth factor and expression of its low affinity receptor (p75–NGFr) in male rat brain. *J. Neurosci. Res.* 1997; 47 (2): 198–207.

24. Wu, M.F., H.L. Chang, and J. Tseng. Dehydroepiandrosterone induces the transforming growth factor-beta production by marine macrophages. *Int. J. Tissue React.* 1997; 19 (3–4): 141–148.

25. Rasika, S., A. Alvarez-Buylla, and F. Nottebohm. BDNF mediates the effects of testosterone on the survival of new neurons in an adult brain. *Neuron* 1999; 22 (1): 53–62.

26. Yang, L.Y. and A.P. Arnold. BDNF regulation of androgen receptor expression in axotomised SNB motoneurons of adult rats. *Brain Res.* 2000; 852 (1): 127–139.

27. Szarvas, F. [The male climacteric from the practical viewpoint.] *Wien. Med. Wochenschr.* 1992; 142 (5–6): 100–103.

28. Lovejoy, J.C., G.A. Bray, C.S. Greeson, et al. Oral anabolic steroid treatment, but not parenteral androgen treatment, decreases abdominal fat in obese, older men. *Int. J. Obes. Relat. Metab. Disord.* 1995; 19 (9): 614–624.

29. Proctor, D.N., P. Balaopal, and K.S. Nair. Age-related sarcopenia in humans is associated with reduced synthetic rates of specific muscle proteins. *J. Nutr.* 1998; 128 (2 Suppl.): 351S–355S.

30. Hermann, M., and P. Berger. Hormone replacement in the aging male? *Exp. Gerontol.* 1999; 34 (8): 923–933.

31. Bross, R., M. Javanbakht, and S. Bhasin. Anabolic interventions for aging-associated sarcopenia. *J. Clin. Endocrinol. Metab.* 1999; 84 (10): 3420–3430.

32. Casaburi, R. Rationale for anabolic therapy to facilitate rehabilitation in chronic obstructive pulmonary disease. *Baillieres Clin. Endocrinol. Metab.* 1998; 12 (3): 407–418.

33. Morley, J.E., and H.M. Perry. Androgen deficiency in aging men. *Med. Clin. North Am.* 1999; 83 (5): 1279–1289.

34. Lund, B.C., K.A. Bever-Stille, and P.J. Perry. Testosterone and andropause: the feasibility of testosterone replacement therapy in elderly men. *Pharmacothrapy* 1999; 19 (8): 951–956.

35. Roubenoff, R. Sarcopenia: a major modifiable cause of frailty in the elderly. *J. Nutr. Health Aging* 2000; 4 (3): 140–142.

36. Castelo-Branco, C., J.J. Vicente, F. Figueras, et al. Comparative effects of estrogens plus androgens and tibolone on bone, lipid pattern and sexuality in postmenopausal women. *Maturitas* 2000; 34 (2): 161–168.

37. Ferrando, A.A. Anabolic hormones in critically ill patients. *Curr. Opin. Clin. Nutr. Metab. Care* 1999; 2 (2): 171–175.

38. Creutzberg, E.C., and A.M. Schols. Anabolic steroids. *Curr. Opin. Clin. Nutr. Metab. Care* 1999; 2 (3): 243–253.

39. Tenover, J.S. Effects of testosterone supplementation in the aging male. *J. Clin. Endocrinol. Metab.* 1992; 75 (4): 1092–1098.

40. Carter, W.J. Effect of anabolic hormones and insulin-like growth factor-1 on muscle mass and strength in elderly patients. *Clin. Geriatr. Med.* 1995; 11 (4): 735–748.

41. Reid, I.R., D.J. Wattie, M.C. Evans, et al. Testosterone therapy in glucocorticoid treated men. *Arch. Intern. Med.* 1996; 156 (11): 1173–1177.

42. Tenover, J.S. Androgen replacement therapy to reverse and/or prevent age-associated sarcopenia in men. *Baillieres Clin. Endocrinol. Metab.* 1998; 12 (3): 419–425.

43. Grinspoon, S., C. Corcoran, H. Askari, et al. Effects of androgen administration

in men with the AIDS wasting syndrome. A randomized, double-blind, placebo-controlled trial. *Ann. Intern. Med.* 1998; 129 (1): 18–26.

44. Strawford, A., T. Barbieri, M. van Loan, et al. Resistance exercise and supraphysiologic androgen therapy in eugonadal men with HIV-related weight loss: a randomized controlled trial. *JAMA* 1999; 281 (14): 1282–1290.

45. Sattler, F.R., S.V. Jaque, E.T. Schroder, et al. Effects of pharmacological doses of nandrolone decanoate and progressive resistance training in immunodeficient patients infected with human immunodeficiency virus. *J. Clin. Endocrinol. Metab.* 1999; 84 (4): 1268–1276.

46. Giorgi, A., R.P. Weatherby, and P.W. Murphy. Muscular strength, body composition and health responses to the use of testosterone enanthate: a double blind study. *J. Sci. Med. Sport* 1999; 2 (4): 341–355.

47. Ferrando, A.A. Anabolic hormones in critically ill patients. *Cur. Opin. Clin. Nutr. Metab. Care* 1999; 2 (2): 171–175.

48. Lye, M.D., and A.E. Ritch. A double-blind trial of an anabolic steroid (stanozolol) in the disabled elderly. *Rheumatol. Rehabil.* 1977; 16 (1): 62–69.

49. Bakhshi, V., M. Elliot, A. Gentili, et al. Testosterone improves rehabilitation outcomes in ill older men. *J. Am. Geriatr. Soc.* 2000; 48 (5): 550–553.

50. Casson, P.R., N. Santoro, K. Eldind-Hirsch, et al. Postmenopausal dehydroepiandrosterone administration increases free insulin-like growth factor-1 and decreases high-density lipoprotein: a six month trial. *Fertil. Steril.* 1998; 70 (1): 107–110.

51. Legrain, S., C. Massien, N. Lahlou, et al. Dehydroepiandrosterone replacement administration: pharmacokinetic and pharmacodynamic studies in healthy elderly subjects. *J. Clin. Endocrinol. Metab.* 2000; 85 (9): 3208–3217.

52. Baulieu, E.E., G. Thomas, S. Legrain, et al. Dehydroepiandrosterone (DHEA), DHEA sulfate, and aging: contribution of the DHEAge Study to a sociobiomedical issue. *Proc. Natl. Acad. Sci. USA* 2000; 97 (8): 4279–4284.

53. Sheffield-Moore, M. Androgens and the control of skeletal muscle protein synthesis. *Ann. Med.* 2000; 32 (3): 181–186.

54. Kovanenko, A.N., and V.G. Kostiuchenko. [Gonadal and gonadotrophic function of late middle-aged men and women with sequelae of ischemic stroke.] *Zh. Nervopatol. Psikhiatr. Im. S.S. Korsakova* 1987; 87 (1): 29–33.

55. Elwan, O., M. Abdallah, I. Issa, et al. Hormonal changes in cerebral infarction in the young and elderly. *J. Neurol. Sci.* 1990; 98 (2–3): 235–243.

56. Dash, R.J., B.K. Sethi, K. Nalini, et al. Circulating testosterone in pure motor stroke. *Funct. Neurol.* 1991; 6 (1): 29–34.

57. Johansson, A., B. Ahren, B. Nasman, et al. Cortisol axis abnormalities early after stroke — relationships to cytokines and leptin. *J. Intern. Med.* 2000; 247 (2): 179–187.

58. Casson, P.R., K.E. Elkind-Hirsh, J.E. Buster, et al. Effect of postmenopausal estrogen replacement on circulating androgens. *Obstet. Gynecol.* 1997; 90 (6): 995–998.

59. Spratt, D.I., C. Longcope, P.M. Cox, et al. Differential changes in serum concentrations of androgens and estrogens (in relation to cortisol) in postmenopausal women with acute illness. *J. Clin. Endocrinol. Metab.* 1993; 76 (6): 1542–1547.

60. Harper, A.J., J.E. Bruster, and P.R. Casson. Changes in adrenocortical function with aging and therapeutic implications. *Semin. Reprod. Endocrinol.* 1999; 17 (4): 327–338.

61. Zeitz, B., R. Reber, M. Oertel, et al. Altered function of the hypothalamic stress axis in patients with moderately active systemic lupus erythematosus. II. Dissociation between androstenedione, cortisol, or dehydroepiandrosterone and interleukin-6 or tumor necrosis factor. *J. Rheumatol.* 2000; 27 (4): 911–918.

62. Obut, T.A. [Dehydroepiandrosterone, reticular area of adrenal cortex and resistance to stress and disease.] *Vestin. Ross Akad. Med. Nauk.* 1998; 10: 18–22.

63. Scheepens, A., E. Sirimanne, E. Beilharz, et al. Alterations in the neural growth hormone axis following hypoxic-ischemic brain injury. *Brain Res. Mol. Brain Res.* 1999; 68 (1–2): 88–100.

64. Casson, P.R., N. Santoro, K. Elkiind-Hirsch, et al. Postmenopausal dehydroepiandrosterone administration increases free insulin-like growth factor-1 and decreases high-density lipoproteins: a six month trial. *Fertil. Steril.* 1998; 70 (1): 107–110.

65. Arvat, E., F. Broglio, and E. Ghigo. Insulin-like growth factor 1: implications in aging. *Drugs Aging* 2000; 16 (1): 29–40.

66. Schwab, S., M. Spranger, S. Krempien, et al. Plasma insulin-like growth factor 1 and IGF binding protein 3 levels in patients with acute cerebral ischemic injury. *Stroke* 1997; 28 (9): 1744–1748.

67. Loddick, S.A., X.J. Liu, Z.X Liu, et al. Displacement of insulin-like growth factors from their binding proteins as a potential treatment for stroke. *Proc. Nat'l. Acad. Sci. USA* 1998; 95 (4): 1894–1898.

68. Gluckman, P.D., J. Guan, C. Williams, et al. Asphyxial brain injury — role of the IGF system. *Mol. Cell. Endocrinol.* 1998; 140 (1–2): 95–99.

69. Eakman, G.D., J.S. Dallas, S.W. Ponder, et al. The effects of testosterone and dihydrotestosterone on hypothalamic regulation of growth hormone secretion. *J. Clin. Endocrinol. Metab.* 1996; 81 (3): 1212–1223.

70. Morales, A.J., J.J. Nolan, J.C. Nelson, et al. Effects of replacement dose of dehydroepiandrosterone in men and women of advancing age. *J. Clin. Endocrinol. Metab.* 1994; 78 (6): 1360–1367.

71. Hobbs, C.J., S.R. Plymate, C.J. Rosen, et al. Testosterone administration increases insulin-like growth factor-1 levels in normal men. *J. Clin. Endocrinol. Metab.* 1993; 77 (3): 776–779.

72. Morales, A.J., R.H. Haubrich, J.Y. Hwang, et al. The effect of six months' treatment with 100mg daily dose of dehydroepiandrosterone (DHEA) on circulating sex steroids, body composition and muscle strength in age-advanced men and women. *Clin. Endocrinol. (Oxf.)* 1998; 49 (4): 421–434.

73. Casson, P.R., N. Santoro, K. Elkind-Hirsch, et al. Postmenopausal dehydroepiandrosterone administration increases free insulin-like growth factor-1 and decreases high density lipoprotein: a six month trial. *Fertil. Steril.* 1998; 70 (1): 107–110.

74. Gelato, M.C., and R.A. Frost. IGFBP-3. Functional and structural implications in aging and wasting syndromes. *Endocrine* 1997; 7 (1): 81–85.

75. Eakman, G.D., J.S. Dallas, S.W. Ponder, et al. The effects of testosterone and dihydrotestosterone on hypothalamic regulation of growth hormone secretion. *J. Clin. Endocrinol. Metab.* 1996; 81 (3): 1217–1223.

76. Abbasi, A., D.E. Matson, M. Ciusiner, et al. Hyposomatomedinemia and hypogonadism in hemiplegic men who live in nursing homes. *Arch. Phys. Med. Rehabil.* 1994; 75 (5): 594–599.

77. Jeppensen, L.L., H.S. Jorgensen, H. Nakayama, et al. Decreased serum testosterone in men with acute ischemic stroke. *Arterioscler. Thromb. Vasc. Biol.* 1996; 16 (6): 749–754.

78. Schwab, S., M. Spranger, S. Krempien, et al. Plasma insulin-like growth factor 1 and IGF binding protein 3 levels in patients with acute cerebral ischemic injury. *Stroke* 1997; 28 (9): 1744–1748.

79. Abbasi, A., D.E. Mattson, M. Ciusinier, et al. Hyposomatomedinemia and hypogonadism in hemiplegic men who live in nursing homes. *Arch. Phys. Med. Rehabil.* 1994; 75 (5): 594–599.

80. Lapchak, P.A., D.F. Chapman, S.Y. Nunez, et al. Dehydroepiandrosterone sulfate is neuroprotective in a reversible spinal cord ischemia model: possible involvement of GABA (A) receptors. *Stroke* 2000; 31 (8): 1953–1956.

81. Lu, A.G., D.A. Otero, M. Hiraiwa, et al. Neuroprotective effect of retro-inverso Prosaptide D5 on focal cerebral ischemia in rat. *Neuroreport* 2000; 11 (8): 1791–1794.

82. Scheepens, A., E. Sirimanne, E. Beilharz, et al. Alterations in the neural growth hormone axis following hypoxic-ischemic brain injury. *Brain Res. Mol. Brain Res.* 1999; 68 (1–2): 88–100.

83. Gluckman, P.D., J. Guan, C. Williams, et al. Asphyxial brain injury — the role of the IGF system. *Mol. Cell. Endocrinol.* 1998; 140 (1–1): 95–99.

84. Loddick, S.A., X.J. Liu, Z.X. Lu, et al. Displacement of insulin-like growth factors from their binding proteins as a potential treatment for stroke. *Proc. Natl. Acad. Sci. USA* 1998; 95 (4): 1894–1898.

85. Winkler, U.H. Effects of androgens on haemostasis. *Maturitas* 1996; 24 (3): 147–155.

86. Porsova-Dutoit, I., J. Sulcova, and L. Starka. Does DHEA/DHEAS play a protective role in coronary heart disease? *Physiol. Res.* 2000; 49 (Suppl. 1): S43–56.

87. Thogersen, A.M., J.H. Jansson, K. Boman, et al. High plasminogen activator inhibitor and tissue plasminogen activator levels in plasma precede a first acute myocardial infarction in both men and women: evidence for the fibrinolytic system as an independent primary risk factor. *Circulation* 1998; 98 (21): 2241–2247.

88. Axuma, T., T. Matsubara, Y. Shima, et al. Neurosteroids in cerebral spinal fluid in neurologic disorders. *J. Neurol. Sci.* 1993; 120 (1): 87–92.

89. Glueck, C.J., H.I. Glueck, D. Stroop, et al. Endogenous testosterone, fibrinolysis, and coronary heart disease risk in hyperlipidemic men. *J. Lab. Clin. Med.* 1993; 122 (4): 412–420.

90. Caron, P., A. Bennet, R. Carare, et al. Plasminogen activator inhibitor in plasma is related to testosterone in men. *Metabolism* 1989; 38 (10): 1010–1015.

91. Bonithon-Kopp, C., P.Y. Scarabin, L. Bara, et al. Relationship between sex hormones and haemostatic factors in healthy middle-aged men. *Atherosclerosis* 1988; 71 (1): 71–76.

92. Davidson, J.F., G.A. McDonald, and G.P. McNicol. Fibrinolytic enhancement by stanozolol: a double-blind trial. *J. Clin. Pathol.* 1972; 25 (7): 639.

93. Davidson, J.F., G.A. McDonald, and J.A. Conkie. Fibrinolytic enhancement by stanozolol — a two year study. *Br. J. Haematol.* 1972; 22 (5): 639–640.

94. Jarrett, P.E., M. Morland, and N.L. Browse. Idiopathic recurrent superficial thrombophlebitis: treatment with fibrinolytic enhancement. *Br. Med. J.* 1977; 1 (6066): 933–934.

95. Small, M., B.M. McArdle, G.D. Lowe, et al. The effect of intramuscular stanozolol on fibrinolysis and blood lipids. *Thromb. Res.* 1982; 28 (1): 27–36.

96. Verheijen, J.H., D.C. Rijken, G.T. Chang, et al. Modulation of rapid plasminogen activator inhibitor in plasma by stanozolol. *Thromb. Haemost.* 1984; 51 (3): 396–397.

97. Kluft, C., F.E. Preston, R.G. Malia, et al. Stanozolol-induced changes in fibrinolysis and coagulation in healthy adults. *Thromb. Haemost.* 1984; 51 (2): 157–164.

98. Small, M., C. Kluft, A.C. MacCuish, et al. Tissue plasminogen activator inhibition in diabetes mellitus. *Diabetes Care* 1989; 12 (9): 655–658.

99. Cooper, R.G., Mitchell, W.S., and K.J. Illingworth. Fibrinolytic enhancement with stanozolol fails to improve symptoms and signs in patients with post-surgical back pain. *Scand. J. Rheumatol.* 1991; 20 (6): 414–418.

100. Vogel, G., R. Huyke, and G. Lauten. [Modification of hypofibrinolytic states by dehydrochloromethyltestosterone.] *Folia Haematol. Int. Mag. Klin. Morphol. Blutforsh* 1984; 111 (4): 536–566.

101. Rizzo, S.C., G. Grignani, G. Gamba, et al. Fibrinolysis induced by danazol. *Blut.* 1986; 53 (4): 351–352.

102. Ford, I., T.C. Li, I.D. Cooke, et al. Changes in hematological indicies, blood viscosity and inhibitors of coagulation during treatment of endometriosis with danazol. *Thromb. Haemost.* 1994; 72 (2): 218–221.

103. Van Wersch, J.W., J.M. Ubachs, A. van den Ende, et al. The effect of two regimens of hormone replacement therapy on the haemostatic profile in postmenopausal women. *Eur. J. Clin. Chem. Biochem.* 1994; 32 (6): 449–453.

104. Winkler, U.H., R. Altkemper, B. Kwee, et al. Effects of tibolone and continuous combined hormone replacement therapy on parameters in the clotting cascade: a multicenter, double-blind, randomized study. *Fertil. Steril.* 2000; 74 (1): 10–19.

105. Glueck, C.J., R. Freiberg, H.I. Glueck, et al. Idiopathic osteonecrosis, hypofibrinolysis, high plasminogen activator inhibitor, high lipoprotein (a), and therapy with stanozolol. *Am. J. Hematol.* 1995; 48 (4): 213–220.

106. Shepherd, J. Danazol and plasma lipoprotein metabolism. *Int. J. Gynaecol. Obstet.* 1995; 50 (Suppl. 1): S23–26.

107. Winkler, U.H. Effects of androgens on haemostasis. *Maturitas* 1996; 24 (3): 147–155.

108. Bjarnason, N.H., K. Bjarnason, J. Haarbo, et al. Tibolone: influence on markers of cardiovascular disease. *J. Clin. Endocrinol. Metab.* 1997; 82 (6): 1752–1756.

109. Kleinrok, Z., and M. Sieklucka-Dziuba. [Androgens and the brain.] *Ginekol. Pol.* 1994; 65 (1): 45–50.

110. Schumacher, M., P. Robel, E.E. Baulieu, et al. Development and regeneration of the nervous system: role for neurosteroids. *Dev. Neurosci.* 1996; 18 (1–2): 6–21.

111. Schumacher, M., F. Robert, and E.E. Baulieu. [Neurosteroids: trophic effects in the nervous system.] *J. Soc. Biol.* 1999; 193 (3): 285–292.

112. Jordan, C.L. Glia as mediators of steroid hormone action on the nervous system: an overview. *J. Nuerobiol.* 1999; 40 (4): 434–445.

113. Zwain, I.H., and S.S. Yen. Dehydroepiandrosterone: biosynthesis and metabolism in the brain. *Endocrinology* 1999; 140 (2): 880–887.

114. Robel, P., and E.E. Baulieu. Neurosteroids: biosynthesis and function. *Crit. Rev. Neurobiol.* 1995; 9 (4): 383–394.

115. Baulieu, E.E., and R. Robel. Neurosteroids: a new brain function? *J. Steroid Biochem. Mol. Biol.* 1990; 37 (3): 395–403.

116. Celotti, F., P. Negri-Cesi, and A. Poletti. Steroid metabolism in the mammalian brain: 5alpha-reduction and aromatization. *Brain Res. Bull.* 1997; 44 (4): 365–375.

117. Tsutsui, K., K. Ukena, M. Usui, et al. Novel brain function: biosynthesis and actions of neurosteroids in neurons. *Neurosci. Res.* 2000; 36 (4): 261–273.

118. Lambert, J.J., D. Belelli, C. Hill-Venning, et al. Neurosteroid modulation of native and recombinant GABA (A) receptors. *Cell. Mol. Neurobiol.* 1996; 16 (2): 155–174.

119. Spindler, K.D. Interactions between steroid hormones and the nervous system. *Neurotoxicology* 1997; 18 (3): 745–754.

120. Zinder, O., and D.E. Dar. Neuroactive steroids: their mechanism of action and their function in the stress response. *Acta Physiol. Scand.* 1999; 167 (3): 181–188.

121. Park-Chung, M., A. Malayev, R.H. Purdy, et al. Sulfated and unsulfated steroids modulated gama-aminobutyric acid A receptor function through distinct sites. *Brain Res.* 1999; 830 (1): 72–87.

122. Maurice, T., V.L. Phan, A. Urani, et al. Neuroactive neurosteroids as endogenous effectors for the sigma1 (sigma1) receptor: pharmacological evidence and therapeutic opportunities. *JPn. J. Pharmacol.* 1999; 81 (2): 125–155.

123. Green, A.R., A.H. Hainsworth, and D.M. Jackson. GABA potentiation: a logical pharmacological approach for the treatment of acute ischaemic stroke. *Neuropharmacology* 2000; 39 (9): 1483–1494.

124. Baulieu, E.E. Neurosteroids: of the nervous system, by the nervous system, for the nervous system. *Recent Prog. Horm. Res.* 1997; 52: 1–32.

125. Gasior, M., R.B. Carter, and J.M. Witkin. Neuroactive steroids: potential therapeutic use in neurological and psychiatric disorders. *Trends Pharmacol. Sci.* 1999; 20 (3): 107–112.

126. Rupprecht, R., and F. Holsboer. Neuroactive steroids: mechanisms of action and neuropsychopharmacological perspectives. *Trends Neurosci.* 1999; 22 (9): 410–416.

127. Lapchak, P.A., D.F. Chapman, S.Y. Nunez, et al. Dehydroepiandrosterone sulfate is neuroprotective in a reversible spinal cord ischemia model: a possible involvement of GABA (A) receptors. *Stroke* 2000; 31 (8): 1953–1957.

128. Yang, L.Y., and A.P. Arnold. Interaction of BDNF and testosterone in the regulation of adult perineal motoneurons. *J. Neurobiol.* 2000; 44 (3): 308–319.

129. Tarkowski, E., L. Rosengren, B. Blomstrand, et al. Intrathecal release of pro- and anti-inflammatory cytokines during stroke. *Clin. Exp. Immunol.* 1997; 110 (3): 492–499.

130. Kawamata, T., E.K. Speliotes, and S.P. Finklestein. The role of polypetide growth factors in recovery from stroke. *Adv. Neurol.* 1997; 73: 377–382.

131. Kawamata, T., J. Ren, T.C. Chan, et al. Intracisternal osteogenic protein-1 enhances functional recovery following focal stroke. *Neuroreport* 1998; 9 (7): 1141–1145.

132. Sordello, S., N. Bertrand, and J. Plouet. Vascular endothelial growth factor is up-regulated in vitro and in vivo by androgens. *Biochem. Biophys. Res. Commun.* 1998; 251 (1): 287–290.

133. Ay, H., I. Ay, W.J. Koroshetz, et al. Potential usefulness of basic fibroblast growth factor as a treatment for stroke. *Cerebrovasc. Dis.* 1999; 9 (3): 131–135.

134. Touzani, O., H. Boutin, J. Chuquet, et al. Potential mechanisms of interleukin-1 involvement in cerebral ischaemia. *J. Neuroimmunol.* 1999; 100 (1–2): 203–215.

135. Plate, K.H. Mechanism of angiogenesis in the brain. *J. Neuropathol. Exp. Neurol.* 1999; 58 (4): 313–320.

136. Ruocco, A., O. Nicole, F. Docagne, et al. A transforming growth factor-beta agonist unmasks the neuroprotective role of this endogenous cytokine in excitotoxic and ischemic brain injury. *J. Cereb. Blood Flow Metab.* 1999; 19 (12): 1345–1353.

137. Carlson, N.G., W.A. Wieggel, J. Chen, et al. Inflammatory cytokines IL-1 alpha, IL-1 beta, IL-6, and TNF-alpha impart neuroprotection to an excitotoxin through distinct pathways. *J. Immunol.* 1999; 163 (7): 3963–3968.

138. Semkova, I., and J. Krieglstein. Neuroprotection mediated via neurotrophic factors and induction of neurotrophic factors. *Brain Res. Brain Res. Rev.* 1999; 30 (2): 176–188.

139. Cardounel, A., W. Regelson, and M. Kalimi. Dehydroepiandrosterone protects hippocampal neurons against neurotoxin-induced cell death: mechanism of action. *Proc. Soc. Biol. Med.* 1999; 222 (2): 145–149.

140. Marti, H.J., M. Bernaudin, A. Bellail, et al. Hypoxia-induced vascular endothelial growth factor expression precedes neovascularization after cerebral ischemia. *Am. J. Pathol.* 2000; 156 (3): 965–976.

141. Fox, H.S. Sex steroids and the immune system. *Ciba Found. Symp.* 1995; 191: 203–211.

142. Loria, R.M., D.A. Padgett, and P.N. Huynh. Regulation of the immune system by dehydroepiandrosterone and its metabolites. *J. Endocrinol.* 1996; 150 (Suppl.): S209–220.

143. Kanda, N., T. Tsuchida, and T. Tamaki. Testosterone inhibits immunoglobulin production by peripheral blood mononuclear cells. *Clin. Exp. Immunol.* 1996; 106 (2): 410–415.

144. Dalal, M., S. Kim, and R.R. Voskuhl. Testosterone therapy ameliorates experimental autoimmune encephalomyelitis and induces T helper 2 bias in the autoantigen-specific T lympthocyte response. *J. Immunol.* 1997; 159 (1): 3–6.

145. Blanco, C.E., P. Popper, and P. Micevych. Anabolic-androgenic steroid induces alterations in choline acetyltransferase messenger RNA levels of spinal cord motoneurons in the male rat. *Neuroscience* 1997; 78 (3): 873–882.

146. Bebo, B.F., J.C. Schuster, A.A. Vandenbark, et al. Androgens alter the cytokine profile and reduce encephalogenicity of myelin-reactive T cells. *J. Immunol.* 1999; 162 (1): 35–40.

147. Vemters, H.D., Q. Tang, Q. Liu, et al. A new mechanism of neurodegeneration: a proinflammatory cytokine inhibits receptor signaling by a survival peptide. *Proc. Natl. Acad. Sci. USA* 1999; 96 (17): 9879–9884.

148. Verthelyi, D., and D.M. Klinman. Sex hormone levels correlate with the activity of cytokine-secreting cells in vivo. *Immunology* 2000; 100 (3): 384–390.

149. Papdopoulos, A.D., and S.W. Wardlaw. Testosterone suppresses the response of the hypothalamic-pituitary-adrenal axis to interleukin-6. *Neuroimmunomodulation* 2000; 8 (1): 39–44.

150. Schiffito, G., M.P. McDermott, T. Evans, et al. Autonomic performance and dehydroepiandrosterone sulfate levels in HIV-1 infected individuals: relationship to TH1 and TH2 cytokine profile. *Arch. Neurol.* 2000; 57 (7): 1027–1032.

151. Giron-Gonzales, J.A., F.J. Moral, J. Elvira, et al. Consistent production of a higher TH1: TH2 cytokine ratio in stimulated T cells in men compared to women. *Eur. J. Endocrinol.* 2000; 143 (1): 31–36.

152. Barone, F.C., and G.Z. Feurestein. Inflammatory mediators and stroke: new opportunities for novel therapeutics. *J. Cereb. Blood Flow Metab.* 1999; 19 (8): 818–834.

153. Ren, J.M., and S.P. Finklestein. Time window of infarct reduction by intravenous basic fibroblast growth factor in focal cerebral ischemia. *Eur. J. Pharmacol.* 1997; 327 (1): 11–16.

154. Kawamata, T., W.D. Dietrich, T. Schallert, et al. Intracisternal basic fibroblast growth factor enhances functional recovery and up-regulates the expression of a molecular marker of neuronal sprouting following focal cerebral infarction. *Proc. Natl. Acad. Sci. USA* 1997; 94 (15): 8179–8184.

155. Terreni, L., and M.G. De Simoni. Role of the brain in interleukin-6 modulation. *Neuroimmunomodulation* 1998; 5 (3–4): 214–219.

156. Farrarese, C., P. Mascarucci, C. Zoia, et al. Increased cytokine release from peripheral blood cells after acute stroke. *J. Cere. Blood Flow Metab.* 1999; 19 (9): 1004–1009.

157. Marti, H.H., and W. Risau. Angiogenesis in ischemic disease. *Thromb. Haemost.* 1999; 82 (Suppl. 1): 44–52.

158. Saarelainen, T., J.A. Lukkarinen, S. Koponen, et al. Transgenic mice over expressing truncated trkB neurotrophin receptors in neurons show increased susceptibility to cortical injury after focal cerebral ischemia. *Mol. Cell. Neurosci.* 2000; 16 (2): 87–96.

159. Fabian, R.H., J.R. Perez-Polo, and T.A. Kent. Electrochemical monitoring of superoxide anion production and cerebral blood flow: effect of interleukin-1 beta

pretreatment in a model of focal ischemia and reperfusion. *J. Neurosci. Res.* 2000; 60 (6): 795–803.

160. Ali, C., O. Nicole, F. Docagne, et al. Ischemia-induced interleukin-6 as a potential endogenous neuroprotective cytokine against NMDA receptor-mediated excitotoxicity in the brain. *J. Cere. Blood Flow Metab.* 2000; 20 (6): 956–966.

161. Yanamoto, H., I. Nagata, M. Sakata, et al. Infarct tolerance induced by intracerebral infusion of recombinant brain-derived neurotrophic factor. *Brain Res.* 2000; 859 (2): 240–248.

162. Rabuffetti, M., C. Sciorati, G. Tarozzo, et al. Inhibition of caspace-1 like activity by Ac-Try-Val-Ala-Asp-chloromethyl ketone induces long-lasting neuroprotection in cerebral ischemia through apoptosis reduction and decrease proinflammatory cytokines. *J. Neurosci.* 2000; 20 (12): 4398–4404.

163. Ridker, P.M., C.H. Hennekens, J.E. Buring, et al. C-reactive protein and other markers of inflammation in the prediction of cardiovascular disease in women. *N. Engl. J. Med.* 2000; 342 (12): 836–843.

164. Vitkovic, L., J. Bockaert, and C. Jacque. "Inflammatory" cytokines: neuromodulators in normal brain? *J. Neurochem.* 2000; 74 (2): 457–471.

165. Gagliardi, R.J. Neuroprotection, excitotoxicity and NMDA antagonists. *Arq. Neuropsiquiatr.* 2000; 58 (2B): 583–588.

166. Grilli, M., I Barbieri, H. Basudev, et al. Interleukin-10 modulates neuronal threshold of vulnerability to ischaemic damage. *Eur. J. Neurosci.* 2000; 12 (7): 2265–2272.

167. Streit, W.J. Microglial response to brain injury: a brief synopsis. *Toxicol. Pathol.* 2000; 28 (1): 28–30.

168. Niebauer, J., C.D. Pflaum, A.L. Clark, et al. Deficient insulin-like growth factor 1 in chronic heart failure predicts altered body composition, anabolic deficiency, cytokine and neurohormonal activation. *J. Am. Coll. Cardiol.* 1998; 32 (2): 393–397.

169. Bebo, B.F., J.C. Scuster, A.A. Vandenbark, et al. Androgens alter cytokine profile and reduce encephalogenicity of myelin-reactive T cells. *J. Immunol.* 1999; 162 (1): 35–40.

170. Johansson, A., B. Ahren, B. Nasman, et al. Cortisol axis abnormalities early after stroke — relationships to cytokines and leptin. *J. Intern. Med.* 2000; 247 (2): 179–187.

171. Wolkowitz, O.M., V.I. Reus, E. Roberts, et al. Dehydroepiandrosterone (DHEA) treatment of depression. *Biol. Psychiatry* 1997; 41 (3): 311–318.

172. Artl, W., F. Callies, J.C. van Vlijment, et al. Dehydroepiandrosterone replacement in women with adrenal insufficiency. *N. Engl. J. Med.* 1999; 341 (14): 1013–1020.

173. Mehta, J.L., T.G. Saldeen, and K. Rand. Interactive role infection, inflammation and traditional risk factors in atherosclerosis and coronary artery disease. *J. Am. Coll. Cardiol.* 1998; 31 (6): 1217–1225.

174. Mattila, K.J., V.V Valtonen, M.S. Nieminen, et al. Role of infection as a risk factor for atherosclerosis, myocardial infarction, and stroke. *Clin. Infect. Dis.* 1998; 26 (3): 719–734.

175. Appels, A., F.W. Bar, J. Bar, et al. Inflammation, depressive symptomology, and coronary artery disease. *Psychosom. Med.* 2000; 62 (5): 601–605.

176. Wolkowitz, O.M., V.I. Reus, E. Roberts, et al. Dehydroepiandrosterone (DHEA) treatment of depression. *Biol. Psychiatry* 1997; 41 (3): 331–318.

177. Arlt, W., F. Callies, J.C. van Vlijmen, et al. Dehydroepiandrosterone replacement in women with adrenal insufficiency. *N. Engl. J. Med.* 1999; 341 (14): 1013–1020.

178. Stomati, M. S., Rubino, A. Spinetti, et al. Endocrine, neuroendocrine and behavioral effects of oral dehydroepiandrosterone sulfate supplementation in post-

21

Rationale for Anabolic Therapy in Type II Diabetes in Men: Medical Management and Rehabilitation

Introduction: Gender Dimorphism in Type II Diabetes

There is now considerable evidence of a gender dimorphism in Type II diabetes that indicates an inverse association between Type II diabetes and androgens in men and a positive association between Type II diabetes and androgens in women.[1] This gender dimorphism has been shown in both animal models of diabetes[2, 3, 4] and in investigations of Type II diabetics in humans.[5, 6, 7, 8, 9] This gender dimorphism has been shown to represent differences in the disease process between men and women who develop Type II diabetes.

In general, men and women with Type I diabetes and women with Type II diabetes have androgen excess that has been correlated with the pathogenesis of these conditions. Conversely, for Type II diabetes in men, serum androgens are generally low and the development of overt hypoandrogenemia has been shown to be statistically significant in several studies. This hypoandrogenemia contributes significantly and adversely to the overall disease process. In men with Type II diabetes, hypoandrogenemia contributes adversely to the risks for other diabetes-related conditions such as atherogenesis, thromboembolic events, microvascular disease, osteoporosis, sarcopenia, erectile dysfunction, insulin resistance, reduced insulin sensitivity, neuropathy, nephropathy, retinopathy, cytokine imbalance, reduced IGF-1 levels with reduced IGFBP-3 levels, reduced anabolic reserve of tissue growth factors and neurotrophins, depression, reduced sense of well-being, and an overall catabolic state.

Hypoandrogenemia in men with Type II diabetes has been well documented and studied from various epidemiological perspectives. Some authors have offered concluding recommendations that encourage androgen therapy; however, there has been a paucity of medical publications that address the specific issue of androgen therapy in these patients.

There is strong evidence to support the therapeutic use of androgens in men with Type II diabetes undergoing treatment in rehabilitation settings. Many men with Type II diabetes, who have pre-existing hypoandrogenemia and hypercortisolemia,[10] are likely to suffer critical illness and severe injury that require rehabilitation. Pre-existing hypoandrogenemia places these patients in a chronic catabolic state with low anabolic reserves. Then, with the onset of an acute illness and injury conditions, a number of endogenous neuroendocrine changes occur that affect survival and rehabilitative outcomes. One such neuroendocrine change is the catabolic shift towards a prevailing hypercortisolemia that is exacerbated by a resistance to or by a decreased production of anabolic hormones, or both. For some tissues, such as skeletal muscle, bone, brain, and others, these endogenous neuroendocrine alterations induce a predominant and accelerated state of catabolism.

Therefore, in men with Type II diabetes, pre-existing hypoandrogenemia and hypercortisolemia are further exacerbated by the endogenous neuroendocrine shifts that accelerate loss of muscle mass and sarcopenia. The resulting loss of lean body mass compromises the patient's ability to handle acute complications and impairs efforts towards rehabilitation. For these reasons, metabolic and therapeutic efforts should be focused on the restoration of anabolic influences. Recent studies continue to demonstrate that the amelioration of tissue catabolism is possible with anabolic hormonal management.[11]

Androgen therapy in older men has been associated with anabolic effects that reverse catabolic and sarcopenic states by increasing lean body mass, muscle mass, and neuromuscular strength.[12, 13, 14, 15, 16, 17] These findings have provided the physiological evidence that androgens should be considered as pharmacological intervention against losses in lean body mass associated with age, disease, trauma, and burn injury.[18] It has been shown that androgen therapy improves the rehabilitation outcomes in older men with a variety of illnesses.[19]

Therefore, for men with Type II diabetes and hypoandrogenemia who are undergoing traditional rehabilitation modalities, androgen therapy may help correct diabetic metabolic conditions, counteract and reverse existing catabolic mechanisms, and improve overall rehabilitation outcomes. Androgen therapy should be considered an important part of the standard of care for these patients.

Hypoandrogenemia in Men with Type II Diabetes

Numerous studies have linked hypoandrogenemia with the pathogenesis of Type II diabetes in men.[20, 21, 22, 23, 24, 25, 26] In population-based, case-control studies, these diabetic men have been shown to be significantly deficient in a number of androgens including plasma levels of total testosterone, free testosterone, dihydrotestosterone, and dehydroepiandrosterone in comparison to nondiabetic, age-matched men.[27, 28] Results from large epidemiological studies (including the MRFIT Research Group Multiple Risk Factor Intervention Trial) have suggested that declining serum androgen levels in men may constitute part of the prediabetic state that predisposes middle-aged men to Type II diabetes.[29, 30] In a large population-based cross-sectional study of men aged 39 to 70 (the Massachusetts Male Aging Study) it was shown that free testosterone declined by 1.2 percent per year, androstenedione declined by 1.3 percent per year, and dehydroepiandrosterone (DHEA) declined by 3.1 percent per year.[31] Aging men with Type II diabetes have been shown to have a marked decrease in serum testosterone levels, an increase of the waist-to-hip-circumference ratio, and reduced IGF-1 levels compared to age-matched men without a diabetic condition.[32] Results from a large cross-sectional study of 80-year-old men born in 1913 showed that low total and free testosterone levels were an independent risk factor (statistically significant) that predicted Type II diabetes.[33] Other major epidemiological trials have found that low androgen levels in men statistically correlate with Type II diabetes prevalence.[34, 35, 36]

Studies have shown that total testosterone, free testosterone, and DHEA levels are inversely associated in men with serum insulin and glucose concentrations after adjustment for age, obesity, and body fat distributions.[37] It has been shown that low serum testosterone levels are associated with insulin resistance, whereas low concentrations of sex SHBG are related to a reduction in insulin sensitivity.[38] Low SHBG levels and hypoandrogenemia have been shown to constitute part of the prediabetic state in men along with higher glucose and insulin levels.[39] Hyperinsulinemia that is associated with increased insulin resistance or reduced insulin sensitivity, such as in men with Type II diabetes, has been shown to be positively associated with reduced SHBG levels and hypoandrogenemia.[40, 41] This strongly suggests that low levels of testosterone and SHBG play some role in the development of insulin resistance and subsequent Type II diabetes in middle-aged men.[42] Therefore, in men with Type II diabetes, it has been suggested, based on results of experimental work and intervention studies, that hypoandrogenemia and low SHBG may be causally related to insulin resistance and hyperinsulinemia.[43]

It has been postulated that a relative hypogonadism in men might be the primary event in the pathogenesis process of Type II diabetes. The insulin resistance which follows the onset of the disease has been shown to be ameliorated by androgen therapy.[44] The available data indicates that the responsible hypogonadism might be of both central and peripheral origin; however, a peripheral origin is more strongly favored because of the findings of elevated or normal LH levels and concomitant low androgen levels due to testicular dysfunction.[45, 46, 47, 48, 49] It has been shown that men with Type II diabetes have a shift in steroidogenesis, probably within the testes, that causes an elevated progesterone/testosterone ratio (progesterone is a precursor of testosterone production) that contributes to insulin resistance in these men.[50]

It has also been postulated that hyperinsulinemia due to primary abnormalities in the insulin receptors (IRs) is the primary event in Type II diabetes in men. The IR shares structural and functional homology with the IFG-1 receptor (IGF-1R). Hybrid receptors composed of both types are found in tissues that express both insulin and IGF-1. These receptors may preferentially behave as IGF-1R rather that IR. It has been shown that in the skeletal muscle of Type II male diabetics, expression of the hybrid receptors is increased, and correlates with a decrease in IR number and an increase in fasting insulin levels. Increased abundance of hybrid receptors has been positively correlated with insulin levels (statistically significant) and inversely with insulin-mediated glucose uptake (statistically significant). Therefore, this mechanism suggests that in male Type II diabetics, hyperinsulinemia (the primary event) induces IR down-regulation and may lead to the formation of a higher proportion of hybrid IGF-IR receptors and reduced insulin sensitivity.[51] Then, protracted hyperinsulinemia causes some, yet unknown, reduction or alteration in testicular function that results in hypoandrogenemia.

Regardless of the exact primary event that causes Type II diabetes in men, there is a statistically significant correlation with hypoandrogenemia that, in turn, causes significant and pathological alterations in an array of biological markers and factors. Perhaps the most important biochemical alteration associated with hypoandrogenemia in men with Type II diabetes is the reduction of serum levels of IGF-1 (hyposomatomedinemia) and tissue levels of IGF-1.

Hypoandrogenemia Induces Hyposomatomedinemia in Men with Type II Diabetes

It has been well documented that androgens play an influential and stimulatory role in the GHRH-GH-IGF-IGFBP axis and that there is a gender dimorphism in the androgen-related regulatory control of this axis.[52] It has been shown that androgens exert their effect on GH secretion via increased GHRH pulse amplitude.[53]

The reduction in serum IGF-1 levels associated with aging men mainly reflects impaired GH secretion and testicular involution.[54] In men with Type II diabetes, the age-related reductions in IGF-1 are markedly exacerbated by hypoandrogenemia[55] and associated with concomitant reductions in IGFBP-3 and free IGF-1 levels.[56, 57] The reductions in the circulating IGF-1 and IGFBP-3 levels decrease anabolic activities and contribute to the mechanism of catabolism, wasting, and diabetes-related pathologies.[58, 59, 60]

Androgen therapy has been shown to elevate IGF-1 levels in normal, hypogonadal, and aging individuals,[61, 62, 63] increase IGFBP-3 levels and bioavailable IGF-1 levels,[64] elevate IGF-1/IGF-1BP-3 ratios,[65] and augment GH release.[66, 67] Moreover, because correction of androgen and IGF-1 deficiencies improves muscle mass, work capacity, and quality of life, treatment with androgens with or without GH or IGF-1 administration may be a useful adjunct to the traditional rehabilitation protocols.[68]

Androgen therapy has also been shown to stimulate local IGF-1 levels and subsequent anabolic and trophic activities in various tissues and cells.[69, 70, 71, 72] These IGF-1 molecules are essential for the differentiation of many cell types, and have been shown to be powerful protective agents for a number of tissues, including those in the integumentary, musculoskeletal, nervous, immune, and the cardiovascular systems.[73, 74, 75, 76, 77]

Therapy with recombinant IGF-1 has been shown to increase the sensitivity to insulin and improve glucose utilization in men with Type II diabetes.[78, 79] IGF-1 therapy has also been shown to improve, but not completely overcome, insulin resistance in Type II diabetes, indicating that some intrinsic defect or defects responsible for insulin resistance in this disease cannot be overcome by IGF-1 treatment alone.[80] Androgen and IGF-1 combined therapies have also been shown to have exert an additive influence that improves insulin sensitivity.[81] In addition, the combination of recombinant

IGF-1 and IGFBP-3 has been shown to be effective in reducing severe cases of insulin resistance in diabetic patients over a two-week trial period.[82] However, further studies are required to determine the long-term safety and efficacy of IGF-1 administration in Type II diabetes.

Consequences of Hypoandrogenemia and Hyposomatomedinemia in Men with Type II Diabetes

Middle-aged and elderly men with Type II diabetes can have a plethora of biochemical abnormalities and disease processes that are caused by, associated with, or exacerbated by hypoandrogenemia and hyposomatomedinemia. A summary of these abnormalities is given in Table 21-1.

Table 21-1: Hypoandrogenemia and Hyposomatomedinemia in Type II Diabetes in Men: The Associated Biochemical Abnormalities and Elevated Disease Risks

Hypoandrogenemia

Biochemical Abnormalities	*Elevated Disease Risk*
increased fibrinogen levels	thromboembolism and microvascular disease
increased PAI levels	thromboembolism and microvascular disease
decreased Lp(a) levels	accelerated atherogenesis
increased triglyceride levels	accelerated atherogenesis
hypercholesterolemia	accelerated atherogenesis
elevated LDL-C levels	accelerated atherogenesis
reduced GH secretion	sarcopenia, osteoporosis, hyposomatomedinemia
reduced IGF-1 level s	hyposomatomedinemia, low anabolic stimuli
reduced IGFBP-3 levels	hyposomatomedinemia, low anabolic stimuli
altered Th1/Th2 cytokine profiles	inflammation, autoimmune disease, dementia
increased IL-6 levels	osteoporosis, autoimmune disease
reduced SHBG levels	accelerated diabetes pathogenesis
increased insulin requirements	accelerated diabetes pathogenesis
increased serum glucose levels	accelerated diabetes pathogenesis
down-regulated androgen receptors	depression, impotence, dementia, obesity
reduction of tissue IGF-1 levels	reduced anabolic stimuli and anabolic reserves
reduction of cellular neurotrophins	reduced anabolic and trophic cellular activities

Hyposomatomedinemia

Biochemical Abnormalities	*Elevated Disease Risk*
increased insulin requirements	accelerated diabetes pathogenesis
elevated hbA1c	accelerated diabetes pathogenesis
down-regulated IGFR activity	microvascular pathogenesis, insulin resistance
reduction of tissue IGF-1 levels	reduced anabolic reserves & cellular trophic activities

---

Specifically, Type II diabetes in men with hypoandrogenemia has been shown to cause or be associated with a statistically significant elevation in plasminogen activator inhibitor (PAI) and fibrinogen levels,[83] statistically significant elevation of triglyceride levels and low density lipoprotein cholesterol (LDL-C) levels,[84] statistically significant reduction in high density lipoprotein cholesterol (HDL-C), elevation of total cholesterol levels and reduced SHBG levels,[85] elevation of lipoprotein a, Lp(a), levels,[86] and a reduction in serum osteocalcin levels.[87] These biochemical abnormalities play important roles in the pathogenesis of many diabetes-related conditions and diseases.

Available Studies of Androgen Therapy for Type II Diabetes in Men

The potential benefits associated with androgen therapy for patients with diabetes were recognized decades ago. Several reports published in medical and scientific journals outside of the United States indicated that androgen therapy, on an empirical basis, exhibited an array of beneficial effects in diabetic patients, including diabetic retinopathy,[88, 89, 90, 91] diabetic angiopathies,[92, 93] diabetic hyperlipemia,[94] diabetic hypertriglyceridemia and hypercholesterolemia,[95] diabetic erectile dysfunction,[96] diabetic ulcers,[97] and other diabetic metabolic abnormalities.[98] More recent studies have shown that testosterone therapy improved insulin sensitivity, reduced visceral fat mass, and improved sense of well-being in men at risk for Type II diabetes,[99] and another reported on the total remission with testosterone therapy of severe sensory motor polyneuropathy after recognition of hypoandrogenemia.[100]

Recommendations for Anabolic Therapy in Men with Type II Diabetes

Androgen therapy should be a part of the standard of care for men with Type II diabetes and concomitant androgen deficiency. Routine serum androgen levels and LH levels should be part of the biochemical evaluation of middle-aged and elderly men with Type II diabetes. Androgen therapy should assist insulin or other agents in lowering glucose and insulin levels, reducing insulin requirements, improving dyslipidemias, enhancing fibrinolysis, reducing cardiovascular risk factors, maintaining or reversing sarcopenia and osteopenia, elevating mood and libido, improving erectile dysfunction, and perhaps increasing longevity.

Men with Type II diabetes should be evaluated for hypoandrogenemia prior to or during the initial phase of the rehabilitation for acute or chronic illness, thromboembolic events, or injury. An appropriate anabolic stimulus derived from androgen therapy can hasten rehabilitative efforts and improve rehabilitation outcomes. It must be remembered that screening for prostate cancer should be obtained prior to the initiation of androgen therapy even though studies have shown that men with Type II diabetes and hypoandrogenemia have a reduced risk for prostate cancer.[101]

Reasonable choices for androgen therapy for men with Type II diabetes who are undergoing rehabilitation are:

(1) stanozolol (Winstrol) 6–20mg/day orally.
(2) oxandrolone (Anavar) 7.5–20mg/day orally.
(3) nandrolone decanoate (Deca-Durabolin) 200–400mg IM biweekly.
(4) testosterone cypionate (Depo-Testosterone) 200–300mg IM biweekly. Other basic recommendations include routine glucose monitoring that should continue, and doses of hypoglycemic agents should be adjusted accordingly. Routine lipid profiles and other routine diabetic testing protocols should be followed. Dual-energy x-ray absorptiometry (DEXA) scanning for bone mineral density is recommended with men patients with Type II diabetes and hypoandrogenemia.

Notes

1. Goodman-Gruen, D, and E. Barrett-Conner. Sex differences in the association of endogenous sex hormone levels and glucose tolerance status in older men and women. *Diabetes Care* 2000; 23 (7): 912–918.

2. Rossini, A.A., R.M. Williams, M.C. Appel, et al. Sex differences in multiple-dose streptozotocin model of diabetes. *Endocrinology* 1978; 103 (4): 1518–1520.

3. Martin, L., G.A. Keller, D. Liggitt, et al. Male specific beta-cell dysfunction and diabetes resulting from increased expression of a synergeic MHC class 1 protein in the pancreata of transgenic mice. *New. Biol.* 1990; 2 (12): 1101–1110.

4. Efrat, S. Sexual dimorphism of pancreatic beta-cell degeneration in transgenic mice expressing an insulin-ras hybrid gene. *Endocrinology* 1991; 128 (2): 897–901.

5. Simon, D., P. Preziosi, E. Barrett-Conner, et al. Interrelation between plasma testosterone and plasma insulin in healthy adult men: the Telecom Study. *Diabetologia* 1992; 35 (2): 173–177.

6. Haffner, S.M., R.A. Valdez, M.P. Stern, et al. Obesity, body fat distribution and sex hormones in men. *Int. J. Obes. Relat. Metab. Disord.* 1993; 17 (11): 643–649.

7. Haffner, S.M., L. Mykkanen, R.A. Valdez, et al. Relationship of sex hormones to lipids and lipoproteins in nondiabetic men. *J. Clin. Endocrinol. Metab.* 1993; 77 (6): 1610–1615.

8. Andersson, B., P. Martin, L. Lissner, et al. Testosterone concentrations in women and men with NIDDM. *Diabetes Care* 1994; 17 (5): 405–411.

9. Zietz, B., A. Cuk, S. Hugl, et al. Association of increased C-peptide serum levels and testosterone in Type II diabetes. *Eur. J. Intern. Med.* 2000; 11 (6): 322–328.

10. Zietz, B., A. Cuk, S. Hugl. et al. Association of increased C-peptide serum levels and testosterone in Type II diabetes. *Eur. J. Intern. Med.* 2000; 11 (6): 322–328.

11. Ferrando, A.A. Anabolic hormones in critically ill patients. *Curr. Opin. Clin Nutr. Metab. Care* 1999; 2 (2): 171–175.

12. Tenover, J.S. Effects of testosterone supplementation in the aging male. *J. Clin. Endocrinol. Metab.* 1992; 75 (4): 1092–1098.

13. Bross, R., R. Casaburi, T.W. Storer, et al. Androgen effects on body composition and muscle function: implications for the use of androgens as anabolic agents in sarcopenic states. *Baillieres Clin. Endocrinol. Metab.* 1998; 12 (3): 365–378.

14. Bross, R., T. Storer, and S. Bhasin. Aging and muscle loss. *Trends Endocrinol. Metab.* 1999; 10 (5): 194–198.

15. Tenover, J.S. Androgen replacement therapy to reverse and/or prevent age-related sarcopenia in men. *Baillieres Clin. Endocrinol. Metab.* 1998; 12 (3): 419–425.

16. Creutzberg, E.C., and A.M. Schols. Anabolic steroids. *Curr. Opin. Clin. Nutr. Metab. Care* 1999; 2 (3): 243–253.

17. Lund, B.C., K.A. Bever-Stille, and P.l.J. Perry. Testosterone and andropause: the feasibility of testosterone replacement in elderly men. *Pharmacotherapy* 1999; 19 (8): 951–956.

18. Sheffield-Moore, M. Androgens and the control of skeletal muscle protein synthesis. *Ann. Med.* 2000; 32 (3): 181–186.

19. Bashski, V., M. Elliott, A. Gentili, et al. Testosterone improves rehabilitation outcomes of ill older men. *J. Am. Geriatr. Soc.* 2000; 48 (5): 550–553.

20. Ando, S., R. Rubens, and R. Rottiers. Androgen plasma levels in male diabetics. *J. Endocrinol. Invest.* 1984; 7 (1): 21–24.

21. Handelsman, D.J., A.J. Conway, L.M. Boylan, et al. Testicular function and glycemic control in diabetic men. A controlled study. *Andrologia* 1985; 17 (5): 488–496.

22. Murray, F.T., H.U. Wyss, R.G. Thomas, et al. Gonadal dysfunction in diabetic men with organic impotence. *J. Clin. Endocrinol. Metab.* 1987; 65 (1): 127–135.

23. Conte-Delvox, B., C. Olivier, and J.L. Codaccioni. [Hypophyseal-Leydig function in the diabetic.] *Acta Endocrinol. (Paris)* 1988; 49 (4–5): 408–411.

24. Fushimi, H., H. Horie, T. Ioune, et al. Low testosterone in diabetic men and animals: a possible role in testicular impotence. *Diabetes Res. Clin. Pract.* 1989; 6 (4): 297–301.

25. Barrett-Conner, E., K.T. Khaw, and S.S. Yen. Endogenous sex hormone levels in older men with diabetes mellitus. *Am. J. Epidemiol.* 1990; 132 (5): 895–901.

26. Chearskul, S., K. Charoenlarp, V. Thongtang, et al. Study of plasma hormones and lipids in healthy elderly Thais compared to patients with chronic diseases: diabetes mellitus, essential hypertension, and coronary heart disease. *J. Med. Assoc. Thai.* 2000; 83 (3): 266–277.

27. Barrett-Conner, E. Lower endogenous androgen levels and dyslipidemia in men with non-insulin-dependent diabetes mellitus. *Ann. Intern. Med.* 1992; 117 (10): 807–811.

28. Zietz, B., A. Cuk, S. Hugl, et al. Association of increased C-peptide serum levels and testosterone lin Type II diabetes. *Eur. J. Intern. Med.* 2000; 11 (6): 322–328.

29. Haffner, S., J. Shaten, M.P. Stern, et al. Low levels of sex-hormone-binding globulin and testosterone predict the development of non-insulin-dependent diabetes mellitus in men. MRFIT Research Group. Multiple Risk Factor Intervention Trial. *Am. J. Epidemiol.* 1996; 143 (9): 889–897.

30. Tsai, E.C., E.J. Boyko, D.L. Leonetti, et al. Low serum testosterone level as a predictor of increased visceral fat in Japanese-American Men. *Int. J. Obes. Relat. Metab. Disord.* 2000; 24 (4): 485–491.

31. Gray, A., H.A. Feldman, J.B. McKinlay, et al. Age, disease, and changing sex hormone levels in middle-aged men: results of the Massachusetts Male Aging Study. *J. Clin. Endocrinol. Metab.* 1991; 73 (5): 1016–1025.

32. Chang, T.C., C.C. Tung, and Y.L. Hsiao. Hormonal changes in elderly men with non-insulin-dependent diabetes mellitus and the hormonal relationships to abdominal adiposity. *Gerontology*1994; 40 (5): 260–267.

33. Thibblin, G., A. Adlerberth, G. Lindstedt, et al. The pituitary-gonadal axis and health in elderly men: a study of men born in 1913. *Diabetes* 1996; 45 (11): 1605–1609.

34. Defay, R., L. Papoz, S. Barny, et al. Hormonal status and NIDDM in the European and Melanesian populations of New Caledonia: a case-control study. The CALedonia Diabetes Mellitus (CALDIA) Study Group. *Int. J. Obes. Relat. Metab. Disord.* 1998; 22 (9): 927–934.

35. Thomas, N., H.A. Morris, F. Scopacasa, et al. Relationships between age, dehydro-epiandrosterone sulfate and plasma glucose in healthy men.

36. Stellato, R.K., H.A. Feldman, O. Hamdy, et al. Testosterone, sex hormone-binding globulin, and the development of Type II diabetes in middle-aged men: prospective results from the Massachusetts male aging study. *Diabetes Care* 2000; 23 (4): 490–494.

37. Haffner, S.M., R.A. Valdez, L. Mykkanen, et al. Decreased testosterone and dehydroepiandrosterone sulfate concentrations are associated with increased insulin and glucose concentrations in nondiabetic men. *Metabolism* 1994; 43 (5): 599–603.

38. Ebeling, P., U.H. Stenman, M. Seppala, et al. Androgens and insulin resistance in Type I diabetic men. *Clin. Endocrinol. (Oxf.)* 1995; 43 (5): 601–607.

39. Haffner, S.M., J. Shaten, M.P. Stern, et al. Low levels of sex hormone-binding globulin and testosterone predict the development of non-insulin-dependent diabetes mellitus in men. MRFIT Research Group. Multiple Risk Factor Intervention Trial. *Am. J. Epidemiol.* 1996; 143 (9): 889–897.

40. Birkeland, K.I., K. F. Hanssen, P.A. Torjesen, et al. Level of sex-hormone binding globulin is positively correlated with insulin sensitivity in men with Type II diabetes. *J. Clin. Endocrinol. Metab.* 1993; 76 (2): 275–278.

41. Yamaguchi, Y., S. Tanaka, T. Yamakawa, et al. Reduced serum dehydroepiandrosterone levels in diabetic patients with hyperinsulinaemia. *Clin. Endocrinol. (Oxf.)* 1998; 49 (3): 377–383.

42. Stellato, R.K., H.A. Feldman, O. Hamdy, et al. Testosterone, sex hormone-binding globulin, and the development of Type II diabetes in middle-aged men: prospective results from the Massachusetts male aging study. *Diabetes Care* 2000; 23 (4): 490–494.

43. Andersson, B., P. Marin, L. Lissner, et al. Testosterone concentrations in women and men with NIDDM. *Diabetes Care* 1994; 17 (5): 405–411.

44. Tibblin, G., A. Adlerberth, G. Lindstedt, et al. The pituitary axis and health in elderly men: a study of men born in 1913. *Diabetes* 1996; 45 (11): 1605–1609.

45. Ando, S., R. Rubens, and R. Rottiers. Androgen plasma levels in male diabetics. *J. Endocrinol. Invest.* 1984; 7 (1): 21–24.

46. Handelsman, D.J., A.J. Conway, L.M. Boylan, et al. Testicular function and glycemic control in diabetic men. A controlled study. *Andrologia* 1985; 17 (5): 488–496.

47. Murray, F.T., H.U. Wyss, R.G. Thomas, et al. Gonadal dysfunction in diabetic men with organic impotence. *J. Clin. Endocrinol. Metab.* 1987; 65 (1): 127–135.

48. Conte-Delvox, B., C. Olivier, J.L. Codaccioni, et al. [Hypophyseal-Leydig function in the diabetic.] *Ann. Endocrinol. (Paris)* 1988; 49 (4–5): 408–411.

49. Chernyshova, T.E., V.A. Sitnikov, and I.K. Martirosov. [The effect of diabetic

nephropathy on the function of the hypophyseal-gonadal system in men.] *Urol. Nefrol. (Mosk.)* 1991; 1: 54–57.

50. Zietz, B., A. Cuk, S. Hugl, et al. Association of increased C-peptide serum levels and testosterone in Type II diabetes. *Eur. J. Intern. Med.* 2000; 11 (6): 322–328.

51. Federici, M., D. Lauro, M. D'Adamo, et al. Expression of insulin/IGF-1 hybrid receptors is increased in skeletal muscle of patients with chronic hyperinsulinemia. *Diabetes* 1998; 47 (1): 87–92.

52. Jaffe, C.A., B. Ocampo-Lim, W. Guo, et al. Regulatory mechanisms of growth hormone secretion are sexually dimorphic. *J. Clin. Invest.* 1998; 102 (1): 153–164.

53. Eakman, G.D., J.S. Dallas, S.W. Ponder, et al. The effects of testosterone and dihydrotestosterone on hypothalamic regulation of growth hormone secretion. *J. Clin. Endocrinol. Metab.* 1996; 81 (3): 1217–1223.

54. Arvat, E., F. Broglio, and E. Ghigo. Insulin-like growth factor 1: implications in aging. *Drugs Aging* 2000; 16 (1): 29–40.

55. Chang, T.C., T.C. Tung and Y.L. Hsiao. Hormonal changes in elderly men with non-insulin dependent diabetes mellitus and the hormonal relationships to abdominal adiposity. *Gerontology* 1994; 40 (5): 260–267.

56. Clauson, P.G., K. Brismar, K. Hall, et al. Insulin-like growth factor-1 and insulin-like growth factor binding protein-1 in a representative population of Type II diabetic patients in Sweden. *Scand. J. Clin. Lab. Invest.* 1998; 58 (4): 353–360.

57. Frystyk, J., C. Skjaerbaek, E. Vestbo, et al. Circulating levels of free insulin-like growth factors in obese subjects: the impact of Type II diabetes. *Diabetes Metab. Res. Rev.* 1999; 15 (5): 314–322.

58. Gelato, M.C. and R.A. Frost. IGFBP-3. Functional and structural implications in aging and wasting syndromes. *Endocrine* 1997; 7 (1): 81–85.

59. Feldmann, B., G.E. Lang, A. Arnavaz, et al. [Decreased serum level of free bioavailable IGF-1 in patients with diabetic retinopathy.] *Ophthalmologe* 1999; 95 (5): 300–305.

60. Jansswen, J.A., and S.W. Lamberts. Circulating IGF-1 and its protective role in the pathogenesis of diabetic angiopathy. *Clin. Endocrinol. (Oxf.)* 2000; 52 (1): 1–9.

61. Hobbs, C.J., S.R. Plymate, C.J. Rosen, et al. Testosterone administration increases insulin-like growth factor-1 levels in normal men. *J. Clin. Endocrinol. Metab.* 1993; 77 (3): 776–779.

62. Morales, A.J., J.J. Nolan, J.C. Nelson, et al. Effects of replacement dose of dehydroepiandrosterone in men and women of advancing age. *J. Clin. Endocrinol. Metab.* 1994; 78 (6): 1360–1367.

63. Morales, A.J., R.H. Haubrich, J.Y. Hwang, et al. The effect of six months treatment with 100mg daily dose of dehydroepiandrosterone (DHEA) on circulating sex steroids, body composition, and muscle strength in age-advanced men and women. *Clin. Endocrinol. (Oxf.)* 1998; 49 (4): 421–434.

64. Gelato, M.C., and R.A. Frost. IGFBP-3. Functional and structural implications in aging and wasting syndromes. *Endocrine* 1997; 7 (1): 81–85.

65. Casson, P.R., N. Santoro, K. Elkind-Hirsch, et al. Postmenopausal dehydroepiandrosterone administration increases free insulin-like growth factor-1 and decreases high-density lipoprotein: a six month trial. *Fertil. Steril.* 1998; 70 (1): 107–110.

66. Eakman, G.D., J.S. Dallas, S.W. Ponder, et al. The effects of testosterone and dihydrotestosterone on hypothalamic regulation of growth hormone secretion. *J. Clin. Endocrinol. Metab.* 1996; 81 (3): 1212–1223.

67. Span, J.P., G.F. Pieters, C.G. Sweep, et al. Gender difference in insulin-like growth factor 1 response to growth hormone (GH) treatment and GH-deficient adults: role of sex hormone replacement. *J. Clin. Endocrinol. Metab.* 2000; 85 (3): 1121–1125.

68. Abbasi, A., D.E. Mattson, M. Cilusinier, et al. Hyposomatomedinemia and hypogonadism in hemiplegic men who live in nursing homes. *Arch. Phys. Med. Rehabil.* 1994; 75 (5): 594–599.

69. Bitar, M.S., C.W. Pilcher, I. Khan, et al. Diabetes–induced suppression of IGF-1 and its receptor mRNA levels in rat superior cervical ganglia. *Diabetes Res. Clin. Pract.* 1997; 38 (2): 73–80.

70. Gori, F., L.C. Hofbauer, C.A. Conover, et al. Effects of androgens on the insulin-like growth factor system in an androgen-responsive human osteoblastic cell line. *Endocrinology* 1999; 140 (12): 5579–5586.

71. Solerte, S.B., M. Fioravanti, G. Vignati, et al. Dehydroepiandrosterone sulfate enhances natural killer cell cytotoxicity in humans via locally generated immunoreactive insulin-like growth factor-1. *J. Clin. Endocrinol. Metab.* 1999; 84 (9): 3260–3267.

72. Solerte, S.B., R. Gornati, L. Cravello, et al. Dehydroepiandrosterone-sulfate (DHEA-S) restores the release of IGF-1 from natural killer (NK) immune cells in old patients with dementia of Alzheimer's type (DAT). *J. Endocrinol. Invest.* 1999; 22 (10 Suppl.): 32–34.

73. Ren, J., W.K. Samson, and J.R. Sowers. Insulin-like growth factor 1 as a cardiac hormone: physiological and pathophysiological implications in heart disease. *J. Mol. Cell. Cardiol.* 1999; 31 (11): 2049–2061.

74. Smith, L.E., W. Shen, C. Perruzzi, et al. Regulation of vascular endothelial growth factor-dependent retinal neovascularization by insulin-like growth factor-1 receptor. *Nat. Med.* 1999; 5 (12): 1390–1395.

75. Russell, J.W., and E.L. Feldman. Insulin-like growth factor-1 prevents apoptosis in sympathetic neurons exposed to high glucose. *Horm. Metab. Res.* 1999; 31 (2–3): 90–96.

76. Winkler, R., F. Pasleau, N. Boussif, et al. [The IGF system: summary and recent data.] *Rev. Med. Liège.* 2000; 55 (7): 725–739.

77. Blakytny, R., E.B. Jude, J. Martin Gibson, et al. Lack of insulin-like growth factor 1 (IGF1) in the basal keratinocyte layer of diabetic skin and diabetic foot ulcers. *J. Pathol.* 2000; 190 (5): 589–594.

78. Simpson, H.L., A.M. Umpleby, and D.L. Russell-Jones. Insulin-like growth factor-1 and diabetes. A review. *Growth Horm. IGF Res.* 1998; 8 (2): 83–95.

79. Laron, Z. Clinical use of somatomedin-1: yes or no? *Paediatr. Drugs* 1999; 1 (3): 155–159.

80. Cusi, K., and R. DeFronzo. Recombinant human insulin-like growth factor 1 treatment for 1 week improves metabolic control in Type II diabetes by ameliorating hepatic and muscle insulin resistance. *J. Clin. Endocrinol. Metab.* 2000; 85 (9): 3077–3084.

81. Paolisso, G., M.R. Tagliamonte, M.R. Rizzo, et al. [Is aging associated with a diminution of insulin sensitivity? Roles of IGF1 and dehydroepiandrosterone.] *J. Annu. Diabetol. Hotel. Dieu.* 1999; 63–74.

82. Clemmons, D.R., A.C. Moses, M.J. McKay, et al. The combination of insulin-like growth factor 1 and insulin-like growth factor-binding protein-3 reduces insulin requirements in insulin-dependent Type I diabetes: evidence for in vivo biological activity. *J. Clin. Endocrinol. Metab.* 2000; 85 (4): 1518–1524.

83. Small, M., C. Kluft, A.C. MacCuish, et al. Tissue plasminogen activator inhibition in diabetes mellitus. *Diabetes Care* 1989; 12 (9): 655–658.

84. Barrett-Conner, E. Lower endogenous androgen levels and dyslipidemia in men with non-insulin-dependent diabetes mellitus. *Ann. Intern. Med.* 1992; 117 (10): 807–811.

85. Haffner, S.M., L. Mykkanen, R.A. Valdez, et al. Relationship of sex hormones to lipids and lipoproteins in nondiabetic men. *J. Clin. Endocrinol. Metab.* 1993; 77 (6): 1610–1615.

86. Wassef, G.N. Lipoprotein (a) in android obesity and NIDDM: a new member in 'the metabolic syndrome.' *Biomed. Pharmacother.* 1999; 53 (10): 462–465.

87. Kemink, S.A., A.R. Hermus, L.M. Swinkels, et al. Osteopenia in insulin-dependent diabetes mellitus; prevalence and aspects of pathophysiology. *J. Endocrinol. Invest.* 2000; 23 (5): 295–303.

88. Merlin, U. [Treatment of diabetic retinopathy with adrenal cortex hormones and anabolic agents.] *G. Veneto. Sci. Med.* 1965; 20 (3): 129–137.

89. Hunter, P.R., S.G. Cotton, J.H. Kelsey, et al. Controlled trial of methandienone in treatment of diabetic retinopathy. *Br. Med. J.* 1967; 3 (566): 651–653.

90. Hamerski, W. [Durabolin in the treatment of diabetic proliferative angioretinopathy.] *Klin. Oczna* 1974; 44 (5): 461–465.

91. Sobieska-Clarowa, H. [Favorable results of anabolic therapy in cases of retinal degeneration.] *Klin. Oczna* 1975; 45 (7): 811–814.

92. Efimov, A.S., G.V. Limanskaia, A.F. Litvinenko, et al. [Effect and activity of anabolic steroids in diabetic angiopathies.] *Ter. Arkh.* 1970; 42 (6): 81–85.

93. Efimov, A.S., and P.M Karabun. [Mechanisms of action of anabolic steroids in the treatment of diabetes mellitus.] *Ter. Arkh.* 1972; 44 (10: 90–94.

94. Okuno, G. [Effect of oxandrolone, protein anabolic steroid, on hyperlipemia: comparison between cases of hyperlipemia with or without diabetes.] *Naika* 1972; 29 (2): 330–334.

95. Romics, L., M. Bretan, A. Szigeti, et al. Effect of methandrostenolone on serum triglyceride and cholesterol levels in diabetic patients. *Acta Med. Acad. Sci. Hung.* 1975; 32 (1): 27–34.

96. Murray, F.T., H.U. Wyss, R.G. Thomas, et al. Gonadal dysfunction in diabetic men with organic impotence. *J. Clin. Endocrinol. Metab.* 1987; 65 (1): 127–135.

97. Ohonovskyi, V.K., M.D. Podilchak, A.S. Matskiv, et al. [Treatment of purulent and necrotic lesions of the lower extremities in patients with diabetes mellitus.] *Klin. Khir.* 1993; (9–10): 37–40.

98. Small, M., C.D. Forbes, and A.C. MacCuish. Metabolic effects of stanozolol in Type II diabetes mellitus. *Horm. Metab. Res.* 1986; 18 (9): 647–648.

99. Marin, P., S. Holmang, L. Jonsson, et al. The effects of treatment on body composition and metabolism in middle-aged obese men. *Int. J. Obes. Relat. Metab. Disord.* 1992; 16 (12): 991–997.

100. Kabadi, U.M. Severe sensory motor polyneuropathy at the onset of diabetes mellitus. Total remission with testosterone therapy following recognition of associated hypogonadism. *Diabetes Care* 1993; 16 (1): 406–407.

101. Giovannucci, E., E.B. Rimm, M.J. Stampfer, et al. Diabetes mellitus and risk of prostate cancer (United States). *Cancer Causes Control* 1998; 9 (1): 3–9.

22

Rationale for Anabolic Therapy in Chronic Renal Failure

Introduction: Uremic Hypoandrogenemia and Its Dramatic Clinical and Financial Impacts

Chronic renal failure (CRF), acute and chronic dialysis, and pharmacotherapies prior to and after kidney transplantation are associated with hypoandrogenemia and significant hypoandrogenemia-related sequelae.[1] Numerous studies have shown that hypoandrogenemia is associated with many of the comorbid diseases and conditions that afflict patients with CRF. Therefore, in this chapter, the basis and scope for androgen therapy as adjunct to the standard medical care of CRF will be provided.

Androgens have been used for the treatment of the anemia of CRF for over 25 years. However, the use of androgen therapy for the other hypoandrogenemia-related conditions associated with CRF, such as malnutrition, sarcopenia, osteoporosis, hyposomatomedinemia, reduced fibrinolysis, dyslipidemias, depression, and sexual dysfunction has not been fully exploited. Therefore, androgen therapy for many of these conditions has not become universally recommended.[2] Instead, the use of entity-specific agents by various medical specialists has become widespread and generally accepted, but this is an ultraexpensive approach to the management of CRF.[3]

Despite the use of therapeutic strategies to slow or arrest progression of CRF, the number of patients receiving dialysis and entering renal replacement programs is increasing along with the dramatic burden in terms of morbidity, mortality, and resource consumption.[4, 5] For example, therapy with recombinant human erythropoietin (rHuEPO), instead of androgen therapy, for the treatment of the anemia of CRF has resulted in a marked increase in total costs to Medicare and other insurance programs.[6] Studies have indicated that androgen therapy produces an improvement in anemia in hemodialyzed patients similar to that achieved with rHuEPO but at much lower cost, and it also provides other appreciable anabolic effects.[7, 8]

A recent study that considered effectiveness and adverse effects of the use of rHuEPO versus androgens for the approximately 100,000 hemodialysis patients in the U.S. End-Stage Renal Disease program, concluded that the increasing use of rHuEPO projected a marked increased cost to Medicare for managing the anemia of these patients. This study showed that for every 10,000 patients who were to receive rHuEPO instead of androgens, the projected Medicare expenditures would increase by $43 million at the end of one year and $118 million after 5 years.[9]

As another example, therapy with recombinant human growth hormone, instead of androgen therapy, for the malnutrition, sarcopenia, hyposomatomedinemia, and osteoporosis associated with CRF has placed many physicians at odds with managed care payers over therapy goals and outcomes.[10] GH therapy for these conditions can be estimated to be about $20,000 per patient annually.

Extending the Medicare expenditures estimated above for rHuEPO versus androgens, and combining GH therapy for these patients (versus androgens) for the treatment of malnutrition, sarcopenia, and osteoporosis, would generate additional Medicare expenditures of $243 million/10,000 patients at year one and $1.1 billion at the end of five years. For the entire 100,000 patients, therapy with combined rHuEPO and GH rather than androgens would cost Medicare an additional $10 billion over five years!

Androgen therapy has also been shown to be effective in treating other hypoandrogenemia-related conditions that commonly afflict patients with CRF. An estimated cost analysis of androgen therapy versus entity-specific therapies is contained in Table 22-1. Analysis of the information in Table 22-1 should provide convincing evidence to further support the use of androgen therapy for many of the multiple afflictions associated it CRF.

Hypoandrogenemia in Patients with CRF

Hypoandrogenemia, stemming from both abnormal function of the hypothalamic-pituitary-gonadal axis[11, 12] and the hypothalamic-pituitary-adrenal axis,[13] is a well-documented endocrine abnormality commonly seen in patients with CRF.[14, 15] Uremic hypoandrogenemia can occur

Table 22-1. Annual Cost Comparison of Treating Hypoandrogenemia-Related Conditions Associated with Chronic Renal Failure With Androgen Therapy Versus Entity-Specific Therapies

Condition	Androgen Cost	Entity-Specific Therapy
Anemia	$500 Total	rHuEPO $20,000
Sarcopenia & osteoporosis		GH or IGF-1 $20,000
Sexual dysfunction		Viagra $2,000
Depression and/or dysthymia		various drugs $1,000
Reduced fibrinolysis		anti-coagulants $500
Dyslipidemia		lipid-lowering agents $1,000
Pathologic cytokine imbalance		recombinant cytokines ? (not yet available clinically)
Fatigue		amphetamines $500
Depressed immune System		synthetic globulins $5,000

during acute or chronic renal failure,[16, 17, 18] prior to and after renal transplantation (especially during prolonged therapy with corticosteroids),[19] and during short-term and chronic hemodialysis therapy.[20, 21] Elevated estrogen/androgen ratios have also been shown to be associated with hypoandrogenemia in men with CRF.[22]

Hypoandrogenemia-Related Diseases and Conditions in Patients with CRF

Many patients with CRF are afflicted with other diseases and conditions that have been directly or indirectly linked to hypoandrogenemia. Some of these conditions include:

(1) delayed and suboptimal growth, and delayed onset of puberty in children and adolescents.[23, 24, 25]

(2) chronic anemia and reduced sensitivity of the erythroid progenitors to endogenous erythropoietin.[26, 27]

(3) sarcopenia, fatigue, and malnutrition.[28]

(4) hyposomatomedinemia and dysfunction of the GHRH-GH-IGF-IGFBP axis[29, 30] which results in reduced free IGF-1 levels and bioactivities, and elevations in several IGFBPs.[31, 32]

(5) osteoporosis that occurs secondary to multiple factors which include hypogonadism, hypoandrogenemia, reduced osteoblast activity,

corticosteroid therapy, hyperparathyroidism, and immobilization.[33, 34, 35, 36, 37] A recent study has shown that osteoporosis in CRF is significantly higher in whites than blacks.[38] Among women with CRF, despite that high prevalence of osteoporosis risk factors, DEXA screening utilization has been shown to be very low as is therapy with bone protective medications.[39]

(6) atherosclerotic cardiovascular disease and increased levels of pro-inflammatory cytokines that contribute to the high mortality rate observed in CRF patients.[40, 41] The abnormally high incidence of coronary and cerebrovascular occlusive events in CRF patients has been well documented as the leading cause of death.[42] Reported atherogenic lipid profiles include significantly reduced plasma HDL-cholesterol levels and significantly elevated levels of LDL-cholesterol, triglycerides, apoB, Lp(a), and homocysteine.[43]

(7) thromboembolic events from increased fibrinogen and PAI-1 levels and reduced fibrinolysis and plasma tPA activity.[44, 45] These factors, along with the increase in PAI-1 levels in dialysis solutions, may further contribute to the development of thromboses in continuous ambulatory peritoneal dialysis patients and to fibrin deposition.[46]

(8) major psychological and psychiatric illnesses such as depression, dysthymia, anxiety, suicidal ideation, and sexual dysfunctions.[47, 48, 49]

Since hypoandrogenemia plays a role in the pathogenesis of these diseases and conditions, it follows then that androgen therapy should be beneficial for these afflictions. Also, it can be concluded that uremic hypoandrogenemia is a basic biochemical abnormality that affects many systems in the body, including the musculoskeletal, cardiovascular, neuroendocrine, neuroimmune, and neuropsychiatric systems.

Studies with Anabolic Therapy in CRF

Patients receiving dialysis commonly experience malnutrition, sarcopenia, and fatigue for which there has been little or no traditional effective treatment. A few recent studies with anabolic therapy have provided evidence-based results that anabolic agents are effective in treating some of these conditions in patients with CRF. These studies have utilized androgen therapy or GH therapy as anabolic agents, and have indicated:

(1) in a randomized controlled trial of nandrolone decanoate (100mg IM weekly for six months), patients receiving dialysis obtained statistically significant increases in lean body mass and significant improvement in

peak oxygen consumption, exercise performance, and functional capacity compared to the control patients who received dialysis.[50]

(2) in male dialysis patients, androgen therapy (nandrolone decanoate at 100mg IM weekly for 12 weeks) significantly augments the action of rHuEPO by providing a significantly greater increase in hematocrit values and lowering the required rHuEPO doses required for an adequate hematopoietic response.[51]

(3) in boys on routine hemodialysis, low dose androgens can stimulate short-term growth velocity when the basal growth velocity is low.[52]

(4) in adults with chronic renal failure, GH therapy (2–4 IU/m2/day) for six months results in clear anabolic effects and body composition changes, including statistically significant increases in lean body mass and reductions in body fat.[53, 54]

(5) in adults with CRF, GH therapy significantly increases left ventricular muscle mass; however, little or no increase in ejection fraction or cardiac performance during exercise accompanied the cardiac muscle mass changes.[55]

(6) in children with chronic renal failure, GH therapy increases growth velocity, muscle mass, and bone mineral density, and improves overall anabolic and metabolic functions.[56, 57, 58, 59]

Summary

The rationale for anabolic therapy for patients with CRF has been presented in this chapter. CRF is a major catabolic disease that manifests itself with major losses in anabolic potentials that are reflected by hypoandrogenemia and hyposomatomedinemia. Correcting these losses of anabolic potentials with androgen therapy and other anabolic agents is currently underutilized in clinical medicine even though the devastating results of not correcting these conditions are well documented. Hypoandrogenemia has been linked to most of the major CRF-related afflictions, including cardiovascular disease, major thromboembolic events, delayed growth and puberty in children and adolescents, sarcopenia, osteoporosis, malnutrition, depression, and sexual dysfunction.

The management of CRF is one of the most expensive areas in modern medicine and the financial costs to the health care system continue to be a heavy burden. In this arena, only one anabolic therapy has proven to be cost-effective: androgen therapy for CRF-related anemia. Other anabolic therapies, including GH, IGF-1, GHRH, GHRH analogues, and GH secretagogues, will continue to be evaluated in the near future.[60, 61] These agents may ultimately find a place in the overall treatment of patients with CRF.

Current anabolic therapy has many roles in the management of CRF patients. These roles should be integrated with the traditional therapeutic modalities of rehabilitation medicine to provide:

(1) the optimal anabolic stimuli to maintain homeostasis during all phases of renal transplantation.

(2) the optimal anabolic stimuli to prevent and reverse the catabolic state during short-term and long-term dialysis.

(3) the anabolic replacement therapies to counteract hypoandrogenemia to prevent or treat most of the diseases and conditions that are associated with CRF.

(4) the appropriate anabolic stimuli to enhance both the quality of life and longevity of patients with CRF.

Uremic hypoandrogenemia should be suspected, due to its high prevalence in CRF, and it should be treated. Androgen therapy has been the standard of care for CRF-related anemia for three decades, and it should become the first choice for treating the CRF-related conditions that are associated with hypoandrogenemia. Androgen therapy, as an anabolic modality to prevent and treat and comorbid disease, has been significantly underutilized in CRF patients.

Routine androgen therapy for CRF patients could be shown to:

(1) save the health care system billions of dollars annually.

(2) significantly improve the health care, quality of life, and longevity in these patients.

(3) provide a template for the criteria by which other anabolic agents are routinely judged.

(4) provide an evidence-based model to inspect the "upstream" modulating factors which impact the "downstream" factors which influence disease processes. In other words, when hypoandrogenemia is common in a disease, it should be corrected, and, then, the remaining conditions should be studied.

(5) be the standard of care for patients with CRF.

(6) be incorporated into the care of all patients with CRF who are undergoing standard rehabilitative modalities.

Notes

1. Handelsman, D.J., and P.Y. Liu. Androgen therapy in chronic renal failure. *Baillieres Clin. Endocrinol. Metab.* 1998; 12 (3): 485–500.

2. Johnson, C.A. Use of androgens in patients with renal failure. *Semin. Dial.* 2000; 13 (1): 36–39.

3. Mosely, C. Coordination of care in disease management: opportunities and financial issues. *Semin. Dial.* 2000; 13 (6): 346–350.

4. Whittington, R., L.B. Barradell, and P. Benfield. Epoetin: a phramacoeconomic review of its use in chronic renal failure and its effects on quality of life. *Pharmacoeconomics* 1993; 3 (1): 45–82.

5. Nicolucci, A., and D.A. Procaccini. Why do we need outcomes research in end stage renal disease? *J. Nephrol.* 2000; 13 (6): 401–404.

6. Kimmel, P.L., J.W. Greer, R.A. Milam, et al. Trends in erythropoietin therapy in the U.S. dialysis population: 1995–1998. *Semin. Nephrol.* 2000; 20 (4): 335–344.

7. Teruel, J.L., R. Marcen, J. Navarro-Antolin, et al. Androgen versus erythropoietin for the treatment of anemia in hemodialyzed patients: a prospective study. *J. Am. Soc. Nephrol.* 1996; 7 (1): 140–144.

8. Teruel, J.L., A. Aguilera, R. Marcen, et al. Androgen therapy for anemia of chronic renal failure. Indications in the erythropoietin era. *Scand. J. Urol. Nephrol.* 1996; 30 (5): 403–408.

9. Powe, N.R., R.I. Griffiths, and E.B. Bass. Cost implications to Medicare of recombinant erythropoietin therapy for the anemia of end-stage renal disease. *J. Am. Soc. Nephrol.* 1993; 3 (10): 1660–1671,

10. Owens, G.M. Clinician and payer issues in managing growth hormone deficiency. *Am. J. Manag. Care* 2000; 6 (15 Suppl.): S839–S852.

11. Bogicevic, M., and V. Stefanovic. Relationship between parathyroid hormone and pituitary-testicular axis in patients on maintenance hemodialysis. *Exp. Clin. Endocrinol.* 1988; 92 (3): 357–362.

12. Starzky, J. and W. Grzexzczak. [Does a short-term hemodialysis treatment influence function of the pituitary-testicular axis in patients with chronic renal failure?] *Pol. Acrh. Med. Wewn.* 1993; 89 (1): 24–30.

13. Carlstrom, K., A. Pousette, R. Stege, et al. Serum hormone levels in men with end stage renal disease. *Scand. J. Urol. Nephrol.* 1990; 24 (1): 75–78.

14. Akmal, M., D.A. Goldstein, O.A. Kletzky, et al. Hyperparathyroidism and hypotestosteronemia of acute renal failure. *Am. J. Nephrol.* 1988; 8 (2): 166–169.

15. Gambineri, A., and R. Pasquali. Testosterone therapy in men: clinical and pharmacological perspectives. *J. Endocrinol. Invest.* 2000; 23 (3): 196–214.

16. Carlson, H.E., M.L. Graber, M.C. Gelato, et al. Endocrine effects of erythropoietin. *Int. J. Artif. Organs* 1995; 18 (6): 309–314.

17. Akmal, M., D.A. Goldstein, O.A. Kletzky, et al. Hyperparathyroidism and hypotestosteronemia of acute renal failure. *Am. J. Nephrol.* 1988; 8 (2): 166–169.

18. Segarra, A., P. Chacon, M. Vilardell, et al. Prospective case control study to determine the effects of lovastatin on serum testosterone and cortisol concentrations in hyperlipidemic nephrotic patients with chronic renal failure. *Nephron* 1996; 73 (2): 186–190.

19. Handelsman, D.J., and P.Y. Liu. Androgen therapy in chronic renal failure. *Baillieres Clin. Endocrinol. Metab.* 1998; 12 (3): 485–500.

20. Starzyk, J., and W. Grzeszxczak. [Does a short-term hemodialysis treatment influence function of the pituitary-testicular axis in patients with chronic renal failure?] *Pol. Arch. Med. Wewn.* 1993; 89 (1): 24–30.

21. Starzyk, J., and W. Grzeszczak. [The effects of many years of hemodialysis therapy on hypophyseal-gonadal axis function in males with chronic renal insufficiency.] *Pol. Tyg. Lek.* 1996; 51 (6–9): 79–81.

22. Baumann, G., P. Reza, R. Chatterton, et al. Plasma estrogens, androgens, and

von Willebrand factor in men on chronic hemodialysis. *Int. J. Artif. Organs* 1988; 11 (6): 449–453.

23. Van Steenbergen, M.W., J.M. Wit, and R.A. Donckerwolcke. Testosterone esters advance skeletal maturation more than growth in short boys with chronic renal failure and delayed puberty. *Eur. J. Pediatr.* 1991; 150 (9): 676–680.

24. Kassmann, K., R. Rappaport, and M. Broyer. The short-term effect of testosterone on growth in boys on hemodialysis. *Clin. Nephrol.* 1992; 37 (3): 148–154.

25. Handelsman, D.J., and P.Y. Liu. Androgen therapy in chronic renal failure. *Baillieres Clin. Endocrinol. Metab.* 1998; 12 (3): 485–500.

26. Ballal, S.H., D.T. Domoto, D.C. Polack, et al. Androgens potentiate the effects of erythropoietin in the treatment of anemia of end-stage renal disease. *Am. J. Kidney Dis.* 1991; 17 (1): 29–33.

27. Berns, J.S., M.R. Rudnick, and R.M. Cohen. Androgens potentiate the effects of erythropoietin in the treatment of anemia of end-stage renal disease. *Am. J. Kidney Dis.* 1991; 18 (1): 143.

28. Johansen, K.L., K. Mulligan, and M. Schambelan. Anabolic effects of nandrolone decanoate in patients receiving dialysis: a randomized controlled trial. *JAMA* 1999; 281 (14): 1275–1281.

29. Flyvberg, A. The growth hormone/insulin-like growth factor axis in the kidney: aspects in relation to chronic renal failure. *J. Pediatr. Endocrinol.* 1994; 7 (2): 85–92.

30. Hammerman, M.R. The growth hormone-insulin-like growth factor axis in kidney re-revisited. *Nephrol. Dial. Transplant.* 1999; 14 (8): 1853–1860.

31. Frystyk, J., P. Ivarsen. C. Skjaerbaek, et al. Serum-free insulin like growth factor 1 correlates with clearance in patients with chronic renal failure. *Kidney Int.* 1999; 56 (6): 2076–2084.

32. Powell, D.R., F. Liu, B.K. Baker, et al. Effect of chronic renal failure and growth hormone therapy on the insulin-like growth factors and their binding proteins. *Pediatr. Nephrol.* 2000; 14 (7): 579–583.

33. Lindberg, J.S., and S.M. Moe. Osteoporosis in end-stage renal disease. *Semin. Nephrol.* 1999; 19 (2): 115–122.

34. Castillo, A.A., S.Q. Lew, A.M. Smith, et al. Women issues in female patients receiving peritoneal dialysis. *Adv. Ren. Replace. Ther.* 1999; 6 (4): 327–334.

35. Hruska, K.A. New insights related to aging and renal osteodystrophy. *Geriatr. Nephrol. Urol.* 1999; 9 (1): 49–56.

36. Caglar, M., and L. Adeera. Factors affecting bone mineral density in renal transplant patients. *Ann. Nucl. Med.* 1999; 13 (3): 141–145.

37. Binstock, M. Osteoporosis: risk factor prevalence and drug and densitometry utilization. *Obstet. Gynecol.* 2000; 95 (4 Suppl. 1): S50.

38. Stehman-Breen, C.O., D. Sherrard, A. Walker, et al. Racial differences in bone mineral density and bone loss among end-stage renal disease patients. *Am. J. Kidney Dis.* 1999; 33 (5): 941–946.

39. Binstock, M. Osteoporosis: risk factor prevalence and drug and densitometry utilization. *Obstet. Gynecol.* 2000; 95 (4 Suppl. 1): S50.

40. Drueke, T.B. Genesis of atherosclerosis in uremic patients. *Miner. Electrolyte Metab.* 1999; 25 (4–6): 251–257.

41. Stenvinkel, P., B. Lindholm, M. Heimburger, et al. Elevated serum levels of soluble adhesion molecules predict death in pre-dialysis patients: association with malnutrition, inflammation, and cardiovascular disease. *Nephrol. Dial. Transplant.* 2000; 15 (10): 1624–1630.

42. Oda, H., M. Ohno, H. Ohashi, et al. Coagulation and fibrinolysis factors in dialysis patients with and without ischemic heart disease. *Adv. Perit. Dial.* 2000; 16: 152–155.

43. Jungers, P., Z.A. Massy, T.N. Khoa, et al. Incidence and risk factors of atherosclerotic cardiovascular accidents in predialysis chronic renal failure patients: a prospective study. *Nephrol. Dial. Transplant.* 1997; 12 (12): 2597–2602.

44. Oda, H., M. Ohno, and H. Ohashi. Coagulation and fibrinolysis factors in dialysis patients with and without ischemic heart disease. *Adv. Perit. Dial.* 2000; 16: 152–155.

45. Rerolle, J.P. A. Hertig, G. Nguyen, et al. Plasminogen activator inhibitor type 1 is a potential target in renal fibrogenesis. *Kidney Int.* 2000; 58 (5): 1841–1850.

46. Opatrny, K., S. Opatrna, L. Vit, et al. Tissue-type plasminogen activator (tPA) and its inhibitor (PAI-1) in patients with continuous ambulatory peritoneal dialysis. *Am. J. Nephrol.* 1998; 18 (3): 186–192.

47. Cagney, K.A., A.W. Wu, N.E. Fink, et al. Formal literature review of quality-of-life instruments used in end-stage renal disease. *Am. J. Kidney Dis.* 2000; 36 (2): 327–336.

48. Levy, N.B. Psychiatric considerations in the primary medical care of the patient with renal failure. *Adv. Ren. Replace. Ther.* 2000; 7 (3): 231–238.

49. Findelstein, F.O., and S.H. Finkelstein. Depression in chronic dialysis patients: assessment and treatment. *Nephrol. Dial. Transplant.* 2000; 15 (12): 1911–1913.

50. Johansen, K.L., K. Mulligan, and M. Schambelan. Anabolic effects of nandrolone decanoate in patients receiving dialysis: a randomized controlled trial. *JAMA* 1999; 281 (14): 1275–1281.

51. Ballal, S.H., D.T. Domoto, D.C. Polack, et al. Androgens potentiate the effects of erythropoietin in the treatment of anemia of end-stage renal disease. *Am. J. Kidney Dis.* 1991; 17 (1): 29–33.

52. Kassmann, K., R. Rappaport, and M. Broyer. The short-term effect of testosterone on growth in boys on hemodialysis. *Clin. Nephrol.* 1992; 37 (3): 148–154.

53. Mehls, O., and S. Haas. Effects of recombinant human growth hormone in catabolic adults with chronic renal failure. *Growth Horm. IGF Res.* 2000; 10 (Suppl. B): S31–S37.

54. Hansen, T.B., J. Gram, P.B. Jensen, et al. Influence of growth hormone on whole body and regional soft tissue composition in adult patients on hemodialysis. A double-blind, randomized, placebo-controlled study. *Clin. Nephrol.* 2000; 53 (2): 99–107.

55. Jensen, P.B., B. Ekelund, F.T. Nielsen, et al. Changes in cardiac muscle mass and function in hemodialysis patients during growth hormone treatment. *Clin. Nephrol.* 2000; 53 (1): 25–32.

56. Ivanovski, N., Z. Antova, K. Cakararoski, et al. Accelerated growth and improved nutritional status after recombinant human growth hormone (rhGH) therapy in uremic children. *Acta Med. Croatica* 2000; 54 (1): 7–10.

57. van der Sluis, I.M., A.M. Boot, J. Nauta, et al. Bone density and body composition in chronic renal failure: effects of growth hormone treatment. *Pediatr. Nephrol.* 2000; 15 (3–4): 221–228.

58. Hokken-Koelega, A., P. Mulder, R. De Jong, et al. Long-term effects of growth hormone treatment on growth and puberty in patients with chronic renal insufficiency. *Pediatr. Nephrol.* 2000; 14 (7): 701–706.

59. Gipson, D.S., A.T. Kausz, J.E. Striegel, et al. Intraperitoneal administration of recombinant human growth hormone in children with end-stage renal disease. *Pediatr. Nephrol.* 2001; 16 (1): 29–34.

60. Welle, S. Growth hormone and insulin-like growth factor-1 as anabolic agents. *Curr. Opin. Clin. Nutr. Metab. Care* 1998; 1 (3): 257–262.

61. Vijayan, A., T. Behrend, and S. B. Miller. Clinical use of growth factors in chronic renal failure. *Curr. Opin. Nephrol. Hypertens.* 2000; 9 (1): 5–10

23

Rationale for Anabolic Therapy in Muscular Dystrophy and Other Primary Myopathies

Introduction: Many Myopathies Are Associated with Hypoandrogenemia

Primary myopathies, such as muscular dystrophy and myotonic dystrophy and related-myopathies, are a complex and heterogeneous group of muscle-wasting diseases that are defined within the muscular dystrophy umbrella.[1] Many of these conditions are strongly associated with hypoandrogenemia.[2, 3, 4, 5, 6, 7, 8, 9, 10, 11, 12] In general, muscle wasting in these diseases seems to result from decreased anabolic processes rather than from increased catabolism[13] or by an imbalance between muscle protein anabolism and catabolism.[14] The pathologic profile of muscle involvement that is seen with the general cases of hypoandrogenemia have been shown to closely simulate that which is seen in muscular dystrophy and other endocrine myopathies.[15] This similarity has led to current strategies for treating muscular dystrophies and myopathies with anabolic pharmacologic agents, including androgens, growth hormones, and growth factors.[16]

In recent times, there has been considerable research into the "downstream" effects of hypoandrogenemia that are associated with these myopathies, such nitric oxide production abnormalities, androgen receptor polymorphisms,[17] specific genetic abnormalities,[18, 19] abnormal cytokine profiles,[20] and abnormalities of the muscle cell membrane (nuclear envelope disease).[21, 22] These types of downstream research may eventually lead to specific therapies and cures (such as gene therapies). However, much of this downstream research, such as investigations into nitric oxide biochemistry,[23, 24] ultimately leads back to the "upstream" regulation of nitric oxide metabolism in various tissues by androgens.[25, 26, 27, 28, 29, 30] Other research that has implicated downstream pathologic cytokine profiles in muscular dystrophies, and myotonic dystrophies[31] are also modulated by the upstream control of these cytokines by androgens.[32] Presently, hypoandrogenemia remains the most consistent and treatable biochemical abnormality associated with these primary and acquired myopathies.

Anabolic therapy (primarily with androgens) for muscular dystrophies, myotonic dystrophies, and related myopathies has been provided by some physicians for decades with some success.[33, 34, 35, 36, 37, 38, 39, 40] Recent studies and recommendations have echoed the benefits from the earlier studies[41, 42, 43, 44, 45, 46] and suggest that androgen therapy should be considered for primary myopathies.[47] Other recent studies, with animal models and human subjects, have indicated that anabolic therapy with insulin-like growth factor-1 has beneficial effects on muscular dystrophy and related myotonic dystrophies.[48, 49, 50] Notwithstanding the traditional therapy with corticosteroids, a recent review of their use in muscular dystrophy has concluded that there is no evidence that these steroids are associated with prolonged life or long-term improvement of skeletal, myocardial, or pulmonary functions.[51] In addition, it has been shown that androgen therapy provides similar benefits in muscular dystrophy patients that are similar to the benefits of corticosteroid therapy without inducing the catabolic alterations associated with the latter.[52]

Anabolic Therapy for Myopathies

To date, there is no known cure for muscular dystrophy and its related myopathies. However, recent studies with anabolic therapies have shown some beneficial effects. They show:

(1) that androgen therapy increases physical functional benefits for children with Duchenne muscular dystrophy similar to the benefits seen with corticosteroid therapy.[53]

(2) that androgen therapy increases lean body mass, increases muscle mass, and reduces body fat.[54]

(3) that androgen therapy increases amino acid incorporation, increases muscle mass, and enhances muscle protein synthesis rates.[55, 56]

(4) that androgen therapy provides enhancement of daily living and increases muscle strength.[57]

(5) that recombinant IGF-1 therapy provides (statistically significant) increases in lean body mass and neuromuscular functions.[58]

These studies indicate that patients with muscular dystrophy and related myopathies should be considered as candidates for anabolic therapies while more definitive treatments are being researched.

Summary

The rationale for anabolic treatment for patients with primary myopathies, including muscular dystrophy, myotonic dystrophy, and related myopathies has been presented. Anabolic therapies are not a cure for these diseases, but they are the best pharmacologic therapies available to date. Other disease-specific therapies and potential cures are being investigated for each of these diseases.

These diseases are associated with an extraordinarily high incidence of hypoandrogenemia. Numerous studies have linked hypoandrogenemia with hyposomatomedinemia and significantly reduced anabolic functions. Androgen therapy corrects hypoandrogenemia and hyposomatomedinemia and their sequelae.

Patients with primary myopathies are likely candidates for rehabilitation at some point in their lives. Although no studies have been published on the results that incorporate anabolic therapy in conventional physical therapy modalities, it is likely that the combination of these pharmacologic and physical modalities will improve the therapeutic outcomes for these patients. Maintaining the functional abilities of these patients is paramount, since more definitive, and perhaps curative, treatments are imminent.

Notes

1. Dubowitz, V. What is muscular dystrophy? Forty years of progressive ignorance. *J. R. Coll. Physicians Lond.* 2000; 34 (5): 464–468.

2. Harper, P., R. Penny, T.P. Foley, et al. Gonadal function in males with myotonic dystrophy. *J. Clin. Endocrinol. Metab.* 1972; 35 (6): 852–856.

3. Febres, F., H. Scaglia, R. Lisker, et al. Hypothalamic-pituitary-gonadal function in patients with myotonic dystrophy. *J. Clin. Endocrinol. Metab.* 1975; 41 (5): 833–840.

4. Sagel, J., L.A. Distiller, J.E. Morley, et al. Myotonia dystrophica: Studies on gonadal function using luteinizing hormone-releasing hormone (LRH). *J. Clin. Endocrinol. Metab.* 1975; 40 (6): 1110–1113.

5. Carter, J.N., and K.S. Steinbeck. Reduced adrenal androgens in patients with myotonic dystrophy. *J. Clin. Endocrinol. Metab.* 1985; 60 (3): 611–614.

6. Pizzi, A., S. Fusi, G. Forti, et al. Study of endocrine function in myotonic dystrophy. *Ital. J. Neurol. Sci.* 1985; 6 (4): 457–467.

7. Vazquez, J.A., J.A. Pinies, P. Martul, et al. Hypothalamic-pituitary-testicular function in 70 patients with myotonic dystrophy. *J. Endocrinol. Invest.* 1990; 13 (5): 375–379.

8. Zavadenko, N.N. [Study of the hypophyseal-gonadal system in patients with hereditary muscular dystrophy.] *Zh. Nevropatol. Psikhiatr. Im. S.S. Korsakova* 1990; 90 (9): 25–28.

9. Lou, X.Y., Y. Nishi, M. Haji, et al. Reserved Sertoli cell function in the hypogonadic male patients with myotonic dystrophy. *Fukuoka Igaku Zasshi* 1994; 85 (5): 168–174.

10. Mastrogiacomo, I., G. Bonanni, E. Menegazzo, et al. Clinical and hormonal aspects of male hypogonadism in myotonic dystrophy. *Ital. J. Neurol. Sci.* 1996; 17 (1): 59–65.

11. Buyalos, R.P., R.V. Jackson, G.I. Grice, et al. Androgen response to hypothalamic-pituitary-adrenal stimulation with naloxone in women with myotonic muscular dystrophy. *J. Clin. Endocrinol. Metab.* 1998; 83 (9): 3219–3224.

12. Johansson, A., A. Henriksson, B.O. Olofsson, et al. Adrenal steroid dysregulation in dystrophia myotonica. *J. Intern. Med.* 1999; 245 (4): 345–351.

13. Griggs, R.C., D. Halliday, W. Kingston, et al. *Ann. Neurol.* 1986; 20 (5): 590–596.

14. Zdanowicz, M.M., S. Teichberg, M. O'Connor, et al. Metabolic and structural effects of insulin-like growth factor-1 and high-protein diet on dystrophic hamster skeletal muscle. *Proc. Soc. Exp. Biol. Med.* 1997; 215 (2): 168–173.

15. Chauhan, A.K., B.C. Katiyar, S. Misra, et al. Muscle dysfunction in male hypogonadism. *Acta Neurol. Scand.* 1986; 73 (5): 466–471.

16. Tawil, R. Outlook for therapy in the muscular dystrophies. *Semin. Neurol.* 1999; 19 (1): 81–86.

17. Max, S.R. Cytosolic androgen receptor in skeletal muscle from normal and dystrophic mice. *J. Steroid Biochem.* 1983; 18 (3): 281–283.

18. Meola, G. Myotonic dystrophies. *Curr. Opin. Neurol.* 2000; 13 (5): 519–525.

19. Meola, G. Clinical and genetic heterogenecity in myotonic dystrophies. *Muscle Nerve* 2000; 23 (12): 1789–1799.

20. Spencer, M.J., E. Montecino-Rodriguez, K. Dorshkind, et al. Helper (CD4 (+)) and cytotoxic (CD8 (+)) T cells promote the pathology of dystrophin-deficient muscle. *Clin. Immunol.* 2001; 98 (2): 235–243.

21. Patton, B.L. Laminins of the neuromuscular system. *Microsc. Res. Tech.* 2000; 51 (3): 247–261.

22. Nagano, A., and K. Arahata. Nuclear envelope proteins and associated diseases. *Curr. Opin. Neurol.* 2000; 13 (5): 533–539.

23. Stamler, J.S., and G. Meissner. Physiology of nitric oxide in skeletal muscle. *Physiol. Rev.* 2001; 81 (1): 209–237.

24. Crosbie, R.H. NO vascular control in Duchenne muscular dystrophy. *Nat. Med.* 2001; 7 (1): 27–29.

25. McLachlan, J.A., C.D. Serkin, and O. Bakouche. Dehydroepiandrosterone modulation of lipopolysaccharide-stimulated monocytes cytotoxicity. *J. Immunol.* 1996; 156 (1): 328–335.

26. Hutchinson, S.J., K. Sudhir, T.M. Chou, et al. Sex hormones and vascular reactivity. *Herz.* 1997; 22 (3): 141–150.

27. Reddy, D.S., and S.K. Kulkarni. Possible role of nitric oxide in the nootropic and anitiamnesic effect of neurosteroids on aging- and dizolpine-induced learning impairment. *Brain Res.* 1998; 799 (2): 215–229.

28. Kostic, T.S., S.A. Andric, D. Maric, et al. Involvement of inducible nitric

oxide synthase in stress-impaired testicular steroidogenesis. *J. Endocrinol.* 1999; 163 (3): 409–416.

29. McCarty, M.F. Vascular nitric oxide, sex hormone replacement, and fish oil may help prevent Alzheimer's disease by suppressing synthesis of acute-phase cytokines. *Med. Hypotheses* 1999; 53 (5): 369–374.

30. Singh, R., S. Pervin, J. Shryne, et al. Castration increases and androgens decrease nitric oxide synthase activity in the brain: physiologic implications. *Proc. Natl. Acad. Sci. U.S.A.* 2000; 28; 97 (7): 3672–3677.

31. Johansson, A., K. Carlstrom, B. Aheren, et al. Abnormal cytokine and adrenocortical hormone regulation in myotonic dystrophy. *J. Clin. Endocrinol. Metab.* 2000; 85 (9): 3169–3176.

32. Johansson, A., A. Henriksson, B.O. Olofsson, et al. Adrenal steroid dysregulation in dytrophia myotonica. *J. Intern. Med.* 1999; 245 (4): 345–351.

33. Charash, L. Anabolic steroids in the management of muscular dystrophy. *Pediatrics* 1965; 36 (3): 402–405.

34. Yamamoto, H., H. Sugita, and T. Furukawa. [Combined use of anabolic steroids and digitoxin in progressive muscular dystrophy.] *Iryo* 1966; 20 (7): 704–708.

35. Ernst, K. [On the treatment of progressive muscle dystrophy with an anabolic steroid.] *Z. Arztl. Fortbild. (Jena):* 1966; 60 (7): 389–390.

36. Valente, V.L., C.C. Caprarulo, M.R. Luchetta, et al. [Treatment of progressive muscular dystrophy with anabolics and uridine-5–triphosphoric acid.] *Prensa. Med. Argent* 1996; 53 (20): 1130–1134.

37. Heyck, H., and G. Mertens. [Anabolic therapy in progressive muscular dystrophy.] *Dtsch. Med. Wochenschr.* 1966; 91 (48): 2183–2185.

38. Beckmann, R. [Anabolic steroid hormones and progressive muscular dystrophy.] *Dtsch. Med. Wochenschr.* 1972; 97 (6): 213.

39. Bardelli, M., and E. Simonetti. Experimental progressive muscular dystrophy and its treatment with high dose anabolizing agents. *Ital. J. Orthop. Traumatol.* 1978; 4 (1): 115–127.

40. Walton, S. Anabolic steroids and muscular dystrophy. *Neurology* 1992; 42 (7): 1435–1436.

41. Kingston, W.J., R.T. Moxley, and R.C. Griggs. Effect of testosterone on whole body amino acid utilization in myotonic dystrophy. *Metabolism* 1986; 35 (10): 928–932.

42. Griggs, R.C., S. Pandya, J.M. Florence, et al. Randomized controlled trial of testosterone in myotonic dystrophy. *Neurology* 1989; 39 (2 Pt. 1): 219–222.

43. Welle, S., R. Jozefowicz, G. Forbes, et al. Effect of testosterone on metabolic rate and body composition in normal men and men with muscular dystrophy. *J. Clin. Endocrinol. Metab.* 1992; 74 (2): 332–335.

44. Fenichel, G., A. Pestronk, J. Florence, et al. A beneficial effect of oxandrolone in the treatment of Duchenne muscular dystrophy: a pilot study. *Neurology* 1997; 48 (5): 1225–1226.

45. Sugino, M., N. Ohsawa, T. Ito, et al. A pilot study of dehydroepiandrosterone sulfate in myotonic dystrophy. *Neurology* 1998; 51 (2): 586–589.

46. Tsuji, K., D. Furutama, M. Tagami, et al. Specific binding and effects of dehydroepiandrosterone sulfate (DHEA-S) on skeletal muscle cells: possible implication for DHEA-S replacement therapy in patients with myotonic dystrophy. *Life Sci.* 1999; 65 (1): 17–26.

47. Serrano-Munerac, C., and I. Illa. [Therapeutic advances in neuromuscular diseases.] *Neurologia* 1999; 14 (Suppl. 6): 36–45.

48. Zdanowicz, M.M., J. Moyse, M.A. Wingertzahn, et al. Effect of insulin-like growth factor 1 in murine muscular dystrophy. *Endocrinolgy* 1995; 136 (11): 4880–4886.

49. Welle, S. Growth hormone and insulin-like growth factor-1 as anabolic agents. *Curr. Opin. Clin. Nutr. Metab. Care* 1998; 1 (3): 257–262.

50. Furling, D., A. Marette, and J. Puymirat. Insulin-like growth factor 1 circumvents defective insulin action in human myotonic dystrophy skeletal muscle cells. *Endocrinology* 1999; 140 (9): 4244–4250.

51. Iannaccone, S.T., and Z. Nanjiani. Duchenne muscular dystrophy. *Curr. Treat. Options. Neurol.* 2001; 3 (2): 105–117.

52. Fenichel, G., A. Pestronk, J. Florence, et al. A beneficial effect of oxandrolone in the treatment of Duchenne muscular dystrophy: a pilot study. *Neurology* 1997; 48 (5): 1225–1226.

53. Fenichel, G., A. Pestronk, J. Florence, et al. A beneficial effect of oxandrolone in the treatment of Duchenne muscular dystrophy: a pilot study. *Neurology* 1997; 48 (5): 1225–1226.

54. Welle, S., R. Jozefowicz, G. Forbes, et al. Effect of testosterone on metabolic rate and body composition in normal men and men with muscular dystrophy. *J. Clin. Endocrinol. Metab.* 1992; 74 (2): 332–335.

55. Kingston, W.J., R.T. Moxley, and R.C. Riggs. Effects of testosterone on whole body amino acid utilization in myotonic dystrophy. *Metabolism* 1986; 35 (10): 928–932.

56. Griggs, R.C., S. Pandya, J.M. Florence, et al. Randomized controlled trial of testosterone in myotonic dystrophy. *Neurology* 1989; 39 (2 Pt.1): 219–222.

57. Sugino, M., N. Ohsawa, T. Ito, et al. A pilot study of dehydroepiandrosterone sulfate in myotonic dystrophy. *Neurology* 1998; 51 (2): 586–589.

58. Vlachopapadoupoulou, E., J.J. Zachwieja, J.M. Gertner, et al. Metabolic and clinical response to recombinant human insulin-like growth factor 1 in myotonic dystrophy — a clinical research center study. *J. Clin. Endocrionol. Metab.* 1995; 80 (12): 3715–3723.

24

Rationale for Anabolic Therapy in Spinal Cord Injury

Introduction: Spinal Cord Injury Creates Catabolic Endocrine Abnormalities

Persons with acute and chronic spinal cord injury (SCI) exhibit several metabolic, endocrine, and psychologic disturbances that contribute to the insult and lack of recovery potentials of their physical injury. Although subsequent endogenous anabolic metabolic responses would generally be considered beneficial, the evidence-based information shows that the body, instead of responding in that manner, responds to SCI with endogenous catabolic responses.

There is accumulating evidence that suggests that endogenous anabolic hormone levels are depressed in a significant portion of individuals with SCI.[1, 2] Depression of the hypothalamic-pituitary-gonadal axis and hypothalamic-pituitary-adrenal axis with resulting hypoandrogenemia,[3, 4, 5] and depression of the GHRH-GH-IGF-IGFBP axis[6] with resulting hyposomatomedinemia,[7, 8] may exacerbate the injury condition and promote its ill-health sequelae.[9, 10] The loss of these anabolic potentials, both acutely and chronically,[11, 12, 13] tend to exacerbate the physical injury and reduce rehabilitative efforts.[14] It has been suggested that dysregulation of the neuroimmunoendocrine system, from reduction of anabolic hormones and factors, results in pathologic cytokine profiles that have a role in SCI outcomes.[15] Therefore, the recognition and correction of these metabolic and endocrine abnormalities in patients with SCI are vital as a first step in improving clinical care as well as longevity and quality of life.[16]

As a consequence of the reduction of anabolic hormones and physical activity level, patients with SCI tend to:

(1) develop significant body composition changes including loss of skeletal muscle mass and bone mineral density (BMD), and a relative increase in adiposity that contributes to significant increased risks for sarcopenia, osteoporosis and atherogenesis.[17, 18, 19, 20, 21, 22, 23] These body composition changes may not be improved by exercise therapy alone.[24] However, it has been suggested that anabolic therapy combined with physical training may prevent or reverse these detrimental body composition changes.[25] The rapid reduction in BMD following SCI has been shown to occur both from significantly reduced osteoblast activity and increased osteoclast activity.[26] Neither the musculoskeletal strength nor the well-being of an individual with SCI cannot be overstated. Even relatively minor reductions in strength can lead to significant secondary disabilities and further societal limitations.[27]

(2) develop atherogenic lipid and lipoprotein profiles, insulin resistance and hyperinsulinemia, and reduced fibrinolysis, all of which contribute to a significant increased risk of coronary heart disease (CHD), stroke, and thromboembolic events.[28, 29, 30, 31, 32, 33]

(3) develop sexual dysfunction, infertility, depression, dysthymia, and suicidal ideation.[34, 35, 36, 37] The suicide rate among individuals with SCI has been shown to be nearly five times that of the general population.[38] The successful treatment of sexual dysfunction has been shown to significantly increase the quality of life and psychological profiles in SCI patients.[39]

Studies with Anabolic Therapy in SCI

Despite the highly reduced anabolic potentials in patients with SCI, and the association of hypoandrogenemia and hyposomatomedinemia with the acute and chronic sequelae commonly seen with SCI, only a few studies have been published on anabolic therapy in these patients. The available evidence-based studies, considering both animal models with experimentally induced spinal cord injuries and human SCI patients, have indicated:

(1) that androgen therapy (oxandrolone 20/mg day for 1 month) increases lean body mass, pulmonary function, and a subjective reduction in breathlessness in patients with tetraplegia.[40]

(2) that, in in vitro studies of cultured human spinal cord neurons, that androgens exhibit neuroprotective effects.[41]

(3) that in animal models, androgen therapy increases specific messenger RNAs in motoneuron populations throughout the spinal cord.[42]

(4) that in GH therapy (0.2 mg/kg daily for seven to 13 days) in SCI patients increases IGF-1 levels and other markers of protein anabolism.[43]

(5) that in animal models, GH therapy appears to stimulate regeneration of injured spinal cords.[44]

(6) that in human SCI patients, GH stimulation with baclofen for over six months improves hyposomatomedinemia and may reverse the deleterious effects of paralysis and immobilization on GH physiology.[45]

(7) that in animal models, IGF-1 administration increases the rescuing of motor neurons from death after experimentally induced nerve injury.[46]

From this meager scientific evidence regarding anabolic therapy for SCI, it can be suggested that further experimental work is warranted. This information has just scratched the surface of the potentials of anabolic therapy in SCI and has not evaluated the effects of anabolic therapy, particularly with androgens, on the sequelae associated with SCI.

Summary

In this chapter the rationale for utilizing anabolic therapy for patients with SCI has been presented. Convincing evidence has shown that SCI is often associated with deleterious reduction in anabolic hormones, which has a multifaceted detrimental impact on most of the sequelae. These findings have strongly suggested that anabolic therapy could be beneficial for these patients, especially when combined with traditional rehabilitative modalities.

It is likely that immediate use, during the early postinjury hours, of both androgens and components of the GHRH-GH-IGF-IGFPB axis may supply the appropriate anabolic stimuli to improve neuronal survival and ultimate functional capacity of SCI patients. Use of these anabolic agents throughout all postinjury phases and rehabilitation should be investigated. Finally, prolonged use of anabolic therapies should be evaluated to correct the hypoandrogenemia and hyposomatomedinemia and their sequelae which are commonly seen in these patients.

Notes

1. Morley, J.E., L.A. Distiller, I. Lissoos, et al. Testicular function in patients with spinal cord damage. *Horm. Metab. Res.* 1979; 11 (12): 679–682.

2. Baker, H.W. Reproductive effects of nontesticular illness. *Endocrinol. Metab. Clin. North Am.* 1998; 27 (4): 831–850.

3. Naftchi, N.E., A.T. Vian, G.H. Sell, et al. Pituitary-testicular axis dysfunction in spinal cord injury. *Arch. Phys. Med. Rehabil.* 1980; 61 (9): 402–405.

4. Wang, Y.S., T.S. Huang, and I.N. Lien. Hormone changes in men with spinal cord injuries. *Am. J. Phys. Med. Rehabil.* 1992; 71 (6): 328–332.

5. Huang, T.S., Y.H. Wang, S.H. Lee, et al. Impaired hypothalamus-pituitary-adrenal axis in men with spinal cord injuries. *Am. J. Phys. Med. Rehabil.* 1998; 77 (2): 108–112.

6. Huang, T.S., Y.H. Wang, and I.N. Lien. Suppression of the hypothalamus-pituitary somatotrope axis in men with spinal cord injuries. *Metabolism* 1995; 44 (9): 1116–1120.

7. Shetty, K.R., C.H. Sutton, D.E. Mattson, et al. Hyposomatomedinemia in quadriplegic men. *Am. J. Med. Sci.* 1993; 305 (2): 95–100.

8. Bauman, W.A., A.M. Spungen, S. Flanagan, et al. Blunted growth hormone response to intravenous arginine in subjects with spinal cord injury. *Horm. Metab. Res.* 1994; 26 (3): 152–156.

9. Tsitouras, P.D., V.G. Zhong, A.M. Spungen, et al. Serum testosterone and growth hormone/insulin-like growth factor-1 in adults with spinal cord injury. *Horm. Metab. Res.* 1995; 27 (6): 287–292.

10. Bauman, W.A., and A.M. Spungen. Metabolic changes in persons after spinal cord injury. *Phys. Med. Rehabil. Clin. N. Am.* 2000; 11 (1): 109–140.

11. Claus-Walker, J., M. Scurry, R.E. Carter, et al. Steady state hormonal secretion in traumatic quadriplegia. *J. Clin. Endocrinol. Metab.* 1977; 44 (3): 530–535.

12. Naftchi, N.E., A.T. Vian, G.H. Sell, et al. Pituitary-testicular axis dysfunction in spinal cord injury. *Arch. Phys. Med. Rehabil.* 1980; 61 (9): 402–405.

13. Cortes-Gallegos, V., G. Castaneda, R. Alonso, et al. Diurnal variations of pituitary and testicular hormones in paraplegic men. *Arch. Androl.* 1982; 8 (3): 221–226.

14. Bauman, W.A., A.M. Spungen, R.H. Adkins, et al. Metabolic and endocrine changes in persons aging with spinal cord injury. *Assist. Technol.* 1999; 11 (2): 88–96.

15. Cruse, J.M., J.C. Keith, M.L. Bryant, et al. Immune system-neuroendocrine dysregulation in spinal cord injury. *Immunol. Res.* 1996; 15 (4): 306–314.

16. Bauman, W.A., and A.M. Spungen. Metabolic changes in persons after spinal cord injury. *Phys. Med. Rehabil. Clin. N. Am.* 2000; 11 (1): 109–140.

17. Ragnarsson, K.T., and G.H. Sell. Lower extremity fractures after spinal cord injury: a retrospective study. *Arch. Phys. Med. Rehabil.* 1981; 62 (9): 418–423.

18. Shizgal, H.M., A. Roza, B. Leduc, et al. Body composition in quadriplegic patients. *J. Parenter. Enteral Nutr.* 1986; 10 (4): 364–368.

19. Garland, D.E., C.A. Stewart, R.H. Adkins, et al. Osteoporosis after spinal cord injury. *J. Orthop. Res.* 1992; 10 (3): 371–378.

20. Wilmet, F., A.A. Ismail, A. Heilporn, et al. Longitudinal study of the bone mineral content and soft tissue composition after spinal cord section. *Paraplegia* 1995; 33 (11): 674–677.

21. Demirel, G., H. Yilmaz, N. Paker, et al. Osteoporosis after spinal cord injury. *Spinal Cord* 1998; 36 (12): 822–825.

22. Szollar, S.M., E.M. Martin, D.J. Sartoris, et al. Bone mineral density and indexes of bone metabolism in spinal cord injury. *Am. J. Phys. Med. Rehabil.* 1998; 77 (1): 28–35.

23. Bauman, W.A., A.M. Spungen, R.H. Adkins, et al. Metabolic and endocrine changes in persons aging with spinal cord injury. *Assist. Technol.* 1999; 11 (2): 88–96.

24. Leeds, E.M., K.J. Klose, W. Ganz, et al. Bone mineral density after bicycle ergometry training. *Arch. Phys. Med. Rehabil.* 1990; 71 (3): 207–209.

25. Kannisto, M., H. Araranta, J. Merikanto, et al. Bone mineral status after pediatric spinal cord injury. *Spinal Cord* 1998; 36 (9): 641–646.

26. Roberts, D., W. Lee, R.C. Cuneo, et al. Longitudinal study of bone turnover after acute spinal cord injury. *J. Clin. Endocrinol. Metab.* 1998; 83 (2): 415–422.

27. Goldstein, B. Musculoskeletal conditions after spinal cord injury. *Phys. Med. Rehabil. Clin. North Am.* 2000; 11 (1): 91–108.

28. Petaja, J., P. Myllynen, P. Rokkanen, et al. Fibrinolysis and spinal injury. Relationship to post-traumatic deep vein thrombosis. *Acta Chir. Scand.* 1989; 155 (4–5): 241–246.

29. Shetty, K.R., C.H. Sutton, I.W. Rudman, et al. Lipid and lipoprotein abnormalities in young quadriplegic men. *Am. J. Med. Sci.* 1992; 303 (4): 213–216.

30. Lamb, G.C., M.A. Tomski, J. Kaufman, et al. Is chronic spinal cord injury associated with increased risk of venous thromboembolism? *J. Am. Paraplegia Soc.* 1993; 16 (3): 153–156.

31. Nam, C.C., and I.R. Odderson. Stroke in the spinal cord injured. *J. Am. Paraplegia Soc.* 1994; 17 (1): 36–38.

32. Schmid, A., M. Halle, C. Stuzle, et al. Lipoproteins and free plasma catecholamines in spinal cord injured men with different injury levels. *Clin. Physiol.* 2000; 20 (4): 304–310.

33. Miranda, A.R., and H.I. Hassouna. Mechanisms of thrombosis in spinal cord injury. *Hematol. Oncol. Clin. North Am.* 2000; 14 (2): 401–416.

34. Bracket, N.I., C.M. Lynne, M.S. Weizman, et al. Endocrine profiles and semen quality of spinal cord injured men. *J. Urol.* 1994; 151 (1): 114–119.

35. Sipski, M.L. Sexual functioning in the spinal cord injured. *Int. J. Impot. Res.* 1998; 10 (Suppl. 2): S128–S130.

36. Kennedy, P., B. Rogers, S. Speer, et al. Spinal cord injuries and attempted suicide: a retrospective review. *Spinal Cord* 1999; 37 (12): 847–852.

37. Krause, J.S., B. Kemp, and J. Coker. Depression after spinal cord injury: relation to gender, ethnicity, aging, and socioeconomic indicators. *Arch. Phys. Med. Rehabil.* 2000; 81 (8): 1099–1109.

38. Hartkopp, A., H. Bronnum-Hansen, A.M. Seidenschnur, et al. Suicide in a spinal cord injured population: its relation to functional status. *Arch. Phys. Med. Rehabil.* 1998; 79 (11): 1356–1361.

39. Hultling, C., F. Giuliano, F. Quirk, et al. Quality of life in patients with spinal cord injury receiving Viagra (sildenafil citrate) for the treatment of erectile dysfunction. *Spinal Cord.* 2000; 38 (6): 363–370.

40. Spungen, A.M., D.R. Grimm, M. Strakhan, et al. Treatment with an anabolic agent is associated with improvement of respiratory function in persons with tetraplegia: a pilot study. *Mt. Sinai. J. Med.* 1999; 66 (3): 201–205.

41. Ogata, T., Y. Nakamura, T. Shibata, et al. Steroid hormones protect spinal cord neurons from glutamate toxicity. *Neuroscience* 1993; 55 (2): 445–449.

42. Blanco, C.E., P. Popper, and P. Micevych. Anabolic-androgenic steroid induced alterations in choline acetyltransferase messenger RNA levels of spinal cord motoneurons in the male rat. *Neuroscience* 1997; 78 (3): 873–882.

43. Behrman, S.W., K.A. Kudsk, R.O. Brown, et al. The effect of growth hormone on nutritional markers in enterally fed immobilized trauma patients. *J. Parenter. Enteral. Nutr.* 1995; 19 (1): 41–46.

44. Hanci, M., C. Kuday, and S.A. Oguzogula. The effects of synthetic growth hormone on spinal cord injury. *J. Neurosurg. Sci.* 1994; 38 (1): 43–49.

45. Bauman, W.A., A.M. Spungen, Y.G. Zhong, et al. Chronic baclofen therapy improves the blunted growth hormone response to intravenous arginine in subjects with spinal cord injury. *J. Clin. Endocrinol. Metab.* 1994; 78 (5): 1135–1138.

46. Iwasaki, Y., and K. Ikeda. Prevention by insulin-like growth factor-1 and riluzole of motor neuron death after neonatal axotomy. *J. Neurol. Sci.* 1999; 169 (1–2): 148–155.

25

Rationale for Anabolic Therapy in Alzheimer's Disease and Cognition Deficits

Introduction: Reduced Anabolic Potentials Affect Cognition

There is a growing body of evidence that suggests a link between reduced anabolic potentials and Alzheimer's disease (AD) and other conditions that are associated with cognition dysfunction. Several studies, but not all,[1,2,3,4,5] have shown that cognition dysfunction is associated with decreased sex steroid levels (androgens[6,7,8,9,10,11,12] or estrogens[13,14,15] or both), reduced androgen/estrogen ratios,[16,17] reduced androgen/cortisol ratios,[18,19,20,21,22,23] and reduced GH secretion or reduced circulating IGF-1 and free IGF-1 levels.[24,25,26,27,28,29]

Reduced anabolic potentials tends to cause dysfunction of the neuroimmune and neuroendocrine systems that may allow for a cascade of events which results in increased inflammatory cytokines that attack brain tissues causing the classical morphological brain changes seen with AD: the formation neurofibrillary tangles (NFT) and plaque deposition in and around inflamed brain tissues and cells. Since sex steroids and various anabolic growth factors are known to modulate the immune system, cytokine profiles, and various neurotrophic factors, then it follows that reduced levels of these steroids and growth factors may be involved with the etiopathogenesis of AD.

Alzheimer's disease is a progressive, inflammatory, neurodestructive process of the higher cortex that is characterized by the deterioration of memory and higher cognitive function. To date, AD is a progressive, irreversible brain disorder that is characterized by three major pathogenic findings[30].

(1) the aberrant processing and deposition of beta-amyloid precursor protein (beta APP) to form neurotoxic amyloid (beta A) peptides and an aggregated insoluble polymer of beta A that forms senile plaques.

(2) the establishment of intraneuronal neuritic pathology that results in widespread deposits of NFTs.

(3) the initiation and proliferation of brain-specific inflammatory responses that involve elevated levels of pathogenic cytokines.

These three seemingly disparate attributes of AD etiopathogenesis are linked by the fact that proinflammatory microglia, reactive astrocytes, and their associated cytokines and chemokines are associated with microtubule physiology and pathophysiology, especially during the later stages of the disease.[31] Moreover, these cytokines and chemokines are modulated endogenously, in part, by androgens, estrogens, corticosteroids, IGF-1, and other growth factors.[32, 33, 34] This body of scientific evidence supports the investigational use of anabolic therapies (androgens, GH, and IGF-1) for the prevention and treatment of cognitive dysfunction and Alzheimer's disease. Future investigational studies in cognitive dysfunction states may include the two classes of GH secretagogues (GH-releasing hormone and other GH releasing peptides and their analogues, GHRPs) and gene therapy with genes that secrete various anabolic agents.[35, 36]

Studies with Anabolic Agents in Cognitive Dysfunction and AD

The available information obtained from investigational studies utilizing anabolic therapy for cognitive dysfunction and AD is promising and indicates:

(1) in vitro, that androgen administration has neuroprotective effects on hippocampal neurons and protects against neurotoxin-induced cytotoxicity and cell death.[37, 38]

(2) in vitro, that dehydroepiandrosterone sulfate (DHEAS) administration restores the release of IGF-1 from natural killer cells in older patients with dementia.[39]

(3) in animal studies and in vitro with human brain cells, that androgens, via local nitric oxide regulation, have beneficial and

immunomodulating effects which result in cerebral vasodilatation, correction of cytokine imbalances, and improved antioxidant capacity, and which reverse experimentally induced impairments in learning and memory.[40, 41, 42, 43, 44]

(4) from human studies, that testosterone therapy in men with hypoandrogenemia improves various aspects of cognition and memory.[45, 46]

(5) from human studies, that stimulation of the GHRH-GH-GRF-GRFBP axis (at supraphysiologic levels for up to 2 years) results in increased IGF-1 levels and is associated with improved cognitive performance.[47 48] Cognitive improvements with GH therapy that returns IGF-1 to physiologic levels have not been demonstrated.[49]

Summary

In this chapter the evidence-based rationale for utilizing anabolic therapies for cognitive dysfunction and AD has been presented. It has been shown that both hypoandrogenemia and hyposomatomedinemia (along with their proposed mechanisms of action) are associated with both cognitive deficits and AD. Although it seems prudent and physiologically sound to correct these conditions, only a few investigational studies have been conducted to examine the effects of anabolic therapy for these conditions. Both the immediate clinical use and expansion of investigational studies of anabolic agents to prevent and/or treat cognitive dysfunction are warranted.

The correction of hypoandrogenemia (with androgen therapy) seems appropriate, cost-effective, and safe for these patients. Androgen therapy, which also improves hyposomatomedinemia, corrects the reduction of anabolic stimuli and improves immunomodulation of the pathologic inflammatory and pathogenic cytokine profiles which have been associated with progressive dementia. Androgen therapy, through direct and indirect mechanisms, provides neuroprotective and neuroregenerative effects that have not been demonstrated with any other current therapy.

For those patients with cognitive dysfunction who are undergoing traditional rehabilitative therapies, androgen therapy is likely to demonstrate improved outcomes and shortened rehabilitative periods, and to lessen health care expenditures. Patients with low anabolic potentials are less likely to respond to the applied stressors of rehabilitation in a constructive manner. Therefore, anabolic therapy, especially with androgen therapy, is recommended for these patients, regardless of gender. Future investigational studies should refine the current body of knowledge regarding anabolic therapies for demented states.

Notes

1. Yaffe, K., B. Ettinger, A. Pressman, et al. Neuropsychiatric function and dehydroepiandrosterone sulfate in elderly women: a prospective study. *Biol. Psychiatry* 1998; 43 (9): 694–700.

2. Kahonen, M.H., R.S. Tilvis, J. Jolkkonen, et al. Predictors and clinical significance of declining plasma dehydroepiandrosterone sulfate in old age. *Aging (Milano)* 2000; 12 (4): 308–314.

3. Moffat, S.D., A.B. Zonderman, S.M. Harman, et al. The relationship between longitudinal declines in dehydroepiandrosterone sulfate concentrations and cognitive performance in older men. *Arch. Intern. Med.* 2000; 160 (14): 2193–2198.

4. Wolf, O.T., R. Preut, D.H. Hellhammer, et al. Testosterone and cognition in elderly men: a single testosterone injection blocks the practice effect in verbal fluency, but has no effect on spatial or verbal memory. *Biol. Psychiatry* 2000; 47 (7): 650–654.

5. Morrison, M.F., E. Redei, T. TenHave, et al. Dehydroepiandrosterone sulfate and psychiatric measures in an elderly residential care population. *Biol. Psychiatry* 2000; 47 (2): 144–150.

6. Sternbach, H. Age-associated testosterone decline in men: clinical issues for psychiatry. *Am. J. Psychiatry* 1998; 155 (10): 1310–1318.

7. Plouffe, L., and J.A. Simon. Androgen effects on the central nervous system in the postmenopausal woman. *Semin. Reprod, Endocrinol.* 1998; 16 (2): 135–143.

8. Alexander, G.M., R.S. Swerdloff, C. Wang, et al. Androgen-behavior correlations in hypogonadal men and eugonadal men. II. Cognitive abilities. *Horm. Behav.* 1998; 33 (2): 85–94.

9. Solerte, S.B., R. Gornati, L. Cravello, et al. Dehydroepiandrosterone-sulfate (DHEA-S) restores the release of IGF-1 from natural killer (NK) immune cells in old patients with dementia and Alzheimer's type (DAT). *J. Endocrinol. Invest.* 1999; 22 (10 Suppl.): 32–34.

10. Barrett-Conner, E., and D. Goodman-Gruen. Cognitive function and endogenous sex hormones in older women. *J. Am. Geriatr. Soc.* 1999; 47 (11): 1289–1293.

11. Drake, E.B., V.W. Henderson, F.Z. Stanczyk, et al. Associations between circulating sex steroid hormones and cognition in normal elderly women. *Neurology* 2000; 54 (3): 599–603.

12. Hillen, T., A. Lun, F.M. Reischies, et al. DHEA-S plasma levels and incidence of Alzheimer's disease. *Biol. Psychiatry* 2000; 47 (2): 161–163.

13. Asthana, S., S. Craft, L.D. Baker, et al. Cognitive and neuroendocrine response to transdermal estrogen in postmenopausal women with Alzheimer's disease: results of a placebo-controlled, double-blind, pilot study. *Psychoneuroendocrinology* 1999; 24 (6): 657–677.

14. Yaffe, K., L.Y. Lui, D. Grady, et al. Cognitive decline in women in relation to non-protein-bound oestradiol concentrations. *Lancet* 2000; 356 (9231): 708–712.

15. Drake, F.B., V.W. Henderson, F.Z. Stanczyk, et al. Associations between circulating sex steroid hormones and cognition in normal elderly women. *Neurology* 2000; 54 (3): 599–603.

16. Barrett-Conner, E., D. Goodman-Gruen, and B. Patay. Endogenous sex hormones and cognitive function in older men. *J. Clin. Endocrinol. Metab.* 1999; 84 (10): 3681–3685.

17. Janowsky, J.S., B. Chavez, and E. Orwoll. Sex steroids modify working memory. *J. Cogn. Neurosci.* 2000; 12 (3): 407–414.

18. Leblhuber, F., C. Neubauer, M. Peichl, et al. Age and sex differences of dehydroepiandrosterone sulfate (DHEAS) and cortisol (CRT) plasma levels in normal

controls and Alzheimer's disease (AD). *Psychopharmacology (Berl.)* 1993; 111 (1): 23–26.

19. Kalmijn, S., L.J. Launer, R.P. Stolk, et al. A prospective study on cortisol, dehydroepiandrosterone sulfate and cognitive function in the elderly. *J. Clin. Endocrinol. Metab.* 1998; 83 (10): 3487–3492.

20. Carlson, L.E., and B.B. Sherwin. Relationships among cortisol (CRT), dehydroepiandrosterone sulfate (DHEAS), and memory in a longitudinal study of healthy elderly men and women. *Neurobiol. Aging* 1999; 20 (3): 315–324.

21. Carlson, L.E. B.B. Sherwin, and H.M. Chertkow. Relationship between dehydroepiandrosterone sulfate (DHEA) and cortisol (CRT) plasma levels and everyday memory in Alzheimer's disease patients compared to healthy controls. *Horm. Behav.* 1999; 35 (3): 254–263.

22. Magri, F., T. Terenzi, T. Ricciardi, et al. Association between changes in adrenal secretion and cerebral morphometric correlates in normal aging and senile dementia. *Dement. Geriatr. Cog. Disord.* 2000; 11 (2): 90–99.

23. Murialdo, G., A. Barreca, F. Nobili, et al. Dexamethasone effects on cortisol secretion in Alzheimer's disease: some clinical and hormonal features in suppressor and nonsuppressor patients. *J. Endocrinol. Invest.* 2000; 23 (3): 178–186.

24. Rollero, A., G. Murialdo, S. Fonzi, et al. Relationship between cognitive function, growth hormone and insulin-like growth factor 1 plasma levels in aged subjects. *Neurospychobiology* 1998; 38 (2): 73–79.

25. Aleman, A., H.J., Verhaar, E.H. De Haan, et al. Insulin-like growth factor-1 and cognitive function in healthy older men. *J. Clin. Endocrinol. Metab.* 1999; 84 (2): 471–475.

26. Dore, S., S. Kar, W.H. Zheng, et al. Rediscovering good old friend IGF-1 in the new millennium: possible usefulness in Alzheimer's disease and stroke. *Pharm. Acta Helv.* 2000; 74 (2–3): 273–280.

27. Kalmijn, S., J.A. Janssen, H.A. Pols, et al. A prospective study on circulating insulin-like growth factor-1 (IGF-1), IGF-binding proteins, and cognitive function in the elderly. *J. Clin. Endocrinol. Metab.* 2000; 85 (12): 4551–4555.

28. van Dam, P.S., A. Aleman, W.R. de Vries, et al. Growth hormone, insulin-like growth factor 1 and cognitive function in adults. *Growth Horm. IGF Res.* 2000; 10 (Suppl. B): S69–S73.

29. Aleman, A., W.R. de Vries, E.H. de Haan, et al. Age-sensitive cognitive function, growth hormone and insulin-like growth factor 1 plasma levels in healthy older men. *Neuropsychobiology* 2000; 41 (2): 73–78.

30. Lukiw, W.J., and N.G. Bazan. Neuroinflammatory signaling upregulation in Alzheimer's disease. *Neurochem. Res.* 2000; 25 (9–10): 1173–1184.

31. Luterman, J.D., V. Haroutunian, S. Yemul, et al. Cytokine gene expression as a function of the clinical progression of Alzheimer disease dementia. *Arch. Neurol.* 2000; 57 (8): 1153–1160.

32. Cardinali, D.P., R.A. Cutrera, and A.I. Esquifino. Psychoimmune neuroendocrine integrative mechanisms revisited. *Biol. Signals. Recept.* 2000; 9 (5): 215–230.

33. Durany, N., T. Michel, J. Kurt, et al. Brain-derived neurotrophic factor and neurotrophin-3 levels in Alzheimer's disease brains. *Int. J. Dev. Neurosci.* 2000; 18 (8): 807–813.

34. Morley, J.E. Andropause, testosterone therapy, and quality of life in aging men. *Cleve. Clin. J. Med.* 2000; 67 (12): 880–882.

35. Merriam, G.R., D.M. Buchner, P.N. Prinz, et al. Potential applications of GH secretagogues in the evaluation and treatment of the age-related decline in growth hormone secretion. *Endocrine* 1997; 7 (1): 49–52.

36. Smith, R.G. The aging process: were are the drug opportunities? *Curr. Opin. Chem. Biol.* 2000; 4 (4): 371–376.

37. McLachlan, J.A., C.D. Serkin, and O. Bakouche. Dehydroepiandrosterone modulation of lipopolysaccharide-stimulated monocyte cytotoxicity. *J. Immunol.* 1996; 156 (1): 328–335.

38. Cardounel, A., W. Regelson, and M. Kalimi. Dehydroepiandrosterone protects hippocampal neurons against neurotoxin-induced cell death: mechanism of action. *Proc. Soc. Exp. Biol. Med.* 1999; 222 (2): 145–149.

39. Solerte, S.B., R. Gornati, L. Cravello, et al. Dehydroepiandrosterone-sulfate (DHEA-S) restores the release of IGF-1 from natural killer (NK) immune cells in old patients with dementia of Alzheimer's type (DAT). *J. Endocrinol. Invest.* 1999; 22 (10 Suppl.): 32–34.

40. Reddy, D.S., and S.K. Kulkarni. Possible role of nitric oxide in the nootropic and antiamnestic effects of neurosteroids on aging- and dizocilpine-induced learning impairment. *Brain Res.* 1998; 799 (2): 215–229.

41. McCarty, M.F. Vascular nitric oxide, sex hormone replacement, and fish oil may help to prevent Alzheimer's disease by suppressing synthesis of acute-phase cytokines. *Med. Hypotheses* 1999; 53 (5): 369–374.

42. Kipper-Galperin, M., R. Galilly, H.D. Danenberg, et al. Dehydroepiandrosterone selectively inhibits production of tumor necrosis factor alpha and interleukin-6 in astrocytes. *Int. J. Dev. Neurosci.* 1999; 17 (8): 765–775.

43. Bastianetto, S., C. Ramassamy, J. Poirier, et al. Dehydroepiandrosterone (DHEA) protects hippocampal cells from oxidative stress-induced damage. *Brain Res. Mol. Brain Res.* 1999; 66 (1–2): 35–41.

44. Singh, R., S. Pervin, J. Shryne, et al. Castration increases and androgens decrease nitric oxide synthase activity in the brain: physiological implications. *Proc. Natl. Acad. Sci. USA* 2000; 97 (7): 3672–3677.

45. Alexander, G.M., R.S. Swerdloff, C. Wang, et al. Androgen-behavior correlations in hypogonadal men and eugonadal men. II. Cognitive abilities. *Horm. Behav.* 1998; 33 (2): 85–94.

46. Janowsky, J.S., B. Chavez, and E. Orwoll. Sex steroids modify working memory. *J. Cogn. Neurosci.* 2000; 12 (3): 407–414.

47. Deijen, J.B., H. de Boer, and E.A. van der Veen. Cognitive changes during growth hormone replacement in adult men. *Psychoneuroendocrinology* 1998; 23 (1): 45–55.

48. Aleman, A., W.R. de Vries, E.H. de Haan, et al. Age-sensitive cognitive function, growth hormone and insulin-like growth factor 1 plasma levels in healthy older men. *Neurospychobiology* 2000; 41 (2): 73–78.

49. Baum, H.B., L. Katznelson, J.C. Sherman, et al. Effects of physiological growth hormone (GH) therapy on cognition and quality of life in patients with adult-onset GH deficiency. *J. Clin. Endocrinol. Metab.* 1998; 83 (9): 3184–3189

26

Rationale for Anabolic Therapy in Osteoarthritis

Introduction: Reduced Anabolic Processes Result in Joint Destruction

Articular chondrocytes maintain cartilage health and homeostasis throughout life by replacing lost or damaged matrix with freshly synthesized materials. Under normal biochemical conditions, matrix synthesis activity is upregulated well above basal levels in response to cartilage injury. Such responses suggest that anabolic synthesis activity is linked to the rate of matrix loss by endogenous "damage control" mechanisms.[1] Anabolic factors involved with these damage control mechanisms depend on both systemic and local tissue anabolic hormones, growth factors, and peptides that modulate or counteract destructive and catabolic activities of various cytokines, chemokines, and other catabolic molecules.[2, 3] Several arthritic disorders result from a disruption of the equilibrium between the synthesis and degradation of synovial tissue matrix macromolecules.[4] Disruption of these anabolic and growth factor functions creates an imbalance in effector cascades, feedback loops, and intracellular, intercellular events, all of which leads to catabolic effects on articular cartilage and subchondral bone structure and function.[5, 6]

Systemic and Local Anabolic Losses in Osteoarthritis

Decades ago, systemic anabolic endocrine abnormalities were associated with various arthropathies.[7] However, the prevailing and previously held view that the pathogenesis of idiopathic osteoarthritis (OA) originated in the synovial joint and was not influenced by systemic metabolic disturbances in the patient, has been shown to be inconsistent with recent data that demonstrate abnormalities in the GHRH-GH-IGF-IGFBP axis in symptomatic OA patients.[8] The most consistent dysfunctions of this axis, that occur at the systemic and local levels in OA patients, indicate that serum GH levels tend to be elevated (up to thrice normal values), but serum IGF-1 levels are normal or reduced.[9, 10, 11, 12, 13, 14]

Despite the dampened IGF-1 response to elevated or normal GH levels in OA patients, in vitro studies of the articular cartilage and synovial fluid, with assays and immunohistochemical techniques, have indicated that the articular IGF-1 levels tend to be significantly elevated.[15] The elevated synthesis of IGF-1 by adult human OA chondrocytes occurs through a mechanism that is independent of the GHRH-GH-IGF-IGFBP axis.[16] However, elevated local IGFBP-3 levels,[17] reduced IGFBP enzymatic degradation,[18] reduced IGF-1/IGFBP ratios,[19, 20] and elevated IGF-1 binding affinities for IGFBPs[21] have been shown to have the net effect of reduced IGF-1 bioavailability and bioactivity and loss of potential anabolic stimuli in joint tissues.[22] In this manner, human osteoarthritic chondrocytes become hyporesponsive to the anabolic stimulation by IGF-1.[23, 24]

In addition, age-related and zone-related synovial decreases in IGF-1 receptor concentrations and activities may contribute to the reduction of anabolic functions in cartilage in OA.[25, 26] Besides being an endocrine mediator of GH, IGF-1 also plays a prominent role in the regulation of immunity and inflammation in OA.[27 28]

Other anabolic endocrine alterations include serum androgen production and its binding globulin. Several studies have shown an association of hypoandrogenemia and low circulating sex hormone binding globulin (SHBG) in some OA patients,[29, 30, 31, 32] while other data have indicated normal or elevated androgen levels.[33] It has been suggested that when hypoandrogenemia is present in patients with OA, it correlates with the severity of the inflammatory-degenerative processes in the joints.[34]

Studies with Anabolic Therapy in Osteoarthritis

Despite the considerable progress in understanding the cascade of events involved with the pathogenesis of OA, very few published studies have examined anabolic therapies that may counteract the catabolic events in articular cartilage and underlying bone. One older study has indicated that androgen therapy (nandrolone decanoate) has some beneficial effects in the management of OA.[35] Animal studies have indicated the cartilage protective and regeneration effects of anabolic therapy with recombinant IGF-1 in vitro[36] and when administered via intra-articular injection.[37] Further clinical use and clinical studies are warranted.

Summary

In this chapter the supportive evidence-based rationale for the use of anabolic agents has been provided. Although OA is a catabolic and destructive condition of the joints, little is known about the application of anabolic agents to prevent or treat this condition. Considerable research has been conducted to define the catabolic mechanisms in OA and much progress has been made. The exact cause of OA continues to be elusive; perhaps it is multifaceted. Many important questions remain to be answered including:

(1) is there a pre-existing loss of systemic anabolic potential that predisposes an individual to OA when an injurious, infectious, or age-related process occurs to the joint-related tissues?

(2) can anabolic therapies be administered to one or more joints—therapies which re-establish anabolic and regenerative processes?

(3) is OA an autoimmune disease or is it a normal process of aging and age-related reductions in systemic and local anabolic potentials?

(4) are there specific genetic factors that predispose individuals to OA?

(5) will maximizing anabolic potentials in aging individuals prevent OA? From these questions, it is easily seen that more research is required, but answers must be provided. General recommendations for anabolic therapy, although it may be indicated and prescribed on a case-by-case basis, cannot be given at present.

Notes

1. Martin, J.A., M.B. Scherb, L.A. Lembke, et al. Damage control mechanisms in articular cartilage: role of the insulin-like growth factor 1 axis. *Iowa Orthop.* 2000; 20: 1–10.

2. van den Berg, W.B. The role of cytokines and growth factors in cartilage destruction in osteoarthritis and rheumatoid arthritis. *Z. Rheumatol.* 1999; 58 (3): 136–141.

3. van der Kraan, P.M., and W.B. van den Berg. Anabolic and destructive mediators in osteoarthritis. *Curr. Opin. Clin. Nutr. Metab. Care* 2000; 3 (3): 205–211.

4. Tavera, C., T. Abribat, P. Reboul, et al. IGF and IGF-binding protein system in the synovial fluid of osteoarthritic and rheumatic arthritic patients. *Ostoarthritis Cartilage* 1996; 4 (4): 263–274.

5. Trippel, S.B. Growth factor actions on articular cartilage. *J. Rheumatol. Suppl.* 1995; 43: 129–132.

6. Hilal, G., J. Martel-Pelletier, J.P. Pelletier, et al. Abnormal regulation of urokinase plasminogen activator by insulin-like growth factor 1 in human osteoarthritic subchondral osteoblasts. *Arthritis Rheum.* 1999; 42 (10): 2112–2122.

7. Johanson, N.A. Endocrine arthropathies. *Clin. Rheum. Dis.* 1985; 11 (2): 297–323.

8. Denko, C.W., and C.J. Malemud. Metabolic disturbances and synovial joint responses in osteoarthritis. *Front. Biosci.* 1999; 4: D686–693.

9. Denko, C.W., B. Boja, and R.W. Moskowitz. Growth promoting peptides in osteoarthritis: insulin, insulin-like growth factor-1, and growth hormone. *J. Rheumatol.* 1990; 17 (9): 1217–1221.

10. Moskowitz, R.W., B. Boja, and C.W. Denko. The role of growth factors in degenerative joint disorders. *J. Rheumatol. Suppl.* 1991; 27: 147–148.

11. McAlindon, T.E., J.D. Teale, and P.A. Dieppe. Levels of insulin related growth factor 1 in osteoarthritis of the knee. *Ann. Rheum. Dis.* 1993; 52 (3): 229–231.

12. Hochberg, M.C., M. Lethbridge-Dejku, W.W. Scott, et al. Serum levels of insulin-like growth factor in subjects with osteoarthritis of the knee. Data from the Baltimore Longitudinal Study of Aging. *Arthritis Rheum.* 1994; 37 (8): 1177–1180.

13. Lloyd, M.E., D.J. Hart, D. Nandra, et al. Relation between insulin-like growth factor-1 concentrations, osteoarthritis, bone density, and fractures in the general population: the Chingford study. *Ann. Rheum. Dis.* 1996; 55 (12): 870–874.

14. Fraenkel, L., Y. Zhang, S.B. Trippel, et al. Longitudinal analysis of the relationship between serum insulin-like growth factor-1 and radiographic knee osteoarthritis. *Osteoarthritis Cartilage* 1998; 6 (5): 362–367.

15. Schneiderman, R., N. Rosenberg, J. Hiss, et al. Concentration and size distribution of insulin-like growth factors in human normal and osteoarthritic synovial fluid and cartilage. *Arch. Biochem. Biophys.* 1995; 324 (1): 173–188.

16. Dore, S., T. Abribat, N. Rousseau, et al. Increased insulin-like growth factor 1 production by human osteoarthritic chondrocytes is not dependent on growth hormone action. *Arthritis Rheum.* 1995; 38 (3): 413–419.

17. Tardif, G., P. Reboul, J.P. Pelletier, et al. Normal expression of type 1 insulin-like growth factor receptors in human osteoarthritic chondrocytes with increased expression and synthesis of insulin-like growth factor binding proteins. *Arthritis Rheum.* 1996; 39 (6): 968–978.

18. Fernihough, J.K., M.E. Billingham, S. Cwyfan-Hughes, et al. Local disruption of the insulin-like growth factor system in the arthritic joint. *Arthritis Rheum.* 1996; 39 (9): 1556–1565.

19. Tavera, C., T. Abribat, R. Reboul, et al. IGF and IGF-binding protein system in the synovial fluid of osteoarthritic and rheumatoid arthritic patients. *Osteoarthritis Cartilage* 1996; 4 (4): 263–274.

20. Fernihough, J.K., M.E. Billingham, S. Cwyfan-Hughes, et al. Local disruption of the insulin-like growth factor system in the arthritic joint. *Arthritis Rheum.* 1996; 39 (9): 1556–1565.

21. Dore, S., J.P. Pelletier, J.A. DiBattista, et al. Human osteoarthritic chondrocytes possess an increased number of insulin-like growth factor 1 binding sites but are unresponsive to stimulation. Possible role of IGF-1 binding proteins. *Arthritis Rheum.* 1994; 37 (2): 253–263.

22. Whellams, E.J., L.A. Maile, J.K. Fernihough, et al. Alterations in insulin-like growth factor binding protein-3 proteolysis and complex formation in the arthritic joint. *J. Endocrinol.* 2000; 165 (3): 545–556.

23. Tardif, G., P. Reboul, J.P. Pelletier, et al. Normal expression of type 1 insulin-like growth factor receptor in human osteoarthritic chondrocytes with increased expression and synthesis of insulin-like growth factor binding proteins. *Arthritis Rheum.* 1996; 39 (6): 968–978.

24. Martel-Pelletier, J., J.A. Battista, D. Lajeunesse, et al. IGF/IGFBP axis in cartilage and bone in osteoarthritis pathogenesis. *Inflamm. Res.* 1998; 47 (3): 90–100.

25. Verschure, P.J., J.V. Marle, L.A. Joosten, et al. Localization of insulin-like growth factor-1 receptor in human normal and osteoarthritic cartilage in relation to proteoglycan synthesis and content. *Br. J. Rheumatol.* 1996; 35 (11): 1044–1055.

26. Loeser, R.F., G. Shanker, C.S. Carlson, et al. Reduction in the chondrocytes response to insulin-like growth factor-1 in aging and osteoarthritis: studies in non-human primate model of naturally occurring disease. *Arthritis Rheum.* 2000; 43 (9): 2110–2121.

27. Pelletier, J.P., and J. Martel-Pelletier. [Role of synovial inflammation, cytokines and IGF-1 in the physiopathology of osteoarthritis.] *Rev. Rhum. Ed. Fr.* 1994; 61 (9 Pt.2): 103S-108S.

28. Heemskerk, V.H., M.A. Daemen, and W.A. Buurman. Insulin-like growth factor-1 (IGF-1) and growth hormone (GH) on immunity and inflammation. *Cytokine Growth Factor Rev.* 1999; 10 (1): 5–14.

29. Spector, T.D., L.A. Perry, and R.W. Jubb. Endogenous sex steroid levels in women with generalized osteoarthritis. *Clin. Rheumatol.* 1991; 19 (3): 316–319.

30. De la Torre, B., M. Hedman, E. Nilsson, et al. Relationship between blood and joint tissue DHEAS levels in rheumatoid arthritis and osteoarthritis. *Clin. Exp. Rheumatol.* 1993; 11 (6): 597–601.

31. Sowers, M.F., M. Hochberg, J.P. Crabbe, et al. Association of bone mineral density and sex hormone levels with osteoarthritis of the hand and knee in premenopausal women. *Am. J. Epidemiol.* 1996; 143 (1): 38–47.

32. Siniachenko, O.V., E.F. Barinov, A.S. Rudnev, et al. [Sex and gonadotrophic hormones in the blood in joint diseases in coal miners.] *Lik. Sprava.* 1996; (7–9): 92–95.

33. Cauley, J.A., C.K. Kwoh, G. Egeland, et al. Serum sex hormones and severity of osteoarthritis of the hand. *J. Rheumatol.* 1993; 20 (7): 1170–1175.

34. Siniachenko, O.V., E.F. Barinov, A.S. Rudnev, et al. [Sex and gonadotrophic hormones in the blood in joint diseases in coal miners.] *Lik. Sprava.* 1996; (7–9): 92–95.

35. Caniggia, A. [A multicenter study on the effectiveness of non-steroidal anti-inflammatory agents associated with nandrolone decanoate in the management of osteoarthritis and rheumatoid arthritis.] *Minerva Med.* 1983; 74 (45–46): 2737–2799.

36. Frisbie, D.D., and A.J. Nixon. Insulin-like growth factor 1 and corticosteroid modulation of chondrocytes' metabolic and mitogenic activities in interleukin 1 conditioned equine cartilage. *Am. J. Vet. Res.* 1997; 58 (5): 524–530.

37. Rogachefsky, R.A., D.D. Dean, D.S. Howell, et al. Treatment of canine osteoarthritis with insulin-like growth factor (IGF-1) and sodium pentosan polysulfate. *Osteoarthritis Cartilage* 1993; 1 (2): 105–114

27

Rationale for Anabolic Therapy in Prolonged Immobilization, Microgravity, and Extended Space Travel

Introduction: Dramatic Losses of Anabolic Potentials

Prolonged immobilization and weightlessness are interrelated parts of a continuum which results in profound biochemical and body composition changes in the human body. These conditions induce profound antianabolic and catabolic reactions. The major metabolic aspects of these conditions are hypoandrogenemia, hyposomatomedinemia, and reduced erythropoietin (EPO) production.[1, 2, 3, 4] These metabolic changes result in an array of clinical conditions, including sarcopenia, osteoporosis, anemia, reduced cardiac contractility and aerobic capacity, detrimental changes in the immune system, dyslipidemias, and reduced fibrinolysis.[5, 6, 7, 8, 9, 10, 11, 12] These effects have been shown in immobilized patients, animal models that simulate weightlessness, and in humans exposed to microgravity conditions during space travel. To account for these biochemical alterations, it has been proposed that gravity receptors or gravity-sensitive receptors may be present in the hypothalamus and other organs that respond to reduced gravity and mimic conditions and responses similar to that of a fetus in utero (as shown in Table 28-1).[13]

Table 28-1. Human Conditions Suggesting the Presence of
Hypothalamic and Renal Receptors for Reduced Gravity Conditions

Human Condition	Hormonal Response
Fetal stage (in utero)	low androgen levels low growth hormone (GH) levels low erythropoietin (EPO) levels
Prolonged immobilization	reduced androgen levels reduced GH levels reduced EPO levels
Microgravity conditions	dramatically reduced androgen levels dramatically reduced GH levels dramatically reduced EPO levels

Studies with Anabolic Therapy for Immobilization and Microgravity Conditions

To date, studies specifically designed to treat the well-documented catabolic responses to immobilization or microgravity conditions in humans have not been published. A few animal studies that model these conditions have shown that androgen therapy has the expected beneficial effects[14, 15] that echo some of the findings from an early Russian study with humans.[16]

The reduced levels of anabolic hormones and EPO which have been documented in both prolonged immobilization and microgravity conditions have obvious therapeutic implications. To counteract these conditions, the following quotation from a prominent microgravity researcher, may help define the goals.[17]

"There needs to be applied research utilizing animal and human models in conjunction with modern molecular probes coupled with novel physical activity, hormonal, and pharmacological experimental treatments. This work is important because the transformations having impact on muscle during weightlessness are often similar to those transformations occurring with chronic inactivity, immobilization, and aging on Earth. A major challenge facing society will be to maintain the functional integrity of an ever aging population with an inherent proneness to injury and incapacitation."

It has been shown that pronounced losses of anabolic potentials in humans reduces their long-term spaceflight capabilities.[18] Also, it is well known that prolonged bed rest results in similar losses in anabolic potentials that can have detrimental outcomes on the recovery phases of patients with other treatable conditions. This can be demonstrated by the following true case.

Case Example

A 75-year-man, who was previously healthy, an active golfer, and lived independently, slips from a stairway and sustains a crush injury to his left acetabular region. After surgical repair of his pelvis, the man is placed in a rehabilitation unit where he is exposed to prolonged bed rest while limited physical therapy treatments and the necessary restrictions are applied. His ability to bear weight and ambulate is restricted for several weeks. Meanwhile, he suffers from a major loss in anabolic potentials (from hypoandrogenemia, hyposomatomedinemia, and reduced EPO production) which limits his capacity to recover from his injury; he suffers from reduced bone-healing function, sarcopenia, osteoporosis, anemia, depression, and increased risk for thromboembolism. Even though the science-based information has shown that androgen therapy reverses these conditions, it is not prescribed for him. His outcome is poor and he has to sell his home, enter an assisted living facility, lose his previously independent life, and stop playing golf. The lack of anabolic therapy for patients can result in harm and poor outcomes. To date, such an absence of treatment is the standard of care for a patient with this type of injury.

Summary

In this chapter, the available evidence-based information regarding the substantial losses in anabolic potentials during prolonged immobilization and microgravity conditions has been presented. Although the conditions of hypoandrogenemia, hyposomatomedinemia, and reduced EPO production are known to be associated with these conditions, there have been no published scientific studies with anabolic therapy for individuals undergoing these conditions.

The efficacy of anabolic therapy in the treatment of these conditions should provide a substantial stimulus for both its clinical use and scientific investigation of it. A case study has been provided to exemplify both the current standard of care (that does not use anabolic therapy) and the need for anabolic therapy for patients who have treatable conditions and who are immobilized for prolonged periods of time.

Anabolic therapy for immobilized patients is likely to provide a safe and beneficial treatment, especially when combined with traditional rehabilitative modalities. Further research efforts are warranted.

Notes

1. Baldwin, K.M. Effect of spaceflight on the functional, biochemical, and metabolic properties of skeletal muscle. *Med. Sci. Sports Exerc.* 1996; 28 (8): 983–987.

2. Strollo, F., G. Riondino, B. Harris, et al. The effect of microgravity on testicular androgen secretion. *Aviat. Space Environ. Med.* 1998; 69 (2): 133–136.

3. Wimalawansa, S.M., M.T. Chapa, J.N. Wei, et al. Reversal of weightlessness-induced musculoskeletal losses with androgens: quantification by MRI. *J. Appl. Physiol.* 1999; 86 (6): 1841–1846.

4. Vandenburgh, H., J. Chromiak, J. Shansky, et al. Space travel directly induces skeletal muscle atrophy. *FASEB J.* 1999; 13 (9): 1031–1038.

5. Hargens, A.R., and D.E. Watenpaugh. Cardiovascular adaptation to spaceflight. *Med. Sci. Sports Exerc.* 1996; 28 (8): 977–982.

6. Tipton, C.M., J.E. Greenleaf, and C.G.R. Jackson. Neuroendocrine and immune system responses with spaceflights. *Med. Sci. Sports Exerc.* 1996; 28 (8): 988–998.

7. Covertino, V.A. Exercise as a countermeasure for physiological adaptation to prolonged spaceflight. *Med. Sci. Sports Exerc.* 1996; 28 (8): 999–1014.

8. Tipton, C.M., and A. Hargens. Physiological adapatations and countermeasures associated with long-duration spaceflights. *Med. Sci. Sports Exerc.* 1996; 28 (8): 974–976.

9. Zerwekh, J.E., L.A. Ruml, F. Gotschalk, et al. The effects of twelve weeks of bed rest on bone histology, biochemical markers of bone turnover, and calcium homeostasis in eleven normal subjects. *J. Bone Miner. Res.* 1998; 13 (10): 1594–1601.

10. Wimalawansa, S.M., and S.J. Wimalawansa. Simulated weightlessness-induced attenuation of testosterone production may be responsible for bone loss. *Endocrine* 1999; 10 (3): 253–260.

11. Vandenburgh, H., J. Chromiak, J. Shansky, et al. Space travel induces skeletal muscle atrophy. *FASEB J.* 1999; 13 (9): 1031–1038.

12. Inoue, M., H. Tanaka, T. Moriwake, et al. Altered biochemical markers of bone turnover in humans during 120 days of bed rest. *Bone* 2000; 26 (3): 281–286.

13. Taylor, W.N. *Anabolic Steroids and the Athlete,* second edition. Jefferson, N.C.: McFarland & Company, Inc., Publishers, 2002.

14. Wimalawansa, S.M., and S.J. Wimalawansa. Simulated weightlessness attenuation of testosterone production may be responsible for bone loss. *Endocrine* 1999; 10 (3): 253–260.

15. Wimalawansa, S.M., M.T. Chapa, J.N. Wei, et al. Reversal of weightlessness-induced musculoskeletal losses with androgens: quantification by MRI. *J. Appl. Physiol.* 1999; 86 (6): 1841–1846.

16. Sgibnev, A.K., V.K. Filosofov, and N. V. Pisarenko. [Effect of anabolic steroids on performance characteristics of a human operator exposed to space flight factors.] *Kosm. Biol. Med.* 1973; 7 (5): 65–68.

17. Baldwin, K.M. Effect of spaceflight on the functional, biochemical, and metabolic properties of skeletal muscle. *Med. Sci. Sports Exerc.* 1996; 289 (8): 983–987.

18. Vandenburgh, H., J. Chromiak, J. Shansky, et al. Space travel directly induces skeletal muscle atrophy. *FASEB J.* 1999; 13 (9): 1031–1038

28

Rationale for Anabolic Therapy with Nutritional Replacement Treatments

Introduction: Critical Illness Is Associated with Profound Catabolism and Reduced Recuperative Abilities

Critically ill, traumatized, and postsurgical patients characteristically exhibit a pronounced catabolism in addition to a *down-regulation of normal endogenous anabolic activities*, leading to major complications from the marked loss of body protein stores and synthesis.[1] Depression of the hypothalamic-pituitary-gonadal, alterations of the hypothalamic-pituitary-adrenal,[2] and depression of the GHRH-GH-IGF-IGFBP axes[3, 4, 5] have been documented in patients with various critical illnesses and account for the endogenous down-regulation of anabolic potentials. This anabolic down-regulation usually results in hypoandrogenemia and hyposomatomedinemia at a time when the body needs to upregulate these anabolic mechanisms by producing more androgens and growth factors. Hormonal responses to major trauma and critical illness trigger a cascade of metabolic adjustments leading to catabolism and substrate mobilization.[6] Moreover, some types of alimentation programs have been shown to further reduce serum levels of anabolic hormones in both animal and human subjects.[7, 8, 9, 10, 11]

It has been a long-held view that maximizing dietary metabolites, via hyperalimentation or transcutaneous parenteral nutrition (TPN) alone would prove adequate in counteracting the catabolic responses of the body to critical illness or surgery. Unfortunately, nutritional support alone usually does not reverse a catabolic state and thereby induce a positive protein balance.[12] In the early catabolic phase of severe injury and illness, conventional nutritional support alone is inadequate to reverse negative nitrogen balance and an additional anabolic stimulus has been shown to be both required and effective for overcoming the body's catabolic responses.[13, 14] Administration of anabolic agents with special nutrition has become a novel strategy that can improve outcomes in critically ill patients.[15]

With critical illness the body responds with predominantly endogenous catabolic responses that overwhelm the body's anabolic attempts to restore homeostasis and repair itself. This response results in marked losses in lean body mass and functional body proteins which have detrimental impacts on the body's endocrine, neuroendocrine, and neuroimmune systems. As a result, the body has a reduced ability to recuperate and defend itself from further insults due to a compromise in the immune system and the production of acute-phase proteins that include catabolic cytokines and other proteins.[16]

Recent investigations have established that anabolic therapy with anabolic hormones and factors is essential for counteracting the endogenous catabolic responses promoted by critical illness and major surgical interventions even when the most advanced nutritional support is provided. This fact has provided the impetus for investigational studies that utilize anabolic agents in conjunction with adequate nutritional support for critically ill patients. These studies have included anabolic therapy with testosterone and its analogues (anabolic steroids), GH, and other components of or stimulators of the GHRH-GH-IGF-IGFBP axis. Some studies have suggested that combinations of anabolic agents may prove to provide the greatest benefit with patients on TPN.[17, 18]

Therefore, the beneficial degree to which critically ill patients respond to optimal nutritional support depends on the biochemical condition of the patient which can be improved by the concurrent use of anabolic agents.[19] Providing an appropriate anabolic stimulus increases the efficacy of hyperalimentation or TPN therapy by improving the utilization of the nutrients provided.

Studies with Anabolic Agents and Nutritional Support

Anabolic Therapy with Androgens

Since the 1940s, androgen therapy has been known to improve nitrogen balance in surgical and critically ill patients.[20] However, the earlier investigational results with androgen therapy combined with nutritional support were mixed.[21, 22, 23, 24] Unfortunately, when the clinical trials of androgen therapy as adjuvant treatment were conducted, the assessment markers and tools were less advanced than those that are currently utilized. The most recent study of androgen therapy with TPN has concluded that androgen therapy (with nandrolone decanoate given intramuscularly at 200mg at the onset of TPN therapy) significantly improves the efficacy of TPN, resulting in a more rapid correction of the catabolic state.[25] Recent studies, utilizing modern markers of anabolism, have proven the efficacy of androgen therapy for increasing anabolism[26, 27] and for reversing the catabolism associated with catabolic states alone and with catabolic states treated with nutritional support.[28, 29, 30] Androgen therapy has been shown to restore appetite,[31] enhance wound-healing time,[32, 33] correct acute-phase cytokine abnormalities, correct anemia, enhance fibrinolysis, and prevent bone mineral losses that are commonly associated with short-term and long-term alimentation therapy. Both short-term and long-term total parenteral nutrition has been associated with a predisposition to thromboembolic events due to reduced fibrinolysis,[34] bone mineral density losses,[35, 36] and anemia.[37, 38] Androgen therapy has been shown to treat these conditions (see specific chapters regarding these issues).

Androgen therapy has a primary role as adjuvant therapy for critically ill patients undergoing nutritional support treatment, especially in those patients with comorbid or concomitant conditions, such as:

(1) hypoandrogenemia.
(2) reduced fibrinolysis.
(3) osteoporosis.
(4) anemia.
(5) cytokine profile abnormalities.
(6) compromised immune system functioning.
(7) cognitive deficits.

Anabolic Therapy with GHRH-GH-IGF-IGFBP Axis Components

Numerous studies have indicated that coadminstration of various components of the GHRH-GH-IGF-1-IGFBP axis improves the efficacy of TPN in both animal models and patients.[39, 40, 41, 42, 43, 44, 45, 46, 47, 48, 49, 50, 51, 52, 53, 54, 55, 56] The results from animal models indicate that cotherapy with these components further optimizes the beneficial effects of TPN therapy. In the near future, it is likely that GHRH analogues and GH secretagogues will be evaluated in investigational studies.

Although components of the GRHR-GH-IGF-IGFBP axis provide anabolic stimuli to the body and enhance the efficacy of TPN, there are some inadequacies with these anabolic agents. They do not correct the reduced fibrinolysis, anemia, acute phase cytokine abnormalities, and immunodepression that are often seen in critically ill patients who require TPN. This evidence provides the appropriate rationale to include androgens with these agents to correct such concurrent conditions. Future studies should be directed at utilizing androgen therapy to improve the effectiveness of the total anabolic stimulus, and at the same time, reducing the doses of the GHRH-GH-IGF-IGFBP components to improve cost-effectiveness.

Summary

In this chapter the rationale for the use of anabolic therapy in critically ill and postsurgical patients has been provided. The appropriate nutrients and the appropriate anabolic stimuli to biochemically use these nutrients are intertwined. Patients who are deemed to be candidates for TPN are also candidates for anabolic therapy. Anabolic therapy with androgens, along with components of the GHRH-GH-IGF-IGFBP axis, is indicated to correct the full spectrum of catabolic responses that take place in critically ill patients. Androgens (in rapid-acting and mildly supraphysiologic doses) remain the most efficient and cost-effective therapy for these patients. Combinations of anabolic agents for critically ill patients should be investigated.

Notes

1. Chang, D.W., L. DeSanti, and R.H Demling. Anticatabolic and anabolic strategies in critical illness: a review of the current treatment modalities. *Shock* 1998; 19 (3): 155–160.

2. Jeevanadam, M., N.J. Holaday, and S.R. Petersen. Posttraumatic hormonal environment during total parenteral nutrition. *Nutrition* 1993; 9 (4): 333–338.

3. Burgess, E.J. Insulin-like growth factor 1: a valid nutritional indicator during parenteral feeding of patients suffering an acute phase response. *Ann. Clin. Biochem.* 1992; 29 (2): 137–144.

4. Petersen, S.R., M. Jeevanandam, and N.J. Holaday. Adjuvant recombinant human growth hormone stimulates insulin-like growth factor binding protein-3 secretion in critically ill trauma patients. *J. Trauma* 1995; 39 (2): 295–300.

5. Bjarnason, R., R. Wickelgren, M. Hermansson, et al. Growth hormone treatment prevents the decrease in insulin-like growth factor 1 gene expression in patients undergoing abdominal surgery. *J. Clin. Endocrinol. Metab.* 1998; 83 (5): 1566–1572.

6. Jeevanandam, M., N.J. Holaday, and S.R. Peterson. Posttraumatic hormonal environment during total parenteral nutrition. *Nutrition* 1993; 9 (4): 333–338.

7. Tcholakian, R.K., and R.J. Keating. In vivo patterns of circulating steroids in adult male rats. IV. Evidence for rapid oscillations in testosterone in normal and total parenterally nourished animals. *Steroids* 1978; 32 (2): 269–278.

8. Keating R.J, and R.K. Tcholakian. In vivo patterns of circulating steroids in adult male rats. III. Effect of total parenteral nutrition on the diurnal variation of testosterone. *Endocr. Res. Commun.* 1979; 6 (2): 95–105.

9. Tulikoura, I., K. Liewendahl, M.R. Taskinen, et al. Effect of parenteral nutrition on the blood levels of insulin, glucagon, growth hormone, thyroid hormones and cortisol in catabolic patients. *Acta Chir. Scand.* 1982; 148 (4): 315–322.

10. Rosenbaum, M., Y.M. Fong, D.G. Hesse, et al. Intravenous refeeding blocks growth hormone (GH)-provoked increase in serum free fatty acids and blunting of somatotroph response to GH-releasing hormone in normal men. *J. Clin. Endocrinol. Metab.* 1989; 69 (2): 310–316.

11. Ney, D.M., H. Yang, S.M. Smith, et al. High-calorie total parenteral nutrition reduces hepatic insulin-like growth factor-1 mRNA and alters serum levels of insulin-like growth factor-binding protein-1, -3, -5, and –6 in the rat. *Metabolism* 1995; 44 (2): 152–160.

12. Gjerde, S., H. Flaatten, and K. Svanes. [Use of growth hormone during catabolic state in a patient in postoperative intensive care.] *Tidsskr. Nor. Laegeforen* 1995; 115 (24): 3028–3030.

13. Peterson, S.R., N.J. Holaday, and M. Jeevanandam. Enhancement of protein synthesis efficiency in parenterally fed trauma victims by adjuvant recombinant human growth hormone. *J. Trauma* 1994; 36 (5): 726–733.

14. Jeevanandam, M., N.J. Holaday, and S.R. Petersen. Integrated nutritional, hormonal, and metabolic effects of recombinant human growth hormone (rhGH) supplementation in trauma patients. *Nutrition* 1996; 12 (11–12): 777–787.

15. Zeigler, T.R. Growth hormone administration during nutritional support: what is to be gained? *New Horiz.* 1994; 2 (2): 244–256.

16. Petersen, S.R., M. Jeevanandam, L.M. Shahbazian, et al. Reprioritization of liver protein synthesis resulting from recombinant human growth hormone supplementation in parenterally fed trauma patients: the effect of growth hormone on the acute-phase response. *J. Trauma* 1997; 42 (6): 987–995.

17. Ney, D.M. Effects of insulin-like growth factor-1 and growth hormone in models of parenteral nutrition. *J. Parenter. Enteral Nutr.* 1999; 23 (6 Suppl.): S184–S189.

18. Jackson, N.C., P.V. Carroll, D.L. Russell-Jones, et al. Effects of glutamine supplementation, GH, and IGF-1 on glutamine metabolism in critically ill patients. *Am. J. Physiol. Endcrinol. Metab.* 2000; 278 (2): E226–E233.

19. Mattox, T.W., K.E. Bertch, J.M. Mirtallo, et al. Recent advances: parenteral nutrition support. *Ann. Pharmacother.* 1995; 29 (2): 174–180.

20. Yule, A.G., J. Macfie, and G.L. Hill. The effect of an anabolic steroid on body composition in patients receiving intravenous nutrition. *Aust. N.Z. J. Surg.* 1981; 5 (3): 280–284.

21. Johnson, P.C., and J. Shaw. A vitamin, anabolic, stimulant mixture. Is this form of medication advantageous for debilitated geriatric patients? *J. Am. Geriatr. Soc.* 1966; 14 (5): 525–532.

22. Yule, A.G., J. Macfie, and G.L. Hill. Effect of anabolic steroid on body composition in patients receiving intravenous nutrition. *Aust. N.Z. Surg.* 1981; 51 (3): 280–284.

23. Lewis, L., M. Dahn, and J.R. Kirkpatrick. Anabolic steroid administration

during nutritional support: a therapeutic controversy. *J. Parenter. Enteral Nutr.* 1981; 5 (1): 64–66.

24. Young, G.A., A.G. Yule, and G.L. Hill. Effects of an anabolic steroid on plasma amino acids, proteins, and body composition in patients receiving intravenous hyperalimentation. *J. Parenter. Enteral Nutr.* 1983; 7 (3): 221–225.

25. Shizgal, H.M. Anabolic steroids and total parenteral nutrition. *Wien. Med. Wocheschr.* 1993; 143 (14–15): 375–380.

26. Demling, R.H., and L. De Santi. Oxandrolone, an anabolic steroid, significantly increases the rate of weight gain in the recovery phase after major burns. *J. Trauma* 1997; 43 (1): 47–51.

27. Wolfe, R., A. Ferrando, M. Sheffield-Moore, et al. Testosterone and muscle protein metabolism. *Mayo Clin. Proc.* 2000; 75 (Suppl.): S55–S59.

28. Demiling, R.H. Comparison of the anabolic effects and complications of human growth hormone and the testosterone analogue, oxandrolone, after severe burn injury. *Burns* 1999; 25 (3): 215–221.

29. Sheffield-Moore, M., R.R. Wolfe, D.C. Gore, et al. Combined effects of hyperaminoacidemia and oxandrolone on skeletal muscle protein synthesis. *Am. J. Physiol. Endocrinol. Metab.* 2000; 278 (2): E273–279.

30. Demling, R.H., and L. De Santi. The rate of restoration of body weight after burn injury, using the anabolic agent oxandrolone, is not age dependent. *Burns* 2001; 27 (1): 46–51.

31. Krasner, D.L., and A.E. Belcher. Oxandrolone restores appetite. An increase in weight helps heal wounds. *Am. J. Nurs.* 2000; 100 (11): 53.

32. Demling, R., and L. De Santi. Closure of the "non-healing wound" corresponds with correction of weight loss using the anabolic agent oxandrolone. *Ostomy Wound Manage.* 1998; 44 (10): 58–62.

33. Demling, R.H., and D.P. Orgill. The anticatabolic and wound healing effects of the testosterone analogue oxandrolone after severe burn injury. *J. Crit. Care* 2000; 15 (1): 12–17.

34. Fernandez Ruiz, M., and J. Lasierra Cirujeda. [The fibrinolytic system and total parenteral nutrition.] *Nur. Hosp.* 1993; 8 (9): 574–579.

35. Foldes, J., B. Rimon, M. Muggia-Sullam, et al. Progressive bone loss during long-term home total parenteral nutrition. *J. Parenter. Enteral Nutr.* 1990; 14 (2): 139–142.

36. Nomura, K., Y. Noguchi, T. Yoshikawa, et al. Long-term total parenteral nutrition and osteoporosis. *Surg. Today* 1993; 23 (11): 1027–1031.

37. Dudrick, S.J., J.J. O'Donnell, R.G. Matheny, et al. Stimulation of hematopoiesis as an alternative to transfusion. *South. Med. J.* 1986; 79 (6): 669–673.

38. Burns, D.L., E.A. Mascioli, and B.R. Bistrian. Effect of iron-supplemented total parenteral nutrition in patients with iron deficiency anemia. *Nutrition* 1996; 12 (6): 411–415.

39. Ziegler, T.R., L.S. Young, E. Ferrari-Baliviera, et al. Use of human growth hormone combined with nutritional support in a critical care unit. *J. Parenter. Enteral Nutr.* 1990; 14 (6): 574–581.

40. Suchner, U., M.M. Rothdopf, G. Stanislaus, et al. Growth hormone and pulmonary disease. Metabolic effects in patients receiving parenteral nutrition. *Arch. Intern. Med.* 1990; 150 (6): 1225–1230.

41. Ponting, G.A., H.C. Ward, D. Halliday, et al. Protein and energy metabolism with biosynthetic human growth hormone in patients on full intravenous nutritional support. *J. Parenter. Enteral Nutr.* 1990; 14 (5): 437–441.

42. Takagi, K., T. Tashiro, Y Mashima, et al. [The effect of human growth hormone

on protein metabolism in surgically stressed rats.] *Nippon Geka Gaddai Zasshi* 1991; 92 (11): 1545–1551.

43. Koea, J.B., R.G. Douglas, B.H. Brier, et al. Synergistic effect of insulin-like growth factor-1 administration improves the protein-sparing effects of total parenteral nutrition in fasted lambs. *Endocrinology* 1992; 131 (2): 643–648.

44. Hammarqvisst, F., C. Stromberg, A. von der Decken, et al. Biosynthetic human growth hormone preserves both muscle protein synthesis and the decrease in muscle-free glutamine, and improves whole-body nitrogen economy after operation. *Ann. Surg.* 1992; 216 (2): 184–191.

45. Guerrero, J.A., J.M. Capitan, J. Rosell, et al. [Effect of growth hormone and parenteral nutrition on the catabolic phase following major digestive surgery.] *Rev. Esp. Enferm. Dig.* 1992; 81 (6): 379–382.

46. Ma, E.L. [Changes of protein turnover in perioperative patients and effect of recombinant human growth hormone.] *Zhonghua Wai Ke Za Zhi* 1992; 30 (10): 631–634.

47. Manson, J.M., R.J. Smith, and D.W. Wilmore. Growth hormone stimulates protein synthesis during hypocaloric parenteral nutrition. Role of hormonal-substrate environment. *Ann. Surg.* 1988; 202 (2): 136–142.

48. Mjaaland, M., K. Unneberg, T. Bjoro, et al. Growth hormone treatment after abdominal surgery decreased carbohydrate oxidation and increased fat oxidation in patients on total parenteral nutrition. *Metabolism* 1993; 42 (2): 185–190.

49. Vara-Thorbeck, R., J.A. Guerrero, J. Rosell, et al. Exogenous growth hormone: effects on the catabolic response to surgically produced acute stress and on post-operative immune function. *World J. Surg.* 1993; 17 (4): 530–537.

50. Voerman, B.J., R.J. Strack van Schijndel, H. de Boer, et al. Effects of human growth hormone on fuel utilization and mineral balance in critically ill patients on full intravenous nutritional support. *J. Crit. Care* 1994; 9 (3): 143–150.

51. Wong, W.K., K.C. Soo, R. Nambiar, et al. The effect of recombinant growth hormone on nitrogen balance in malnourished patients after major abdominal surgery. *Aust. N.Z. Surg.* 1995; 65 (2): 109–113.

52. Jeevanandam, M., M.R. Ali, N.J. Holaday, et al. Adjuvant recombinant human growth hormone normalizes plasma amino acids in parenterally fed trauma patients. *J. Parenter. Enteral Nutr.* 1995; 19 (2): 137–144.

53. Vara-Throbeck, R., E. Ruiz-Reguena, and J.A. Guerrero-Fernandez. Effects of human growth hormone on the catabolic state after surgical trauma. *Horm. Res.* 1996; 45 (1–2): 55–60.

54. Jeevanandam, M., N.J. Holaday, and S.R. Petersen. Adjuvant recombinant human growth hormone does not augment endogenous glucose production in total parenteral nutrition-fed multiple trauma patients. *Metabolism* 1996; 45 (4): 450–456.

55. Koea, J.B., B.H. Breier, R.G. Douglas, et al. Anabolic and cardiovascular effects of recombinant human growth hormone in surgical patients with sepsis. *Br. J. Surg.* 1996; 83 (2): 196–202.

56. Berman, R.S., L.E. Harrison, D.B. Pearlstone, et al. Growth hormone, alone and in combination with insulin, increases whole body and skeletal muscle protein kinetics in cancer patients after surgery. *Ann. Surg.* 1999; 229 (1): 1–10.

29

Rationale for Anabolic Therapy in Dermatological Maladies and Wound Healing

Introduction: Loss of Anabolic Potentials Delays Wound Healing

There is a growing body of evidence that delayed dermal wound healing, such as with decubitus and diabetic ulceration, is often associated with decreased anabolic potentials.[1, 2] These anabolic losses can stem from hypoandrogenemia, hyposomatomedinemia, and other reductions in various local tissue growth factors. It has been recommended that systemic anabolic evaluation, along with local tissue anabolic considerations of ulcerated areas, is an important method of managing dermal ulcers and other conditions that delay wound healing.[3] Additional factors which are important for evaluation of wound-healing potential include fibrinolytic ability and other factors that influence microcirculation.[4, 5]

There is also significant evidence that anabolic steroids, which are derived from testosterone and have markedly fewer androgenic activities, promote dermal tissue growth and enhance tissue repair.[6] Some of the mechanisms of action of androgen therapy on dermal homeostasis and regeneration have been recently identified. Anabolic therapy has been shown to be beneficial in a variety of dermatological afflictions including hereditary angioedema, urticaria, generalized vitiligo, psoriasis, Raynaud's phenomenon, cryofibrinogenemia, lipodermatosclerosis, ulceration, and delayed wound-healing conditions.[7, 8, 9, 10, 11, 12, 13, 14, 15, 16, 17]

Anabolic Therapy and Mechanisms of Action for Wound Healing

Anabolic therapy, particularly with androgens that possess a high anabolic/androgenic ratio (therapeutic index) such as stanozolol and oxandrolone, has been shown to enhance dermal wound healing by several mechanisms. These mechanisms, identified from utilizing animal models and from in vitro and in vivo human studies, indicate that androgen therapy:

(1) elevates the transcutaneous oxygen tension delivered to injured or ulcered tissues.[18]

(2) upregulates collagen synthesis through the action of transforming growth factor-beta 1 stimulation.[19, 20]

(3) enhances microvascular blood flow to damaged or vasospastic dermal tissues.[21]

(4) enhances fibrinolysis[22, 23] and reduces the pericapillary fibrin deposition that restores the proper physiologic circulatory exchanges between blood and dermal tissues, all of which results in enhanced healing.[24, 25, 26]

(5) increases the circulating and local IGF-1 levels that enhance anabolic and healing properties[27] (see Chapter 3 for full discussion).

(6) provides an overall anabolic stimulus to the body that enhances protein metabolism via a dual receptor mechanism that involves both local androgen and IGF-1 receptors (see Chapter 3 for full discussion).

Summary

In this chapter the available rationale for utilizing anabolic therapy for non-healing dermal wounds and other dermatological conditions has been presented. The evidence-based information suggests that androgen therapy, especially with stanozolol or oxandrolone, is beneficial, via a number of mechanisms, for accelerating wound closure and managing other microvascular and dermal conditions. Androgen therapy for these conditions is currently underutilized in these conditions and the various other therapeutic modalities for these conditions have proven to be less than satisfactory. Both the immediate clinical use and further research studies are recommended at this time. Stanozolol or oxandrolone (10–20mg per day) therapy is recommended for dermal wound healing in both genders. Adverse effects of short-term androgen therapy are mostly dose-related and are preventable with appropriate follow-up.[28]

Notes

1. Falabella, A.F. American Academy of Dermatology 1998 Awards for Young Investigators in Dermatology. The anabolic steroid stanozolol upregulates collagen synthesis through the action of transforming growth factor-beta 1. *J. Am. Acad. Dermatol.* 1998; 39 (2 Pt. 1): 272–273.

2. Bitar, M.S. Insulin and glucocorticoid-dependent suppression of the IGF-1 system in diabetic wounds. *Surgery* 2000; 127 (6): 687–695.

3. Falanga, V., and W.H. Eaglstein. A therapeutic approach to venous ulcers. *J. Am. Acad. Dermatol.* 1986; 14 (5 Pt. 1): 777–784.

4. Falanga, V., and W.H. Eaglstein. A therapeutic approach to venous ulcers. *J. Am. Acad. Dermatol.* 1986; 14 (5 Pt. 1): 777–784.

5. Colgan, M.P., D.J. Moore, and D.G. Shanik. New approaches in the medical management of venous ulceration. *Angiology* 1993; 44 (2): 138–142.

6. Falanga, V., A.S. Greenberg, L. Zhou, et al. Stimulation of collagen synthesis by the anabolic steroid stanozolol. *J. Invest. Dermatol.* 1998; 111 (6): 1193–1197.

7. Choudhury, S.N. Preliminary observation of the effect of anabolic steroids in psoriasis. *Indian J. Dermatol.* 1965; 10 (4): 137.

8. Alvarez, O.M., K.D. Levendorf, R.V. Smerbeck, et al. Effect of topically applied steroidal and nonsteroidal anti-inflammatory agents on skin repair and regeneration. *Fed. Proc.* 1984; 43 (13): 2793–2798.

9. Stacey, M.C., K.G. Burnand, G.T. Layer, et al. Transcutaneous oxygen tensions in assessing the treatment of healed venous ulcers. *Br. J. Surg.* 1990; 77 (9): 1050–1054.

10. Falanga, V., R.S. Kirsner, W.H. Eaglstein, et al. Stanozolol in treatment of leg ulcers due to cryofibrinogenaemia. *Lancet* 1991; 338 (8763): 347–348.

11. Elnicki, D.M. Hereditary angioedema. *South. Med. J.* 1992; 85 (11): 1084–1090.

12. Kirsner, R.S., W.H. Eaglstein, M.H. Katz, et al. Stanozolol causes rapid pain relief and healing of cutaneous ulcers caused by cryofibrinogenemia. *J. Am. Acad. Dermatol.* 1993; 28 (1): 71–74.

13. Helfman, T., and V. Falanga. Stanozolol as a novel therapeutic agent in dermatology. *J. Am. Acad. Dermatol.* 1995; 33 (2 Pt. 1): 254–258.

14. Muto, M., H. Furumoto, A. Ohmura, et al. Successful treatment of vitiligo with a sex steroid-thyroid hormone mixture. *J. Dermatol.* 1995; 22 (10): 770–772.

15. Falanga, V., A.S. Greenberg, L. Zhou, et al. Stimulation of collagen synthesis by the anabolic steroid stanozolol. *J. Invest. Dermatol.* 1998; 111 (6): 1193–1197.

16. Renton, A.M. Pharmacologic treatments for venous leg ulcer. *J. Wound Care* 1999; 8 (4): 385–387.

17. Demling, R.H. Oxandrolone, an anabolic steroid, enhances the healing of a cutaneous wound in the rat. *Wound Repair Regen.* 2000; 8 (2): 97–102.

18. Stacey, M.C., K.G. Burnand, G.T. Layer, et al. Transcutaneous oxygen tensions in assessing the treatment of healed venous ulcers. *Br. J. Surg.* 1990; 77 (9): 1050–1054.

19. Falabella, A.F. American Academy of Dermatology 1998 Awards for Young Investigators in Dermatology. The anabolic steroid stanozolol upregulates collagen synthesis through the action of transforming growth factor-beta 1. *J. Am. Acad. Dermatol.* 1998; 39 (2 Pt. 1): 272–273.

20. Falanga, V., A.S. Greenberg, L. Zhou, et al. Stimulation of collagen synthesis by the anabolic steroid stanozolol. *J. Invest. Dermatol.* 1998; 111 (6): 1193–1197.

21. Kirsner, R.S., W.H. Eaglstein, M.H. Katz, et al. Stanozolol causes rapid pain relief and healing of cutaneous ulcers caused by cryofibrinogenemia. *J. Am. Acad. Dermatol.* 1993; 28 (1): 71–74.

22. Lowe, G.D. Anabolic steroids and fibrinolysis. *Wien. Med. Wochenschr.* 1993; 143 (14–15): 383–385.

23. Winkler, U.H. Effects of androgens on haemostasis. *Maturitas* 1996; 24 (3): 147–155.

24. Falanga, V., and W.H. Eaglstein. A therapeutic approach to venous ulcers. *J. Am. Acad. Dermatol.* 1986; 14 (5 Pt. 1): 777–784.

25. Falanga, V., R.S. Kirsner, W.H. Eaglstein, et al. Stanozolol in the treatment of leg ulcers due to cryofibrinogenaemia. *Lancet* 1991; 338 (8763): 347–348.

26. Helfman, T., and V. Falanga. Stanozolol as a novel therapeutic agent in dermatology. *J. Am. Acad. Dermatol.* 1995; 33 (2 Pt. 1): 254–258.

27. Solerte, S.B., M. Firavanti, G. Vignati, et al. Dehydroepiandrosterone sulfate enhances natural killer cell cytotoxicity in humans via locally generated immunoreactive insulin-like growth factor 1. *J. Clin. Endocrinol. Metab.* 1999; 84 (9): 3260–3267.

28. Helfman, T., and V. Falanga. Stanozolol as a novel therapeutic agent in dermatology. *J. Am. Acad. Dermatol.* 1995; 33 (2 Pt. 1): 254–258.

30

Rationale for Anabolic Therapy in Miscellaneous Ill-Health Conditions

Introduction: Loss of Anabolic Potential Can Result in a Variety of Ill-Health Conditions

There are several ill-health and traumatic conditions that may benefit from maximizing anabolic potentials with anabolic therapies. Unfortunately, the clinical investigations have lagged far behind the established need for anabolic therapy in these conditions. Selected conditions for which anabolic therapies could be beneficial are included in this chapter, and for each, the available science-based information will be presented.

Fibromyalgia

The specific cause or causes of fibromyalgia (FM) remain uncertain. Patients with FM experience many clinical features such as diminished energy levels, dysphoria, cognition impairments, poor general health, osteoporosis, reduced fibrinolysis, cytokine imbalances, sleep disturbances, depression, anxiety, angina, reduced exercise tolerance, muscle weakness, cold intolerance with Raynaud's phenomenon, and chronic pain with multiple musculoskeletal trigger points.[1, 2, 3, 4, 5, 6, 7] A growing body of evidence has linked reduced anabolic potentials to many of these signs and symptoms.[8]

Fibromyalgia afflicts about 2 percent of the general population and about 20 percent of a typical rheumatology outpatient practice.[9] There is a strong gender dimorphism in FM with the female to male ratio 9 to 1.[10]

Although FM is much less common in men, the clinical course of the disease can be more severe in men.[11]

Depressed hypothalamic-pituitary-gonadal,[12] hypothalamic-pituitary-adrenal,[13, 14, 15, 16, 17, 18, 19] and GHRH-GH-IGF-IGFBP [20, 21, 22, 23, 24, 25, 26, 27] axes have been identified in a significant number of patients with FM. Depression of these axes results in hypoandrogenemia and hyposomatomedinemia, which correlates with much of the poor health status and chronic pain in FM.[28, 29] Recently, it has been suggested that anabolic therapy should be evaluated in patients with FM.[30, 31]

To date, only one study has been published utilizing anabolic therapy in patients with FM. Fifty women with FM and low IGF-1 levels were enrolled in a randomized, placebo-controlled, double-blind study to access the efficacy of GH therapy over nine months' duration. In this study, the treatment group showed statistically significant improvements in their overall symptomatology and number of tender points. Discontinuing GH therapy was also associated with worsening symptomatology.[32]

No studies with androgen therapy in FM patients have been published. However, it is likely that optimizing anabolic potentials with therapy with androgens and a component of or stimulator of the GHRH-GH-IGF-IGFBP axis should prove to provide the greatest benefits. Future clinical trials are warranted.

Skeletal Muscle Contusions and Injuries

It has been a long-held view that anabolic therapy could have a beneficial effect on the healing rate and strength of damaged skeletal muscle tissues. Recent animal studies have indicated that androgen therapy aids the healing of severe muscle contusion and ischemic injury and accelerates the recovery of force-generating capacity.[33, 34, 35] It has been suggested that androgen therapy in the treatment of muscle injuries warrants further research.[36, 37, 38]

Major Joint Replacement: Preoperational and Rehabilitation

Elderly women and men who require total joint replacement of the hip and knee are an increasing group of patients in many countries. These joint replacements usually result from severe arthritic changes (where elective surgery is common) or from osteoporotic fractures. In both of these situations recent studies have indicated that many of these patients have reduced anabolic potentials prior to surgery, postsurgically, and for up to six months of the rehabilitation phase.[39] Both bone mass and muscle strength have been shown to be decreased from reduced levels of anabolic hormones, including androgens, GH, and IGF-1.[40]

To date, there are no published clinical trials that have utilized anabolic therapy for patients undergoing total knee or hip replacement. In vitro studies of human osteoblastlike cells taken from patients undergoing total hip replacement are stimulated by androgen administration.[41] One study has investigated the effects of GH-loaded polymethylmethacrylate (PMMA) implants and found that local GH and IGF-1 levels, but not systemic levels, are elevated postoperatively, which indicates an improved local anabolic milieu.[42]

Clinical trials utilizing anabolic therapies for elective and postfracture total arthroplasties are warranted. It is likely that postsurgical function and reduced rehabilitation periods can be shown.

Traumatic Brain Injury

Traumatic brain injury (TBI) can result in immediate and prolonged reductions of anabolic potentials. Dysfunctions of the anabolic axis following TBI have been shown to result in hypoandrogenemia and hyposomatomedinemia, both acutely and for up to six years postinjury.[43, 44, 45] Reduced anabolic hormone levels may inhibit recovery and rehabilitative outcomes in patients with TBI and further exacerbate brain damage via cytokine imbalances in other metabolites that are mediated by anabolic hormones.[46] It has been shown that infusion of recombinant IGF-1 and aggressive early intravenous nutrition have beneficial effects on the immunologic response of patients with TBI.[47] Further clinical studies utilizing single and multiple anabolic agents are warranted both acutely and during rehabilitation for patients with TBI.

Summary

Optimizing anabolic stimuli, via pharmacologic and anabolic agents, for many ill-health and injury conditions is in its infancy. It can be expected that anabolic therapies will find their places in the treatment and management of many of these and other conditions.

Notes

1. Murkerji, B., V. Mukerji, M.A. Alpert, et al. The prevalence of rheumatic disorders in patients with chest pain and angiographically normal coronary arteries. *Angiology* 1995; 46 (5): 425–430.

2. Moldofsky, H. Sleep, neuroimmune and neuroendocrine functions in fibromyalgia and chronic fatigue syndrome. *Adv. Neuroimmunol.* 1995; 5 (1): 39–56.

3. Swezey, R.L., and J. Adams. Fibromyalgia: a risk factor for osteoporosis. *J. Rheumatol.* 1999; 26 (12): 2642–2644.

4. Pay, S., M. Calguneri, S. Caliskaner, et al. Evaluation of vascular injury with proinflammatory cytokines, throbomodulin and fibronectin in patients with primary fibromyalgia. *Nagoya J. Med. Sci.* 2000; 63 (3–4): 115–122.

5. Hakkinen, A., K. Hakkinen, P. Hannonen, et al. Strength training induced adaptations in neuromuscular function in premenopausal women with fibromyalgia: comparison with healthy women. *Ann. Rheum. Dis.* 2001; 60 (1): 21–26.

6. Glass, J.M., and D.C. Park. Cognitive dysfunction in fibromyalgia. *Curr. Rheumatol. Rep.* 2001; 3 (2): 123–127.

7. McBeth, J., and A.J. Silman. The role of psychiatric disorders in fibromyalgia. *Curr. Rheumatol. Rep.* 2001; 3 (2): 157–164.

8. Neeck, G., and W. Riedel. Hormonal perturbations in fibromyalgia syndrome. *Ann. N.Y. Acad. Sci.* 1999; 876: 325–338.

9. Cathebras, P., A. Lauwers, and H. Rousset. [Fibromayalgia. A critical review.] *Ann. Med. Interne. (Paris)* 1998; 149 (7): 406–414.

10. Yunus, M.B. The role of gender in fibromyalgia syndrome. *Curr. Rheumatol. Rep.* 2001; 3 (2): 128–134.

11. Buskila, D., L. Neumann, A. Alhoashle, et al. Fibromyalgia syndrome in men. *Semin. Arthritis Rheum.* 2000; 30 (1): 47–51.

12. Riedel, W., H. Layka, and G. Neeck. Secretory pattern of GH, TSH, thyroid hormones, ACTH, cortisol, FSH, and LH in patients with fibromyalgia syndrome following systemic injection of the relevant hypothalamic-releasing hormones. *Z. Rheumatol.* 1998; 57 (Suppl. 2): 81–87.

13. McCain, G.A., and K.S. Tilbe. Diurnal hormone variation in fibromyalgia syndrome: a comparison with rheumatoid arthritis. *J. Rheumatol. Suppl.* 1988; 19: 154–157.

14. Griep, E.N., J.W. Boersma, and E.R. de Kloet. Altered reactivity of the hypothalamic-pituitary-adrenal axis in the primary fibromyalgia syndrome. *J. Rheumatol.* 1993; 20 (3): 469–474.

15. Crofford, L.J., S.R. Pillemer, K.T. Kalogeras, et al. Hypothalamic-pituitary-adrenal axis perturbations in patients with fibromyalgia. *Arthritis Rheum.* 1994; 37 (11): 1583–1592.

16. Lentjes, E.G., E.N. Griep, J.W. Boersma, et al. Glucocorticoid receptors, fibromyalgia and low back pain. *Psychoneuroendocrinology* 1997; 22 (8): 603–614.

17. Griep, E.N., J.W. Boersma, E.G. Lentjies, et al. Function of the hypothalamic-pituitary-adrenal axis in patients with fibromyalgia and low back pain. *J. Rheumatol.* 1998; 25 (7): 1374–1381.

18. Adler, G.K., B.T. Kinsley, S. Hurwitz, et al. Reduced hypothalamic-pituitary and sympathoadrenal responses to hypoglycemia in women with fibromyalgia syndrome. *Am. J. Med.* 1999; 106 (6): 534–543.

19. Torpy, D.J., D.A. Papanicolaou, A.J. Lotsikas, et al. Responses of the sympathetic nervous system and the hypothalamic-pituitary-adrenal axis to interleukin-6: a pilot study in fibromyalgia. *Arthritis Rheum.* 2000; 43 (4): 872–880.

20. Griep, E.N., J.W. Boersma, and E.R. de Kloet. Pituitary release of growth hormone and prolactin in the primary fibromyalgia syndrome. *J. Rheumatol.* 1994; 21 (11): 2125–2130.

21. Ferraccioli, G., P. Guerra, V. Rizzi, et al. Somatomedin (insulin-like growth factor 1) levels decrease during acute changes of stress related hormones. Relevance for fibromyalgia. *J. Rheumatol.* 1994; 21 (7): 1332–1334.

22. Bennett, R.M., D.M. Cook, S.R. Clark, et al. Hypothalamic-pituitary-insulin-like growth factor-1 axis dysfunction in patients with fibromyalgia. *J. Rheumatol.* 1997; 24 (7): 1384–1389.

23. Bennett, R.M., S.C. Clark, and J. Walczyk. A randomized, double-blind, placebo-controlled study of growth hormone in the treatment of fibromyalgia. *Am. J. Med.* 1998; 104 (3): 227–231.

24. Bennet, R.M. Disordered growth hormone secretion in fibromyalgia: a review of recent findings and a hypothesized etiology. *Z. Rheumatol.* 1998; 57 (Suppl.2): 72–76.

25. Berwaerts, J., G. Moorkens, and R. Abs. Secretion of growth hormone in patients with chronic fatigue syndrome. *Growth Horm. IGF Res.* 1998; 8 (Suppl. B): 127–129.

26. Leal-Cerro, A., J. Povedano, R. Asorga, et al. The growth hormone (GH)-releasing hormone-GH-insulin-like growth factor-1 axis in patients with fibromyalgia syndrome. *J. Clin. Endocrinol. Metab.* 1999; 84 (9): 3378–3381.

27. Disner, R., T. Halama, and A. Hoffmann. Stringent endocrinological testing reveals subnormal growth hormone secretion in some patients with fibromyalgia syndrome but rarely severe growth hormone deficiency. *J. Rheumatol.* 2000; 27 (10): 2482–2488.

28. Dessein, P.H., E.A. Shipton, B.I. Joffe, et al. Hyposecretion of adrenal androgens and the relation of serum adrenal steroids, serotonin and insulin-like growth factor-1 to clinical features in women with fibromyalgia. *Pain* 1999; 83 (2): 313–319.

29. Neeck, G. Neuroendocrine and hormonal perturbations and relations to the serotonergic system in fibromyalgia patients. *Scand. J. Rheumatol.* 2000; 113: 8–12.

30. Bagge, E., B.A. Bengtsson, L. Carlson, et al. Low growth hormone secretion in patients with fibromyalgia — a preliminary report on 10 patients and 10 controls. *J. Rheumatol.* 1998; 25 (1): 145–148.

31. Leal-Cerro, J. Povendano, R. Astorga, et al. The growth hormone (GH)-releasing hormone-GH-insulin-like growth factor-1 axis in patients with fibromyalgia syndrome. *J. Clin. Endocrinol. Metab.* 1999; 84 (9): 3378–3381.

32. Bennett, R.M., S.C. Clark, and J. Walczyk. A randomized, double-blind, placebo-controlled study of growth hormone in the treatment of fibromyalgia. *Am. J. Med.* 1998; 104 (3): 227–231.

33. Lohman, R., R. Yowell, S. Barton, et al. Dehydroepiandrosterone protects muscle flap microcirculatory hemodynamics from ischemia/reperfusion injury: an experimental in vivo study. *J. Trauma* 1997; 42 (1): 74–80.

34. Beiner, J.M., P. Jokl, J. Cholewicki, et al. The effect of anabolic steroids and corticosteroids on healing of muscle contusion injury. *Am. J. Sports Med.* 1999; 27 (1): 2–9.

35. Ferry, A., P. Noirez, C.L. Page, et al. Effects of anabolic/androgenic steroids on regeneration of skeletal muscles in the rat. *Acta. Physiol. Scand.* 1999; 166 (2): 105–110.

36. Beiner, J.M., P. Jokl, J. Cholewicki, et al. The effects of anabolic steroids and corticosteroids on healing of muscle contusion injury. *Am. J. Sports Med.* 1999; 27 (1): 2–9.

37. Ferrando, A.A. Effects of inactivity and hormonal mediators on skeletal muscle during recovery from trauma. *Curr. Opin. Clin. Nutr. Metab. Care* 2000; 3 (3): 171–175.

38. Sheffield-Moore, M. Androgens and the control of skeletal muscle protein synthesis. *Ann. Med.* 2000; 32 (2): 181–186.

39. Hedstrom, M., M. Saaf, and N. Dalen. Low IGF-1 levels in hip fracture patients. A comparison of 20 coxarthrotic and 23 hip fracture patients. *Acta Orthop. Scand.* 1999; 70 (2): 145–148.

40. Hedstrom, M. Hip fracture patients, a group of frail elderly people with low

bone mineral density, muscle mass and IGF-1 levels. *Acta Physiol. Scand.* 1999; 167 (4): 347–350.

41. Bruch, H.R., L. Wolf, R. Budde, et al. Androstenedione metabolism in cultured human osteoblast-like cells. *J. Clin. Endocrinol. Metab.* 1992; 75 (1): 101–105.

42. Prichett, J.W. Human growth hormone in polymethyl methacrylate. A controlled study of 15 hip arthroplasties. *Acta Orthop. Scand.* 1992; 63 (5): 520–522.

43. Hackl, J.M. [Metabolic disorders in severe head injuries.] *Fortschr. Med.* 1981; 99 (38): 1562–1566.

44. Lenzen, J., G. Hildebrand, A. Laun, et al. Function tests on the neuroendocrine hypothalamo-pituitary system following acute midbrain syndrome, with special reference to computertomographical and magnetic resonance results. *Neurosurg. Rev.* 1993; 16 (3): 183–187.

45. Cernak, I., V.J. Savic, A. Lazarov, et al. Neuroendocrine responses following graded traumatic brain injury in male adults. *Brain Inj.* 1999; 13 (12): 1005–1015.

46. Feurestein, G.Z., X. Wang, and F.C. Barone. The role of cytokines in the neuropathology of stroke and neurotrauma. *Neuroimmunomodulation* 1998; 5 (3–4): 143–159.

47. Kudsk, K.A., C. Mowatt-Larssen, J. Bukar, et al. Effect of recombinant human insulin-like growth factor 1 and effect of total parenteral nutrition on immune depression following severe head injury. *Arch. Surg.* 1994; 129 (1): 66–70.

Afterword: Hypoandrogenemia Is the Most Commonly Missed Disorder in Modern Medicine

The information provided in this book has documented the wide array of diseases and ill-health conditions associated directly or indirectly with hypoandrogenemia and other reductions in anabolic hormones and agents. However, physicians have been exceedingly slow to accept that these reductions in anabolic hormones are linked with many disease processes. Moreover, physicians have been even slower in prescribing these agents for their patients who can benefit from them.

A number of misconceptions about anabolic therapy, particularly with androgens, are still prevalent in the medical community. Some of these misconceptions include:

(1) androgens are male hormones and the prevalence of hypoandrogenemia in aging men is very low.

(2) androgens are male hormones and have a little role in the health and welfare of women.

(3) androgen therapy is ineffective and causes significant adverse effects, especially in women patients.

(4) androgens cause prostate cancer.

(5) androgens promote heart disease.

(6) androgen therapy is talked about in medical circles but should not be prescribed to patients.

With these misconceptions as a prevalent backdrop, there is little doubt that hypoandrogenemia is the most missed medical condition in modern medicine.

Education and re-education of physicians, and altering physicians' attitudes regarding anabolic therapies, have been suggested by several authors as the largest hurdles to overcome if adequate anabolic therapies are to be provided for the large number of patients who can benefit from them. This book has provided a comprehensive benchmark to begin these educational processes for the betterment of patient care.

Index

About the Author

William N. Taylor, M.D., is a leading expert in the field of anabolic hormones.

He wrote the first medical book on the athletic use and abuse of anabolic steroids and growth hormones, *Anabolic Steroids and the Athlete*, published in 1982. He chronicled the progression of the anabolic steroid epidemic in America in his book *Hormonal Manipulation: A New Era of Monstrous Athletes* (1985) that became an influential part of the congressional hearings and records that eventually led to the reclassification of anabolic steroids as controlled substances in the United States. In his book *Macho Medicine: A History of the Anabolic Steroid Epidemic* (1991), Dr. Taylor provided a comprehensive history of the social abuse of anabolic hormones and the federal regulations that have been imposed to curb their abuse. A recent resurgence of the social abuse of these drugs and the need for further solutions to this problem have prompted an updated edition of his 1982 book *Anabolic Steroids and the Athlete* in 2002. Other recent books written by Dr. Taylor have focused on the medical use of anabolic agents for therapies in patients who can benefit from these include: *Osteoporosis: Medical Blunders and Treatment Strategies* (1996).